# NUTRITION AND THE BRAIN

*Volume 2*

# Nutrition and the Brain

## *Volume 2*

## Control of Feeding Behavior

### and

## Biology of the Brain in Protein-Calorie Malnutrition

Editors

Richard J. Wurtman, M.D.
*Professor of Endocrinology*
*  and Metabolism*
*Department of Nutrition and*
*  Food Science*
*Massachusetts Institute of Technology*
*Cambridge, Massachusetts*

Judith J. Wurtman, Ph.D.
*Research Associate*
*Department of Nutrition and*
*  Food Science*
*Massachusetts Institute of Technology*
*Cambridge, Massachusetts*

Raven Press ■ New York

**Raven Press, 1140 Avenue of the Americas, New York, New York 10036**

Made in the United States of America

International Standard Book Number 0-89004-046-X
Library of Congress Catalog Card Number 75-14593

—

# Preface

The brain requires a number of substances that it cannot make. Some of these nutrients are synthesized in other organs and delivered to the brain by the circulation; a larger number cannot be made anywhere in the body, and must be obtained from foods. The study of the brain's nutrition encompasses all of the processes—metabolic and behavioral—that influence the extent to which nutrients become available to neuronal tissue; the goal of "Nutrition and the Brain" is to illuminate these processes.

The first volume of this series discussed some of the factors that, under normal conditions, control the brain's nutritional state. Its chapters described the natural feeding patterns of man and other primates, and analyzed in some detail the mechanisms that govern the delivery to brain of particular nutrients, including energy substrates, amino acids, methyl groups, and B vitamins. The present, second, volume addresses two phenomena: the control (by brain) of eating behavior, and the changes in brain structure and function that can be caused by protein-calorie malnutrition.

All of the brain's nutrients that cannot be synthesized elsewhere in the body become available to it because of its capacity to direct a particular type of behavior: eating. The brain is responsible for sensing the body's nutritional needs, deciding that the individual should eat, directing the search for appropriate foods, and initiating the process by which foods enter the digestive tract. Exactly how the brain monitors the body's nutritional status and utilizes this information to determine when and what the individual should eat remains obscure. However—as described in Chapter One—its sources of data probably include circulating factors, extrinsic olfactory and visual cues, intrinsic time-sense, and neural signals from the gut. The varieties of foods which man and other mammals generally consume are influenced by where the individual happens to reside and by numerous social and cultural factors. It remains unclear as to whether the brain can discern needs for particular components of foods (such as proteins, vitamins, or minerals), or whether eating behavior is largely directed toward the acquisition of calories or of bulk. The brain loci upon which drugs, nutrients, and hormones act to modify food consumption are gradually becoming known, although the generalizations that characterize this field remain tenuous.

The changes in the central nervous system that result from protein-calorie malnutrition are described from the perspectives of three disciplines: neuroanatomy, biochemistry, and behavior. A central question pervading all three approaches concerns the possibility that, at certain periods early in development, the brain might be especially susceptible to damage as a result of malnutrition, and might suffer irreparable harm as a consequence. It seems clear that the general acceptance of this view is far stronger than the evidence that supports it. As Chapter Four concludes, only in the most severe forms of clinical malnutrition is there clear evidence that protein deficiency can be associated with lasting behavioral deficits. (Clearly, we should all be thankful that it is so difficult to "prove" that perinatal malnutrition causes lasting damage to the brain.) In the absence of compelling evidence that malnutrition has major effects on brain structure and chemical composition, the authors of the chapters on brain anatomy and biochemistry have addressed the question of how one would know, i.e., what studies should be done in the future to determine *if* malnutrition really affects brain structure or composition. They have described the processes by which the normal brain develops, and considered how one might do research to discover whether particular steps in these processes are especially vulnerable to the effects of protein-calorie malnutrition. Future volumes in this series will consider ways in which the scarcity of nutrients other than protein or calories, or the ingestion of unusually large quantities of particular nutrients, can affect the brain and behavior.

Richard J. Wurtman
Judith J. Wurtman
Cambridge, Massachusetts

# Contents

# Contents of Volume 1

# Contributors

**Floyd E. Bloom**
*Arthur Vining Davis Center for Behavioral Neurobiology, The Salk Institute, San Diego, California 92112*


**Loy D. Lytle**
*Department of Nutrition and Food Science, Massachusetts Institute of Technology, Cambridge, Massachusetts 02139*


**Hamish N. Munro**
*Physiological Chemistry Laboratories, Department of Nutrition and Food Science, Massachusetts Institute of Technology, Cambridge, Massachusetts 02139*


**Thaddeus S. Nowak, Jr.**
*Physiological Chemistry Laboratories, Department of Nutrition and Food Science, Massachusetts Institute of Technology, Cambridge, Massachusetts 02139*


**Ernesto Pollitt**
*Department of Nutrition and Food Science, Massachusetts Institute of Technology, Cambridge, Massachusetts 02139*


**William J. Shoemaker**
*Arthur Vining Davis Center for Behavioral Neurobiology, The Salk Institute, San Diego, California 92112*


**Carol Thomson**
*Department of Nutrition and Food Science, Massachusetts Institute of Technology, Cambridge, Massachusetts 02139*

*Nutrition and the Brain,* Vol. 2, edited by R. J. Wurtman and J. J. Wurtman. Raven Press, New York © 1977.

# Control of Eating Behavior

## Loy D. Lytle

*Massachusetts Institute of Technology, Department of Nutrition and Food Science, Cambridge, Massachusetts 02139*

## I. INTRODUCTION

Among the responses in the behavioral repertoire of mammals, those involved in the acquisition of food are the most important. The motor responses underlying eating behavior are merely the end points of a complicated biological control system that enables animals to regulate closely the body levels of nutrients and energy, and thus promote growth, reproduction, health, and survival. In the final analysis, the survival of any species depends on its ability to achieve a balanced energy and nutrient exchange with the environment. Small discrepancies in the rates at which energy or nutrients are acquired or expended produce striking changes in the physicochemical makeup of the organism. Large discrepancies are usually fatal.

Probably more is known about various aspects of eating behavior than about any other behavioral response, although each scientific advancement in our understanding has raised new questions. This chapter summarizes the results of a vast number of experiments aimed at understanding the nature of eating behavior in animals and humans, and describes in some detail the possible environmental, organismic, and physiological factors that may alter its normal expression. Several excellent volumes and review papers are included in the reference list at the end of the chapter, and the interested reader is encouraged to consult them for more comprehensive discussions of specific topics not dealt with in detail here.

## II. THE NATURE OF EATING BEHAVIOR

The precise means by which organisms eat food varies from one species to another, although a few general observations can be made about the feeding habits of almost all animals. Although the factors that influence eating behavior generally become more complex as one ascends the phylogenetic scale, it seems clear that almost without exception all animals eat periodically and cyclically. At any given time an individual animal is either in the process of eating or is not eating. A fundamental question, then, is whether the feeding cycle starts in the eating or the noneating state. If an animal is eating, then any analysis of its feeding behavior must be concerned, at least in part, with the mechanisms involved in terminating the eating response. On the other hand, if the cycle begins in the noneating state, then the analysis must include an understanding of the activating, or initiating, mechanisms involved (42).

A second general observation that appears to hold true across mammalian species is that most animals are able to balance the amounts of energy and nutrients acquired through eating against those that are expended. This observation is supported by the fact that most mature members of a species maintain relatively constant body weights throughout most of their lives. If energy-nutrient intake exceeds expenditure, and the many excess dietary constituents are stored in the body, body weight increases; if the nutrient-energy expenditure is greater than intake, the amount of nutrient-energy stores usually declines and body weight decreases. Although the general outcome resulting from a "positive" or "negative" nutrient-energy balance is unusually similar among most animals, the mechanisms underlying these imbalances may be quite different.

Since body weight in physiologically mature animals remains constant only if the acquisition and expenditure of energy and nutrients are somehow balanced, and since eating food is the primary acquisition process, many investigators (12,42,98) deduced that eating behavior (and nutrient-energy expenditure) must be under rigid control. Simple estimates of annual human caloric intake support this hypothesis. During a single year a normal adult male human ingests somewhat more than one million calories. If only 1% (10,000) of these calories are not expended as energy and are stored in the body, the body weight increases by approximately 1 kg during the year. Hence in the normal situation well over 99% of the calories ingested must be expended if body weight is to remain constant (98). Although the processes that couple energy acquisition and expenditure in humans are unknown, detailed studies of feeding and activity patterns in American males suggest that this coupling does not occur on a moment-by-moment or even on a daily basis (184). Over the long run, however, significant correlations among these variables can be found, although the relationship is not simple (42).

A thorough understanding of eating behavior, then, requires a knowledge of the mechanisms important for meal initiation and termination, as well as a knowledge of how animals are able to maintain constant nutrient-energy balance.

## A. Methods of Measuring Eating Behavior

Feeding behavior has been intensively examined in species as diverse as the blowfly (173), the marine gastropod *Aplysia* (385), rodents (411), primates (629), and humans (562,572,615,644,645,703,801). Of all animals, the laboratory rat has received by far the most empirical study, and this chapter deals largely with the results of experiments conducted with this animal. Generalizations based on a single animal model and applied to the behavior of other animals are always dangerous; in this case especially it is known that factors influencing the eating behavior of animals may not be similar to those that alter human eating behavior. Unlike most animals, human beings are capable of eating food even though they are not hungry and of drinking water even though they are not thirsty. Despite these problems, research based largely on the results gained from the study of laboratory animals has suggested a variety of useful clinical approaches for understanding and treating human eating disorders.

Given that daily food intake is episodic, various investigators (43,304,368, 406,409–411,421,532,534,538,690,749) analyzed eating behavior by quantifying the amount of food eaten over defined time intervals (Table 1). In its most simple analysis, eating behavior can be quantified by measuring the amount

TABLE 1. *Experimental analyses of eating behavior*

---

*Parameters used to infer relative states of "hunger" or "satiety"*
1. Changes in total amount of food eaten in a defined time period
2. Changes in the rate of performing an operant response for food reward
3. Changes in meal patterns
   a. Size of individual meals
   b. Amount of time taken to eat a meal of defined size
   c. Number of meals eaten during a defined time period
   d. Length of time between meals
   f. Number of intermeal intervals during a defined time period
4. Changes in occurrence of "anticipatory" or "postprandial" behaviors

*Measurements of food preferences or aversions*
1. Changes in preference or aversion limens
   a. Amount eaten during simultaneous presentations of food
   b. Relative differences in amounts eaten during successive presentations of food

*Measurements of induced physiological "needs"*
1. Changes in dietary self-selection
   a. Amount eaten during single, successive presentations of foods
   b. Amounts eaten during "cafeteria" presentations of different food

---

eaten during a specified period of time, or it can be broken down into other components aimed at determining changes in meal patterns: meal size (the amount of food consumed during an operationally defined meal), meal length (the time it takes to eat a prescribed amount of food), intermeal intervals (the time that elapses between two meals), the number of daily meals, the number eaten during the light or dark portion of the day-night cycle, etc. In other analyses food "preference" or palatability (816), or the relative ability of animals to select balanced diets to meet daily nutrient requirements, are determined by measuring the amounts of food selected from different types of foodstuffs, from different flavored diets, or from diets that contain different amounts of basic nutrients (carbohydrates, fats, proteins, vitamins, or minerals) (603). The various ways of measuring feeding behavior and assessing meal patterns often lead to differences in the interpretation of how factors influence feeding behavior (411,532).

If one is to characterize the feeding patterns of different animals successfully, it is important to know about the experimental condition under which eating behavior is studied. Almost without exception, feeding behavior is assessed under at least one of the following three experimental conditions: (a) food and water available at all times; (b) varying intervals of food deprivation imposed between meals; or (c) limited numbers of meals allowed per day (195,470). Each of these experimental variables (as well as the conditions under which animals are allowed to obtain food—whether it is freely available or the animal is required to perform an operant response such as bar pressing) can alter the feeding pattern. A few examples will make this clearer. In the free-feeding situation, where there is access to laboratory chow, the size of an individual meal consumed by rats does not correlate well with the length of the fast preceding that particular meal; however, meal size is correlated with the length of time that elapses until the onset of the next meal (412). When animals are placed on restricted feeding schedules, they usually require several days (while they progressively increase individual meal sizes) before they are able to eat enough food per day to maintain their body weight (195). Similarly, rats fed *ad libitum* can usually adjust total daily food consumption rapidly if the caloric density of the diet is altered; in contrast, animals allowed restricted access to food experience great difficulty in adjusting intake to compensate for changes in dietary caloric density (686).

The rather substantial research efforts devoted to establishing reliable methods for measuring feeding behavior have important theoretical ramifications, especially as they relate to a possible understanding of how various factors alter such hypothetical constructs as "hunger" or "satiety." In order to determine to what extent various factors influence hunger or satiety, it is important to know whether animals and humans begin to eat because they are more hungry since their last meal or because they have become less satiated by their last meal. Furthermore, do animals stop eating because they have become less hungry or because they have become more satiated? Stated another way: does a factor influence feeding behavior by altering the hunger-stimulating effects of no food (which intensify with the length of the previous fast) or by altering the satiating effects of food (which lessen with the length of the intermeal interval)? The only means by which these various influences on feeding behavior can be distinguished from one another is by an analysis of changes in feeding pattern. Many theoretical disputes about whether a given factor decreases satiety or increases hunger can be traced to disagreement about the best operational definitions for terms such as a meal or an intermeal interval (411,532). Using one type of statistical criterion for defining a meal, LeMagnen and Tallon (411) found a positive correlation between meal size and the time interval that elapsed between that meal and the subsequent one. They found no correlation, however, between the size of a meal and the time elapsed between that meal and the previous one. In contrast, using other criteria Panskepp (532,538) found no relationship between meal size and postprandial intermeal interval. Instead, he reported that a "satiety ratio" (the ratio of meal size to meal interval, an index of the satiating capacity of food relative to the hunger-inducing capacity of time without food) was a better predictor of meal pattern frequency. Using satiety ratios, it appears that the total amount of food eaten during a meal is important because it alters the amount of hunger that develops during the no-food, intermeal interval that follows. Furthermore, using this criterion it appears that the size of a meal increases the capacity of subsequent meals to inhibit feeding (534). The major obstacle to obtaining agreed-on methods of determining meal size and inter-meal interval is simply that most animals do not eat clearly defined meals with no food consumption between meals. Most mammals appear to be "nib-blers," and while they eat large quantities of food at various times during the day (and night) they also eat less-well-defined, smaller quantities of food throughout a 24-hr period. It appears that the only means by which terms such as hunger and satiety can be adequately defined operationally is to use other indices (e.g., biochemical or hormonal changes) in addition to or in place of statistical analyses of feeding patterns.

## B. The Physiological Disposition of Food

The typical American consumes approximately 800 g of food and 1,200 ml of water each day. Of this total intake, approximately 62% is carbohydrate, 25% protein, and 10% fat by weight. These compounds, the basic energy-yielding nutrients, do not usually exist in the external environment as biologically useful material; foodstuffs must be ingested and broken down (digested). Biologically useful molecules of food remaining after digestion are absorbed across a variety of body membranes and are eventually transported to a number of tissues for storage or use in biochemical reactions. The remaining biologically nonuseful materials are eventually excreted after various salts and water are absorbed from the colon. Owing to differences in metabolism, the energy yield from carbohydrate, protein, and fat is different. Fat is much richer in energy than the other nutrients, and its metabolism yields approximately 9 calories/g; protein and carbohydrate metabolism each yields 4 calories/g.

A detailed description of how foodstuffs are eventually translated into nutrients capable of being utilized by the body is not possible here; however, a brief description of these processes aids in understanding how physiological changes associated with the digestion, absorption, metabolism, utilization, and storage of nutrients are important in the control of eating behavior.

### 1. Anatomy of the Gastrointestinal Tract

Viewed in its most simple terms, the digestive tract is a tube that communicates with other body tissues through nerves, blood vessels, and secretions, and by the absorption of various chemicals across the gastrointestinal (GI) tract membranes. The two prime functions of the GI tract—digestion and absorption of food—are accomplished via two major mechanisms: food movement along the tract and breakdown of foodstuffs into biologically useful material. These two gastric functions—motility and secretion—are mediated in large part by locally active reflex arcs, as well as by nerve fibers from the sympathetic and parasympathetic branches of the autonomic nervous system that enter the digestive tract and form synapses with the internal nerve plexus and with the secretory cells of the tract.

The anatomy of the GI tract is strikingly similar in a wide variety of mammals. The entire GI tract, from the mouth to the anus, is a long tube of variable diameter; the inside (lumen) of the tube is continuous with the external environment. The GI tract can be divided into distinct portions on the basis of functional and anatomical differences: the mouth, pharynx, esophagus, stomach, small intestine, large intestine, and rectum. Despite these distinctions, however, the GI tract has the same general structural features throughout, from the esophagus to the anus. In cross section the lumen of the digestive tract is surrounded by three layers of smooth muscle; the inner muscle layer has cells with a circular orientation, and the outer layer has muscle fibers oriented longitudinally along the lumen. Contraction of the inner muscle layer constricts the tract, decreasing the diameter of the lumen; contraction of the outer muscle layer shortens the tract. A third, and the thinnest layer of smooth muscle (the muscularis mucosa), contains both longitudinal and circular muscle fibers. A layer of cells called the mucosa is situated between the muscularis mucosa and the lumen. This innermost layer of cell contains exocrine cells that secrete compounds that assist in the breakdown and movement of food within the tract, as well as epithelial cells, which are involved in the transport of nutrients from the lumen into the bloodstream and lymph system. The innermost surface of the digestive tract is highly convoluted, an anatomical feature which greatly increases its total surface area. The most extensive convolutions occur in the small intestine— that portion of the digestive tract where absorption of nutrients is greatest. Portions of the digestive tract contain smooth or striated muscle which forms sphincters (the hypopharyngeal, gastroesophageal, pyloric, ileocecal, and internal and external sphincters) that divide the main portions of the digestive tract and are essential in the movement of its contents away from the oral cavity and toward the anus.

## 2. Ingestion and Movement of Food Through the GI Tract

The amount of food taken in the mouth at one time varies considerably from one species to another, as does the extent to which a mouthful of food is chewed and broken down into smaller particles. In most cases the food is mixed with saliva that is secreted reflexively from the submaxillary, sublingual, and parotid glands. Saliva aids the breakdown of carbohydrates and lubricates the food for its subsequent passage through the digestive tract. The act of chewing involves both voluntary and involuntary (reflexive) motor responses; swallowing appears to be a reflexive response. The food is formed into a lump, or bolus, that is propelled by the tongue into the pharynx. The bolus stimulates receptors for the sensory fibers of the glossopharyngeal and vagal nerves; these fibers in turn send efferent discharges through the vagus nerve, initiating muscular contractions which move the bolus past the hypopharyngeal sphincter into the esophagus. Reflexive, peristaltic waves in the esophagus move the bolus toward the stomach, the speed of passage determined by the nature of the bolus (whether it is liquid or solid) and the amount of mucus secreted by the cells lining the lumen of the esophagus. The motor responses involved in the swallowing reflex relax the gastroesophageal sphincter, which allows the bolus to enter the stomach. At all other times the gastroesophageal sphincter remains tonically contracted, preventing the contents of the stomach from being pushed back up the esophagus. This is particularly important since the hydrochloric acid (HCl) in the stomach would irritate the cells lining the esophagus, causing muscle spasms associated with the sensation of heartburn.

The stomach interior is highly convoluted, so that as it fills with food and the smooth muscles lining it relax, the pressure increase is relatively small. The stomach is below the diaphragm, whereas the esophagus is not. The greater atmospheric pressure on the stomach, due to its compression by the contents of the abdominal cavity, would force the bolus back into the esophagus were it not for the tonically contracted gastroesophageal sphincter and the ability of the stomach to relax sufficiently to offset the increase in intragastric pressure associated with the presence of the bolus. The stomach serves two important functions: it secretes acids and enzymes which break down the bolus into smaller molecular particles (called chyme), and it regulates the rate at which the chyme enters the small intestine, where most of the digestive and absorptive processes occur.

The smooth-muscle layers around the portion of the stomach closest to the esophagus (the fundus) are smaller and weaker than the muscles lining the lower portion of the stomach (the antrum). The rate at which the chyme leaves the stomach and is propelled into the small intestine is determined by the rate and strength of contraction of the longitudinal smooth-muscle layer of the stomach. Peristaltic waves originate in the fundus and are directed toward the antrum. The strong antral contraction associated with these waves forces a small amount of chyme into the small intestine when the pyloric sphincter is closed by the contraction. The peristaltic waves, in combination with the antral contraction, mix the gastric contents prior to their entry into the small intestine. The rate at which the contents of the stomach are emptied into the small intestine depends on the rate and force of the muscle contractions of the antrum and pyloric sphincter. These contractions (called gastric motility) are in part related to the physicochemical properties of the chyme in the small intestine. In general, the smaller the size of particles of partially digested food in the chyme, the larger the volume of the chyme or its osmotic pressure, the more dilute the solution of the food, and the less acidic its concentration, the more accelerated is the rate of gastric emptying. Furthermore, high-fat foods leave the stomach more slowly than diets containing a larger proportion of protein or carbohydrate. It appears that chemoreceptors, osmoreceptors, and pressure receptors—all located in the walls of the small intestine—as well as the secretion of hormones by cells in the duodenum affect the activity of gastric smooth muscle. The rate of gastric emptying can also be influenced by efferent nerves from the central nervous system (CNS); intense emotion and physical pain tend to decrease gastric motility.

As the stomach empties, the rate and force of contractions decrease. As fasting continues, the rate of gastric contractions increase. Some investigators (124,126) hypothesize that the increase in gastric motility associated with fasting may provide one of the critical signals to the brain that initiate the process of eating. However, the adequacy of this explanation has been questioned (576).

Stomach cells do not have special transport mechanisms for nutrients, and very little food is absorbed directly from the stomach into the bloodstream. The size and degree of ionization of the particles in gastric chyme does not allow them to diffuse easily across the tissue membranes of the stomach. Some molecules (alcohol and weak acids, e.g., aspirin), however, can be absorbed from the stomach in small quantities.

Most of the digestion and absorption processes occur in the small intestine. Anatomically, the small intestine can be separated into three parts: the duodenum (the short segment of intestine that lies just below the pyloric sphincter), the jejunum (the middle portion of the intestine), and the ileum. Chyme moves so slowly through the duodenum that the residue of one meal is delivered from the ileum to the large intestine as another meal enters the stomach. Pacemaker cells located in the longitudinal smooth muscle of the small intestine generate a rhythmic electrical activity that contracts and relaxes the smooth muscle in various portions of the intestine. These movements, called segmentation, mix the chyme with intestinal secretions of the lumen and repeatedly expose the food mixture to the absorptive surface of the intestine. The frequency of contraction is greater in the upper portion of the small intestine than in the lower portion; chyme is moved through the small intestine with short, weak peristaltic movements that are much less intense and frequent than the muscular contractions associated with gastric emptying. Few contractions occur in the empty intestine; the distention associated with the presence of the chyme contracts the smooth muscles around the chyme and relaxes those muscles that are immediately distal. The small intestine has far greater absorptive capacity than do other parts of the GI tract; the convolutions of its mucosa, combined with the projections of numerous villi and microvilli of epithelial cells into the lumen, greatly increase the total surface area exposed to the chyme.

Heightened gastric motility reflexively increases the contractions of the ileum; these contractions, along with secretion of the hormone gastrin from the small intestine, relax the ileocecal sphincter and allow passage of the residue of a meal from the terminal portions of the ileum into the colon, or large intestine. Distention of the colon contracts the sphincter and prevents further passage of material from the ileum. Very little absorption occurs in the large intestine, whose primary function is to store and concentrate the unabsorbed portion of chyme prior to defecation. Material in the colon is slowly moved and turned over by infrequently occurring, weak contractions of circular smooth muscle. Because of this slow movement, material entering the colon remains there for as long as 18–24 hr after ingestion of a meal. Some of the chyme in the colon is digested by bacterial action, and much of the water is reabsorbed. Marked increases in colon motility generally occur after a meal; this increased motility, during which major sections of the colon contract simultaneously, propels fecal material as much as one-third to three-fourths the length of the colon. The sudden distention of the walls of the rectum arouse the defecation reflex, which consists of rectal muscle contraction, internal and external anal sphincter relaxation, and increased peristaltic activity of the sigmoid colon sufficient to propel the feces through the anus. Reflex relaxation of the external anal sphincter can be modified by voluntary mechanisms, and defecation can be postponed.

The digestive process is associated with biochemical, electrophysiological, and hormonal changes thought by some to provide essential signals regarding relative states of hunger and satiety (for a summary see Table 2).

### 3. Digestion of Food in the GI Tract

The extent to which food is mechanically broken down in the mouth varies from one species to another; in most cases, however, food is mixed with saliva that contains approximately 50% mucins (proteins that lubricate the food particles). The other major digestive protein in saliva is an enzyme, amylase, which initiates the breakdown of carbohydrates. The enzymatic reactions catalyzed by amylase continue until food reaches the stomach, where the secretion of HCl inhibits the enzyme. The digestion of food by compounds secreted in the stomach is not absolutely essential, inasmuch as digestion and absorption still occur in humans with gastrectomies; however, the digestive functions of the stomach certainly aid these processes.

Relatively large amounts of HCl are secreted by the so-called parietal cells of the corpus, or body, of the stomach. HCl reduces large particles of food into smaller ones by denaturing proteins and breaking down other molecular bonds in cells and connective tissue. The acid also kills a large portion of the bacteria present in food and inactivates some of the enzymes secreted by the stomach for digestion. Control of HCl secretion by the parietal cells of the stomach is accomplished by afferent activity of the vagus nerve as well as by the secretion of various hormones from the antrum or the small intestine. The basal secretion of HCl is generally low; it is stimulated by the sight, smell, or taste of food, or by other non-food-related cues, e.g., changes in emotional state (157). The presence of food in the stomach also stimulates the secretion of HCl, apparently by activating local receptors sensitive to gastric distention and by stimulating the release of a hormone, gastrin, from cells located in the walls of the antrum. The amount of gastrin released usually depends on the protein content of the food, although other compounds (e.g., ethanol or caffeine) are also potent stimulants for the release of this hormone (775). In addition to stimulating HCl secretion, gastrin stimulates contraction of the gastroesophageal sphincter, which helps prevent the highly acidic contents of the stomach from reaching the sensitive cells that line the esophagus.

Feedback mechanisms regulate the amount of HCl secreted. As the concentration of hydrogen ions in the stomach increases, the release of gastrin diminishes, in turn reducing the stimulation of HCl secretion. Conversely,

TABLE 2. *Role of the digestive tract in feeding behavior*

| Digestive function | Nature of the signal | Importance for feeding behavior |
| --- | --- | --- |
| Oral cavity | | |
| Mechanical breakdown and lubrication of food; enzymatic catabolism of starches and carbohydrates; transport of food to stomach | Neural; hormonal (?) | Diet selection Food palatability Meal initiation Meal termination |
| Esophagus | | |
| Lubrication of food; transport of food to stomach | Neural | Meal termination |
| Stomach | | |
| Inactivation of upper GI enzymes and bacteria in food; chemical breakdown of foodstuffs; absorption of selected nutrients; transport of food to small intestine | Neural; hormonal (?) | Meal initiation Meal termination |
| Small intestine | | |
| Major role in digestion and absorption of carbohydrates, amino acids, and proteins; transport of food to large intestine | Neural; hormonal | Meal termination |
| Large intestine | | |
| Absorption of water, sodium, vitamins, and small amounts of glucose; lubrication of feces and expulsion of unuseful material | ?? | ?? |

when the concentration of hydrogen ions is decreased by the buffering action of food and protein, gastrin release (and therefore HCl secretion) is increased. Gastric acid secretion is also altered by duodenal reflex mechanisms: Increased duodenal distention or the presence of chyme in the duodenum that is hypertonic or that contains high concentrations of fatty acids, amino acids, or hydrogen ions decreases HCl release in the stomach (157).

The HCl has relatively little destructive effect on the cells lining the stomach because these cells secrete a slightly alkaline mucus which neutralizes the hydrogen ions close to the gastric mucosae. In addition, the mucosal cells are packed closely together, so that relatively little acid reaches deeper tissues of the stomach lining; finally, the cells of the mucosae continually divide and replace themselves to ameliorate their eventual breakdown by the acid.

Other substances secreted in the stomach are pepsins, proteolytic enzymes released from the so-called chief cells of the corpus and antrum. Pepsin catalyzes reactions that break amino acid bonds in the protein chains of foods and reduces these chains to peptide fragments. The secretion of pepsin and the factors that alter its release by the chief cells (distention, gastrin secretion, etc.) are similar to those that alter the release of HCl. The catalytic activity of pepsin depends on a high concentration of hydrogen ions in the stomach; pepsin activity is inhibited when the acid is neutralized by the release of bicarbonate ions from the pancreas into the duodenum.

Most of the processes of digestion and absorption are accomplished after the chyme passes from the stomach into the duodenum. In the small intestine the chyme is mixed with secretions from various other organs as well as with locally secreted hormones. Two hormones, cholecystokinin and secretin, are released by glandular cells in the small intestine, depending on the physico-chemical composition of the chyme and the electrical activity of various neurons that innervate the small intestine. These two hormones profoundly alter the secretion of other hormones, enzymes, proteins, and salts from the pancreas and liver; they also contribute greatly to changes in gastric motility, digestion, and absorption (582).

Cholecystokinin release is dramatically increased in response to high concentrations of certain essential amino acids (tryptophan, phenylalanine, valine), to long-chain fatty acids in the chyme, and to high concentrations of intraluminal hydrogen or calcium ions (582). Cholecystokinin decreases gastric motility and contracts the pyloric sphincter, thus reducing the efflux of chyme from the stomach into the small intestine. At the same time, this hormone markedly increases the release of various enzymes from the pancreas. These enzymes break down proteins, carbohydrates, and fats into amino acids, sugars, and fatty acids, respectively, which are then absorbed from the small intestine into the bloodstream.

Unlike cholecystokinin, which is released by a wide variety of stimuli, secretin release appears to be stimulated selectively by the concentration of acid (hydrogen ions) in the small intestine. Secretin reduces the concentration of acid in the small intestine by contracting the pyloric sphincter and inhibiting further acid secretion in the stomach (by decreasing the release of gastrin). In addition, secretin stimulates intestinal release of alkaline duodenal, biliary, and pancreatic secretions, thus preventing acid damage to the cells lining the lumen and providing an environment in which digestive enzymes secreted from the pancreas into the small intestine can be active (440). Other hormones (enterogastrone, motilin, vasoactive intestinal peptide, and gastric inhibitory peptide) have been isolated from the small intestine, but their precise roles in mediating GI motility, digestion, or absorption remain to be determined (440).

Compounds synthesized in the pancreas and liver are released into the pancreatic and bile ducts, which converge into a single duct entering the duodenum. The compounds released into this duct are absolutely essential for normal intestinal digestion.

Exocrine cells in the pancreas and its duct secrete two solutions—one containing a high concentration of sodium bicarbonate, and the other large concentrations of digestive enzymes. The GI hormones—gastrin, secretin, and cholecystokinin—or the acid-induced release of secretin from the duodenal cells stimulates the release of sodium bicarbonate from cells lining the pancreatic ducts. The bicarbonate ions neutralize acid in the duodenum, providing an appropriate environment for the catalytic activity of food-digesting enzymes released from the pancreas.

The catalytic pancreatic enzymes (trypsin, chymotrypsin, carboxypeptidase, lipase, amylase, and ribo- and deoxyribonuclease) are released from the acinar cells of the pancreas by afferent discharges of the vagus nerve or following the release of the GI hormones. Cholecystokinin appears to be the most important releaser of the pancreatic enzymes, although its effect may be mediated by the vagus nerve inasmuch as the pancreatic response to cholecystokinin is inhibited after extragastric denervation (440). The catalytic actions of the pancreatic enzymes contribute to the digestion of proteins, carbohydrates, and fats in the duodenal chyme: Trypsin and chymotrypsin break the amino acid bonds of protein and form peptide fragments; carboxypeptidase cleaves terminal amino acids from proteins that contain free carboxyl groups; lipase forms free fatty acids (FFAs) and monoglycerides by cleaving triglycerides; pancreatic amylase, similar in structure to salivary amylase, breaks down polysaccharides into glucose and maltose; and the nucleases split nucleic acids into free mononucleotides.

The secretion of bile from the liver is essential for the duodenal breakdown of fats. Bile is a solution that contains relatively large concentrations of salts, the phospholipid lecithin, cholesterol, and various pigments such as bilirubin. The concentration of bile salts and the volume of isotonic fluid in which they are dissolved are controlled by different mechanisms. The rate of bile salt production depends on the concentration of these salts in plasma, which changes as a function of eating, digestion, and reabsorption from the intestine; hence the rate at which liver secretes the salts is low between meals. The secretion of bile by liver cells is stimulated by the release of the three GI hormones or by the activity of the vagus nerve. Secretin appears to be the most potent intestinal hormone associated with the release of bile. Bile is normally secreted by liver cells and is stored in the bile duct. A smooth-muscle sphincter (the sphincter of Oddi) regulates the flow of bile from this duct into the duodenum. Cholecystokinin and vagal nerve activity relax the sphincter; the amount of bile secreted is related to the composition and amount of chyme in the small intestine. A potent stimulus of duodenal cholecystokinin secretion is fat.

When fat accumulates following the initial breakdown of food into chyme, it forms insoluble globules that are emulsified by the bile. The cholesterol contained in bile as well as the globules of fat in the intestine are emulsified primarily via the action of bile salts and lecithin. The bile salts involved in the digestion of fat are absorbed from the intestine into the enterohepatic circulation (which passes through the liver) and allows for their reutilization in liver bile.

Other digestive enzymes involved in the breakdown of food are synthesized, stored, and released by gland cells in the wall of the small intestine. Some of these enzymes—sucrase, maltase, and lactase—break down poly- and disaccharides into the monosaccharides glucose, galactose, and fructose; other enzymes—aminopeptidase and lipase—complete the digestion of proteins and fats, respectively.

By the time the chyme enters the large intestine, most nutrient absorption has occurred, with the exception of sodium, water, and some of the by-products resulting from the action of intestinal bacteria on the chyme. Intestinal bacteria synthesize small amounts of vitamins and produce glucose from the breakdown of cellulose. The vitamins produced are absorbed into the bloodstream but in amounts so small as to be physiologically significant only when the supply of vitamins from exogenous sources is low. The glucose yield from the breakdown of cellulose is not normally absorbed but is used for bacterial growth and reproduction. The only secretion by the large intestine that is significant for the digestive process is mucus, which lubricates the feces for transport through the rest of the colon.

### 4. Absorption of Nutrients from the GI Tract

Most of the absorption of nutrients in the small intestine occurs across the highly convoluted mucosal cells. The folding of the mucosa forms villi, fingerlike protusions made of several epithelial cells that are covered by small, hairlike projections called microvilli. These microstructures combine to increase the total surface area of the intestine approximately 600 times. Each villus contains a fine capillary network through which total blood flow is varied as a function of changes in GI distention. Each villus also contains a centrally located lymph vessel, called a lacteal, as well as several nerve fibers and muscle cells. The transportation of different nutrients across the epithelial cells of the villi and into the bloodstream or lymph system is accomplished by different mechanisms.

When pepsin and other pancreatic enzymes have broken protein chains down into peptide fragments, the fragments are converted into free amino acids by pancreatic carboxypeptidase and by aminopeptidase secreted from the intestinal villi. Several active transport systems, some of which require sodium, then transport the amino acids from the lumen across the epithelial cells of the villi and into the capillary bed. From there the amino acids are distributed to various body tissues.

The monosaccharides glucose and galactose are transported from the lumen of the intestine across the epithelial cells and into the bloodstream by a sodium-dependent, carrier-mediated mechanism in the epithelial cell membrane. Fructose, on the other hand, appears to be transported predominantly by facilitated diffusion. By the time the chyme reaches the end of the jejunum, carbohydrate absorption has been almost completely accomplished.

The absorption of fat is generally a much slower process than that for amino acids or carbohydrates because of the relative difficulty in breaking down fats into transportable FFAs. Lipid droplets arriving in the small intestine are emulsified by bile salts into smaller droplets, which are then broken down by pancreatic lipase into FFAs and mono- and diglycerides. The bile salts aggregate FFAs and monoglycerides into water-soluble particles called micelles. The micelles are in equilibrium with very small pools of fatty acids and monoglycerides. The soluble FFAs diffuse down a concentration gradient into the villi; during their passage through the epithelial cell membrane, the FFAs are resynthesized into triglycerides, which are eventually absorbed into the lacteals and carried throughout the body in the lymph system.

Although most of the vitamins are absorbed from the intestine into the bloodstream by a simple process of diffusion, some, especially the fat-soluble A, D, E, and K vitamins, depend on the secretion of bile salts since their transport is similar to that of fatty acids. Still other vitamins (e.g., vitamin $B_{12}$) appear to depend on a protein-mediated transport system in the ileum.

Although chyme entering the duodenum is usually isotonic, the absorption of amino acids, carbohydrates, fatty acids, vitamins, and salts in the small intestine tends to make the chyme hypotonic. However, the intestinal wall is highly permeable to water, and water diffusing from the hypotonic lumen into the isotonic plasma keeps the contents of the lumen essentially isotonic throughout the process of digestion.

### 5. Metabolism and Storage of Nutrients

*Absorptive state.*

Carbohydrates, proteins, and fats enter the bloodstream or lymph system primarily as monosaccharides, amino acids, and triglycerides, respectively. Most of the monosaccharides and amino acids absorbed into the blood from the digestive tract are transported directly to the liver via the hepatic portal vein. Some of the monosaccharides (e.g., galactose) are immediately converted by liver cells into glucose, which is then transformed into the polysaccharide glycogen for storage or is converted into fat via its breakdown into acetyl-coenzyme A (acetyl-CoA). A portion of the fat synthesized from glucose is stored in the liver cells; most of it, however, is transported into the bloodstream and is eventually stored in adipose tissue. Some of the circulating glucose molecules absorbed from the gut are taken up by adipose tissue and converted directly into fat; other glucose molecules in blood are transported into muscle cells and stored as glycogen. The largest fraction of glucose absorbed after a meal is taken up by an insulin-dependent mechanism into a variety of cells and is ultimately converted into water and carbon dioxide via its metabolism by glycolysis and the Krebs cycle. Energy yielded during these metabolic processes is stored in adenosine triphosphate (ATP) molecules. Hence glucose is the major energy source for cells during the absorptive state (Fig. 1).

A portion of the amino acids is also taken up and deaminated by liver cells. The resulting keto acids either enter the Krebs cycle and are oxidized to provide energy for liver cell function or are converted into fatty acids by the liver. Amino acids not transported into liver cells are either taken up by other cells in the body and used for protein synthesis or are converted into carbohydrate or fat and are stored.

Triglycerides absorbed into the lymph system from the digestive tract are broken down into glycerol and fatty acids, and the fatty acids are taken up by adipose tissue cells and stored primarily during the absorptive state. A small portion of fat is oxidized during this state and utilized for energy.

The secretion of hormones determine in large part the particular metabolic sequences observed during the absorptive state. The pancreatic protein hormone insulin is secreted from $\beta$-cells into the blood; its rate of secretion is controlled directly by the concentration of glucose in the blood circulating through the pancreas, such that reductions in blood glucose are associated with a decreased release of insulin. Insulin stimulates the facilitated diffusion of glucose into cells and increases the availability of carbohydrates for glucose oxidation, fat synthesis, and the formation of glycogen. The transfer of glucose out of the blood and into cells reduces the blood sugar concentration and thus removes the stimulus for insulin secretion. In addition to stimulating cellular glucose uptake, insulin has other anabolic effects associated with the absorptive state: It inhibits the breakdown of triglycerides and decreases their conversion to glycerol and fatty acid, and it increases protein synthesis by stimulating the transport of amino acids into cells and by stimulating ribosomal protein-synthesizing mechanisms.

Other hormones important for nutrient metabolism during the absorptive state are glucagon, epinephrine, and growth hormone (GH). The release of these hormones is related to the concentration of blood glucose and plasma amino acids. $\alpha$-Cells in the pancreas secrete glucagon when the blood glucose concentration falls; similarly, glucoreceptor cells, possibly located in the brain hypothalamic region, activate preganglionic sympathetic fibers that innervate epinephrine-secreting cells of the adrenal medulla. These same hypothalamic glucoreceptors may be involved in the release of GH from the anterior pituitary via their control over hypothalamic releasing factors. The secretion of glucagon and GH also change with fluctuations in the plasma amino acid concentration. An increased concentration of amino acids in blood following the consumption of a protein-rich meal stimulates the release of these two hormones from the pancreas or pituitary gland. Epinephrine, glucagon, and GH increase blood glucose by blocking its uptake and cellular metabolism. (Epinephrine and glucagon increase plasma glucose levels by increasing the breakdown of liver glycogen into glucose and by increasing hepatic gluconeo-

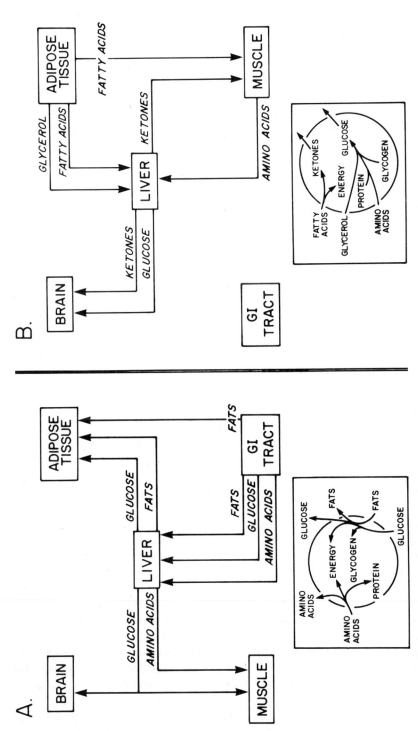

**FIG. 1.** Absorption, storage, and utilization of nutrients. **A:** Changes during the absorptive state. **B:** Changes during the postabsorptive state. (From Friedman and Stricker, ref. 216.)

genesis; all three hormones also increase the concentration of plasma fatty acids and glycerol by increasing the breakdown of triglycerides in adipose tissue.) Because of these reciprocal hormone effects, the quality of the food consumed in a particular meal produces slightly different effects on cellular metabolism depending on the relative amounts of insulin, epinephrine, glucagon, and GH released. For example, the consumption of a high-carbohydrate, low-protein diet is associated primarily with the release of insulin alone caused by the increased concentration of blood glucose; consumption of a low-carbohydrate, protein-rich meal is associated with an increased plasma amino acid level as well as increased secretion of epinephrine, glucagon, and GH, with relatively little change in circulating levels of insulin. Normal meals result in a more balanced release of the hormones involved in cellular metabolism. The release of insulin decreases the net plasma concentration of glucose during the absorptive state. The decreased concentration of plasma glucose as well as the increased concentration of plasma amino acids following the absorption of food stimulate epinephrine and glucagon release. The release of these hormones returns the plasma glucose concentration to a higher level by stimulating gluconeogenesis in the liver and increasing the hepatic breakdown of glycogen into glucose. Hence the hyperglycemic effects of glucagon and epinephrine release during the absorptive state counterbalance the hypoglycemic effects of insulin, and sudden large reductions or increases in the plasma glucose concentration are prevented.

*Postabsorptive state.*

   With one possible exception—the use of ketone bodies for energy during prolonged periods of starvation (121,821)—brain cells are able to derive energy from only one source: the glucose taken up from the bloodstream. Under normal conditions the brain consumes approximately 100 g (66% of the total daily circulating supply) of glucose; inadequate glucose supply for even brief periods is associated with permanent brain damage, coma, and death. During the postabsorptive state, no glucose is absorbed from the GI tract into the bloodstream; although the main reserve for glucose storage in the body is hepatic glycogen, the amount of glycogen readily available for breakdown into glucose is normally not even adequate to satisfy the human brain's glucose requirement for the overnight fast between dinner and breakfast (821). Hence other mechanisms must be available to meet the brain's energy requirements or else mammals would verge on the brink of extinction at each prolonged intermeal interval or each time meals of poor quality were consumed. Mammals utilize a variety of mechanisms to maintain the circulating glucose level during the postabsorptive state. Hepatic and muscle stores of glycogen are broken down, forming sufficient glucose to meet the normal requirement for relatively brief periods. During an extended fast, such as occurs overnight, triglycerides are catabolized in adipose tissue to yield glycerol and fatty acids. Glycerol is taken up by liver cells and is converted to glucose. In addition, especially during prolonged periods of fasting, muscle and other cellular protein stores not absolutely necessary for survival are catabolized, and the resulting amino acids are converted to glucose by the liver. One other very important mechanism ensures that an adequate amount of glucose is available to brain tissue during extended periods of fast; during the postabsorptive state virtually all body organs and tissues, with the exception of nerve cells, decrease the rate at which they oxidize glucose for energy and depend primarily on fat as an energy source. The fatty acids liberated from adipose tissue following the catabolism of triglycerides are transported into other cells and provide the required energy following their oxidation by the Krebs cycle. Some of the fatty acids transported into liver cells during extended periods of fast are converted to acetyl-CoA, which is then metabolized into ketone bodies. These ketone bodies are released into blood, transported into cells (including brain cells if the period of starvation is prolonged), and utilized as energy sources. These various metabolic processes are highly efficient: the circulating level of plasma glucose, even after long periods of starvation, decreases by only a few percentage points (216).

As in the absorptive state, the switchover to the metabolic pathways dominant in the postabsorptive state is accomplished primarily by the release of hormones. When the blood glucose concentration falls after the release of insulin, insulin secretion from the pancreas decreases and the metabolic pattern is shifted such that less glucose is transported into cells and cellular glucose oxidation declines. At the same time, the net catabolism of cellular stores of glycogen, triglycerides, and proteins is increased. The increased availability of amino acids and glycerol stimulates gluconeogenesis in the liver, and increased cellular availability of fatty acids stimulates the production of energy resulting from fatty acid oxidation. Brain tissue is assured of its normal supply of glucose during the postabsorptive state, because its uptake of glucose, in contrast to other cells, is not normally dependent on an insulin-sensitive transport mechanism.

The secretion of epinephrine, glucagon, and GH is increased during the postabsorptive period and during prolonged fasting; similarly, the activity of sympathetic fibers that innervate the adrenal gland and hepatic and adipose tissues is also increased during these times. The metabolic events associated with the postabsorptive state are clearly the direct result of a decreased circulating insulin level acting in combination with the catabolic effects of increased concentrations of epinephrine, glucagon, and GH. Those three hormones are also released following exposure to a variety of environmental stresses, thus facilitating the rapid mobilization of glucose-dependent energy stores.

## C. Classification of Factors that Influence Eating Behavior

Despite the lack of success thus far in arriving at precise definitions of the nature of eating behavior, one point seems clear: Most mammals spend a relatively small portion of each day eating. In addition, it is generally agreed that eating behavior occurs in discrete bouts over a 24-hr period interspersed by occasional periods of nibbling and of complete fast. Analyses of feeding behavior in animals and humans indicate that factors other than previous meal size or the length of the intermeal interval are important in determining the extent to which, and how frequently, animals eat. It is difficult if not impossible to classify all of the factors known to influence feeding behavior into mutually exclusive categories; however, for the purpose of the review that follows, the various factors that influence feeding behavior are discussed under three major classes: (a) "environmental" determinants, including such variables as the physicochemical properties of food, its availability in the environment, and the psychological, social, and cultural values associated with eating behavior; (b) "organismic" determinants, including such constitutional factors as the influence of genetic inheritance, age, feeding habits, and learned food preferences and aversions; and (c) "physiological" determinants that arise from the moment-to-moment biochemical, hormonal, and neural changes associated with the fed or fasted state.

Although experiments aimed at clarifying the factors that might influence human feeding patterns have provided some promising preliminary results, it is especially difficult to isolate the environmental, organismic, and physiological determinants of human eating behavior. For example, there are no techniques to assess adult human food preferences in such a manner that could distinguish the relative importance of "unlearned" food preferences (possibly arising from physiological needs or deficiencies) from those preferences that are learned or created in the marketplace by advertising. The available research suggests that human feeding behavior, at least in adults, is largely determined by environmental factors and by the individual's feeding habits. Until the relative contributions of each of these determinants can be determined, it will not be possible to determine the extent to which human feeding behavior is altered by each of the factors thought to influence the eating behavior of other animals.

## III. ENVIRONMENTAL DETERMINANTS OF EATING BEHAVIOR

Relatively few studies have examined possible environmental influences on the feeding behavior of animals (or even humans) in their natural habitats (for a review of these studies, see Gaulin and Konner, *Volume 1*). Under natural conditions many animals (and humans) do not have a continuously available supply of foodstuffs. It seems clear that many animals have evolved specific biochemical, hormonal, and physiological mechanisms so that they can adapt metabolically to periods of plenty and famine. Hence feeding studies conducted in experimental laboratory settings may be so artificial they entirely miss those adaptive characteristics of the organism most important for the normal control of food intake. Nevertheless, the precision provided by laboratory conditions at the very least offers an opportunity to determine the extent to which possible environmental factors influence feeding behavior.

## A. Food Palatability

The term food palatability usually refers to the organism's response to the physicochemical qualities of foodstuffs. Food qualities important to eating behavior are taste, texture, smell, temperature, and appearance.

The visual cues associated with food play a role in dietary preference inasmuch as most animals rely predominantly on visual as well as olfactory cues to locate food. Chickens (406), rodents (54), and chimpanzees (466) prefer to eat large pieces of food, and mice (45) offered their daily food ration in large pellets increase their total daily food consumption by as much as 20% over the amount consumed of diets presented in small portions. The texture of food also influences total consumption; e.g., rats eat more food if it is oily than if it has a coarse texture (272).

The particular smells associated with food also influence the amount consumed. Olfactory cues seem to affect eating behavior in at least two ways Animals are able to use olfactory cues to select from a variety of diets by a process of learned or unlearned associations with the biological quality of foods (i.e., the food's ability to satisfy nutrient-energy needs), and olfactory cues appear to alter food consumption by providing variety. In a now classic demonstration of the importance of olfactory cues for eating, LeMagnen (403,405) showed that the amount of food eaten by rats consuming a single diet was greatly enhanced if that diet was labeled with four different odors, as opposed to the amount eaten when the diet was labeled with only one of the four. Other experiments indicate that taste quality has a similar magnifying effect on eating behavior (559,560,815,817): Animals reinforced with food for pressing a bar or running a maze perform better when they are allowed to eat the food reinforcement rather than when oropharyngeal sensations are bypassed by placing the food directly in the stomach (65,375,471).

Once established, the taste and olfactory cues associated with particular foods strongly influence subsequent feeding behavior, even if these cues lead the animal to select dietary choices that are metabolically inadequate. For example, vitamin B-deficient rats that had previously learned to select a distinctly flavored diet adequate in the vitamins continued to prefer the flavored diet when it was rendered vitamin-deficient (285,659).

Although counterintuitive, some evidence suggests that food palatability may be more important than calories in determining the amount of food consumed by hungry animals and relatively unimportant in modifying the food intake of satiated animals (331,332,407,408). In many animals pleasant-tasting foods become more preferred and unpleasant tasting foods less preferred when animals are hungry (332,408). This relationship between palatability and hunger is borne out by observations that many animals consume relatively large amounts of a highly palatable diet under minimum conditions of hunger, and relatively small amounts of an unpalatable diet during states of severe hunger (332,408). However, humans may be different, since many of us eat first for palatability and only secondarily for nutritional benefit when food is freely available.

Food palatability clearly plays a large role in the ability of animals to locate foodstuffs; moreover, it appears to be important in dietary selection and contributes to the reinforcing properties of food. However, food palatability factors are not absolutely essential to the control of eating behavior: Humans and animals (187,188,192,703,752,779) are able to maintain relatively constant daily food intake patterns even under experimental or clinical conditions depriving them of the food stimuli associated with eating. Animals that are blind or anosmic or that feed intragastrically still maintain their body weight and grow in a nearly normal fashion. In the final analysis the physicochemical properties of food and their effects on eating behavior are important only in the context of the experiences of the organism; literally, "one man's meat is another man's poison."

### B. Specific Food Preferences and Aversions

Under normal conditions the sensual experiences associated with the diet play a powerful role in influencing the type and amount of food eaten. These influences can arise from either learned or unlearned associations. Animals and humans appear to have innate food preferences that are directly related to food's physicochemical properties, and it can be demonstrated that some taste cues are roughly related to the nutritional composition of the diet. A sweet taste is often associated with a high concentration of carbohydrates; a salty taste most often reveals the presence of a variety of nutrient salts such as sodium; and a bitter taste results from many toxic materials (188,389,406,407, 692). Almost all animals universally prefer the sweet taste over others (692), and many appear to have an innate preference for salt and an aversion to quinine or other bitter-tasting foods (171,625,627). Many food preferences appear to be innate, can be observed early in life, and appear to be relatively unaltered by subsequent learning experiences (5,330,503,557,627,658,816). Moreover, certain preferences (e.g., those for sweet solutions) can be selectively increased or decreased by inbreeding, thus suggesting that there is a strong genetic component to some food preferences and aversions (502,657). The fact that many mammals prefer some food types over others (insectivores, carnivores, herbivores) also lends indirect support to the notion that many food preferences and aversions are inherited (188).

On the other hand, learning strongly influences the selection of food, since odors, textures, volumes, and tastes often bear no clear relationship to nutritional value (406,625,627). For example, many animals (including humans) rapidly decrease their food intake when a new, adequate diet is abruptly substituted for the familiar one (this is called food neophobia); after a period of time, however, the intake increases progressively and eventually becomes stabilized (4,231,625,627). Although the precise mechanisms underlying the gradual acceptance of new foods are not well understood, it seems clear that the initial neophobia must be based largely on the oropharyngeal sensations that arise from eating (4,686).

The preferences or aversions associated with food, whether genetic or learned, and the particular palatability of the diet consumed, profoundly affect the abilities of all animals to select foods that provide nutrients adequate to meet all of their daily requirements. These factors are particularly important in the natural habitat of animals (629), whether it is the African jungle or the streets of New York, since no single natural food source known contains all of the essential nutrients needed by omnivores (389). If the preferences for or aversions to particular foodstuffs do not lead the animal to eat "good" food and avoid "bad" food, then survival can be severely threatened. A great deal of research has focused on determining whether, and to what extent, diet selection (and hence food preferences and aversions) is based on metabolic need. The answer to this question has obvious important practical implications for human eating behavior: If animals (and humans) can accurately select an appropriate diet from a variety of foodstuffs, then social influences on food selection should be minimized. On the other hand, if animals (and humans) are not always capable of selecting the diet best suited to meet physiological needs, nourishment should be scientifically calculated and individuals educated so that their food preferences and aversions allow them to make diet selections compatible with survival (27).

The dispute over whether animals can select appropriate foods to meet physiological needs has raged for more than 50 years without a clear-cut solution. Experiments with laboratory animals indicate that when given a choice animals often select so-called nutritionally adequate diets; moreover, the type of diet selected varies as a function of changes in physiological "needs." However, just as often, experimental animals select diets that are not only incompatible with their physiological needs but are detrimental to survival (389).

The outcomes of such experiments can be influenced by a number of factors that greatly complicate the interpretation of results. For example, the types of diet selected by animals are influenced by each of the following experimental variables: the number of food constituents offered; the ratio of substances offered as liquids or solids; the proportions of the various components offered; the sources, concentrations, and palatability of the substances offered; the strain, age, sex, weight, or number of animals tested; the length of time the experiment is conducted and the previous experiences of animals with dietary self-selection; and even the position of the food offered the animal (389). It is little wonder that the results of dietary self-selection experiments are controversial. Attempts to isolate and determine the effects of each of these variables have been discussed previously and are not reviewed in detail here (389).

The early experiments of Richter and colleagues (596,602,603) stimulated interest in the possibility of appropriate dietary selection by animals, and most of the major questions in this area can be traced to his original studies. Richter et al. showed that when rats were given access to a wide assortment of nutrients, both solids and liquids, and including vitamin, salt, and mineral solutions, they were able to grow and to maintain normal levels of physical activity (596). Furthermore, the types of food selected changed in response to the needs of the animal; protein, fat, and mineral intake increased during pregnancy and lactation in female rats and returned to normal after lactation ceased (599).

The available experimental data suggest that although animals can, under some conditions, recognize and detect certain specific nutrient deficient states and change their dietary preferences to compensate for these deficiencies (526), this wisdom of the body is not infinite; not all nutrient deficiencies can be detected, nor can they be compensated for (285,376,563,611). How are animals able to make appropriate dietary compensations for need states? Do animals have innate recognition systems for monitoring internally each of the nutrient substances necessary for growth and survival? Can these recognition systems be modified by experience so that animals can select foods that are nutritionally adequate to support life? The answer to both questions is yes: Under some conditions animals have innate, specific preferences for and aversions to dietary constituents; other specific food hungers or aversions arise through a process of learning. The two most well-studied hungers—that for sodium and for the B-vitamin thiamine—have contributed substantially to our understanding of how specific hungers and aversions influence feeding behavior.

In the case of sodium, the bulk of the evidence suggests that deficiency of this salt releases an innate preference for foods that contain it. Rats made sodium-deficient show a strong preference for saline solutions immediately upon tasting them for the first time (52,503,595,599,750,818), and animals not sodium-deficient prefer solutions that contain milder concentrations of the salt (52,171,595).

Most of the sodium ions normally circulating in the plasma of animals are not excreted in the urine owing to the effects of the adrenal hormone aldosterone; however, after adrenalectomy, sodium retention is severely impaired and body stores of the salt are eventually depleted. Animals with chronic sodium deficiency are lethargic, anorexic, and eventually die unless they receive dietary replacement doses of the salt. Adrenalectomized animals show a preference for solutions of sodium so concentrated that normal animals will not drink them (600). Although adrenalectomized rats do not immediately ingest large quantities of the salt following the operation, clear sodium preferences can be detected as early as the third postoperative day (191,600). Some investigators hypothesized that time is necessary for adrenalectomized animals to learn that drinking a salt solution makes them "feel better" (42); in contrast, the results of other experiments suggest that this delay is probably related to the time it takes for the operation-induced sodium depletion to reach sufficient magnitude for detection by the animal (191,783). In addition to the adrenalectomy-induced increase in sodium preference, the salt preference also changes following formalin injection (794), during pregnancy (599), or after peritoneal dialysis with glucose (198). Water deprivation causes rats to prefer less concentrated salt solutions (818), as does the injection of hypertonic saline (462) and the consumption of foods with high salt concentrations (596,597). Similarly, intraoral or intragastric injection of a saline solution produces predictable changes in the preference-aversion curves for sodium solutions based on the tonicity of the injected solution (704). Giving rats food with a high concentration of salt, on the other hand, is associated with a large increase in water intake (596,597).

Naive animals prefer a saline solution over water immediately after they are offered a choice for the first time, thus supporting the hypothesis that the preference for sodium is innate (596,597). This innate preference depends on the integrity of afferent and efferent nerves that innervate the tongue and oropharyngeal cavity, inasmuch as animals with damage to the ninth lingual nerve or to the pharyngeal branches of the tenth nerve no longer show clear preferences for saline solutions (597). Hence the salt appetite preference apparently depends on intact nerves that carry gustatory information to the brain or to other peripheral tissues. Brain mechanisms also appear to be involved in the establishment of the sodium preference, inasmuch as lesions of the anterior hypothalamic area diminish salt appetite (151,370) whereas lesions of the arcuate nuclei enhance it (151). Furthermore, lateral hypothalamic lesions diminish the ability of rats to increase sodium intake following injection of 11-deoxycorticosterone acetate (DOCA) (370). The bulk of the evidence, then, indicates that most mammals have an innate preference for sodium, although this appetite can be modified by manipulations that change the physiological needs of the animal.

In contrast, the ability of animals to compensate for an excess or deficient store of the B-vitamin thiamine appears to require learning. Thiamine (vitamin $B_1$) deficiency in humans (beriberi) and animals is associated in the long term with edema, bradycardia, anorexia, nausea, and peripheral neuritis (118,625, 788). The onset of symptoms associated with thiamine deficiency depends in part on the constituents in the diet: animals consuming thiamine-deficient, high-carbohydrate diets become deficient more rapidly because more thiamine is utilized to metabolize carbohydrates (604).

Thiamine levels in the body are not closely regulated, since animals without thiamine deficiency usually select randomly from diets independent of their thiamine concentrations; however, as soon as thiamine deficiency becomes manifest, animals prefer diets that contain the vitamin over diets that do not (624,660). The preferences of thiamine-deficient animals for diets or solutions that contain thiamine are clearly expressed even if these animals are offered a choice of several foodstuffs, although too much variety prevents proper selection (285). In addition, animals appear capable of detecting and compensating for other vitamin deficiencies (i.e., riboflavin or pyridoxine) as well, suggesting that this capacity is not specific only to thiamine (658,659).

Since it seems clear that animals do not normally show an innate preference for solutions or diets that contain thiamine or other vitamins (627,658), as they do for sodium, then how do animals deficient in these vitamins come to select diets that correct these deficiencies? In a detailed analysis of the eating behavior of thiamine-deficient rats, Rozin and colleagues (627,628) reviewed evidence that these animals tend to choose diets that contain adequate amounts of the vitamin only after a trial and error period during which they sample a variety of diets offered them. The deficient animals form an aversion to, and tend to avoid, familiar thiamine-inadequate diets; they also tend to show an enhanced preference for new foods (628). If the new food contains adequate amounts of thiamine, the animal continues to eat it to the exclusion of other food; if the new food does not contain adequate thiamine, the sampling process is continued until an adequate diet is found. The aversions formed to the inadequate diets appear to be relatively long-lasting, and animals continue to avoid eating a previously vitamin-inadequate diet even after it has been supplemented with adequate vitamin (285,587,626). The ability of thiamine-deficient animals to select a new, adequate diet depends on its relative ability to associate the nutrient quality of the diet with its particular smell, flavor, or appearance; after these new associations have been formed, animals tend to prefer to eat the new diet over all others (587,626,627).

Just as animals learn to form new preferences for diets that contain adequate amounts of nutrients, they also form aversions to distinctively flavored diets or solutions that they associate with illness induced experimentally by lithium chloride injection (229–231), irradiation (229,231,232), or injections of other drugs (229,231). These learned aversions can be established even though relatively long periods elapse between the time the food or liquid is consumed and the time the illness is induced; moreover, the learned taste aversions are strong and persist for long periods (231). It appears that aversions cannot be learned to all types of food, however, especially to those that appear to be essential for growth and survival (231,627).

In summary, then, animals learn some food preferences and aversions, but they also have innate, specific preferences and aversions to certain types of food which are relatively unmodifiable by subsequent experiences and which may (as in the case of sodium preference) or may not (as in the case of preferences for sweet-tasting diets and solutions) be essential for survival. Finally, most animals tend to display a neophobic reaction when offered unfamiliar, new diets if the old familiar one contains adequate nutrients and calories for survival. However, animals tend to sample new foodstuffs if the familiar ones are inadequate.

## C. Accessibility of Food

The availability of food influences meal patterns and eventually alters the metabolic disposition of nutrients consumed. When food is freely available, rats eat many small meals, with little or no correlation between meal size and the time that elapses before initiation of the next meal; this is called the preprandial relationship (39,406,410). Significant positive correlations exist, however, between the size of a meal and the intermeal interval that follows— the postprandial relationship (410). This relationship between meal size and intermeal interval changes depending on food accessibility. When placed on restricted-access feeding schedules, rats change their preferred feeding times in response to the new metabolic demands imposed by the feeding schedules. Rats fed *ad libitum* consume approximately 66% of their total daily food ration during the dark portion of the day-night cycle (39,410); in contrast, animals maintained on a daily 22-hr fast with 2-hr access to food eventually eat the same amount of food during the 2-hr period regardless of when it occurs during the light-dark cycle (390,391).

Many animals also appear capable of adjusting food intake in response to learned or unlearned "anticipated needs" imposed by the restricted availability of foods. Certainly the food hoarding and hyperphagia seen in many animals prior to a period of hibernation (461) or migration (521) testifies to the fact that innate mechanisms sensitive to environmental, seasonal triggering stimuli play a strong role in influencing feeding behavior (629). Animals can also learn new feeding habits that maximize survival during periods of limited food availability. In a laboratory test of these abilities, rats were allowed access to food for only three 1-hr periods per day (each 1-hr feeding period was separated by 7 hr of fasting). The food intake of these animals eventually stabilized, so that the amount of food consumed during each of the 1-hr feeding periods was approximately equal. After the stabilization period, one of the daily feeding periods was eliminated. At first the rats increased the amount of food eaten during the meal following the first 15-hr fast; after a period of time, however, the animals readjusted their total food intake, so that they consumed approximately three times as much food during the meal before the fast as during the meal that occurred after it (404). Hence it appeared that these animals were able to anticipate the long daily fast and increased the amount of food consumed in the meal just prior to its onset.

The accessibility of food and the size and frequency of meals may have important consequences for the control of feeding behavior, inasmuch as the patterns for the absorption and metabolism of nutrients change when animals are allowed limited access to food or when they eat following relatively long fasting periods (195,372). The periodic intake of relatively large amounts of food following prolonged fasts is associated with morphological and functional changes in the GI tract. When animals eat a large meal on limited-food-access schedules, the digestive tract becomes enlarged (316), and glucose and fats (but not amino acids) are more rapidly absorbed into the bloodstream (383, 745). Other metabolic changes have been observed in animals consuming fewer and larger meals: Rates of glycogen synthesis and cellular glucose utilization (194,195,745) increase, as does the rate of fatty acid synthesis from glucose—"adaptive hyperlipogenesis" (744,746); fat mobilization and catabolism from adipose tissue stores (195) decreases, leading to a generally increased accumulation of fat relative to lean body mass (138,139,196,573). Each of these metabolic changes favors the enlargement of fat stores in the body, presumably as an adaptive mechanism to ensure an adequate source of cellular energy during periods of fast.

The metabolic changes resulting from intermittent feeding schedules have important ramifications for human nutrition: Humans who eat fewer than the average three meals per day are more likely to be overweight than are individuals who consume more meals (and somewhat surprisingly, slightly greater numbers of total daily calories) per day (97). Hence it appears that many animals have evolved physiological mechanisms most suitable for metabolizing and storing nutrients that are obtained in relatively constant, frequent daily meals; alterations in feeding patterns (whether enforced by environmental constraints or based on voluntary idiosyncrasies) may induce changes that are eventually counterproductive for survival.

In one study aimed at determining the extent to which the accessibility of food might alter the eating behavior of overweight, normal, or underweight human subjects, overweight individuals tended to eat more when a greater supply of food was made available to them than when they were presented with relatively less food. In contrast, normal or underweight subjects tended to consume the same amount of food whether the supply was plentiful or scarce (510). In another study overweight human neonates consumed relatively less of a standard formula diet if they were required to work more for the food (by sucking on a nipple that had small-diameter holes). In contrast, normal or underweight neonates consumed approximately the same amount of the diet regardless of the effort expended in nursing (513). Taken together, then, these data suggest that the food intake of overweight humans might be related in part to the availability of food: When food is easily accessible, overweight humans have a tendency to overeat; under conditions of relative food scarcity, or as in the case of the infant study when more effort must be expended to obtain food, they tend to eat less. Similar findings have been reported in rats made obese with ventromedial hypothalamic (VMH) lesions (144,472). Despite these intriguing preliminary findings, the extent to which differences in food accessibility might alter other aspects of feeding behavior in animals and humans remains to be determined.

## D. Previous Eating Habits

Almost all aspects of human behavior have at one time or another been the focus of psychoanalysis, and eating behavior is no exception. Indeed, since the time of Freud a great deal of interest has been aimed at understanding the possible ways in which early feeding experiences ("oral gratification") might alter subsequent human behavior, and this basic theory still plays a dominant role in current behavioral analyses of human obesity. Crudely stated, the traditional psychoanalytical approach to adult human eating patterns emphasizes the early mother-infant interaction and the attachment of various appropriate or inappropriate impulses to the feeling of hunger in the infant. For example, obesity is thought to result at least in part from the mother's using food, inappropriately, as a "universal pacifier" in response to the varied biological needs of the infant (119). This use of food as a universal, positive reinforcer does not allow the developing infant and adolescent to learn appropriate responses to alleviate specific tensions arising from anxiety, anger, or other emotions. Subsequently, as an adult the obese human tends to use food as a means of alleviating or reducing tensions that are unrelated to nutrient-energy balance. Similar effects of early experience have been hypothesized to underlie the development of anorexia nervosa; this disease occurs predominantly in postpubescent females, is characterized by a refusal to eat with active rejection of food, and is accompanied by acute or chronic weight loss and malnutrition (119,351,662). Even though most of the psychoanalytical theories describing the effects of early experience on human eating disorders are quite attractive and have enjoyed a modest professional and popular interest, little direct empirical evidence supports their validity.

Laboratory studies conducted to determine the extent to which maternal feeding patterns in animals might influence the offspring's behavior have produced mixed results. For example, nocturnal feeding patterns in young and adult rats show diurnal rhythms that may be learned from the mother during the early preweanling period. In one experiment feeding patterns were studied in litters of blinded or sighted offspring reared by blinded or sighted dams (418). Lactating rats with normal vision (e.g., nonpregnant, normally cycling females) eat the majority of their total daily rations of food at night. As might be expected, these diurnal patterns of food intake were blocked in blinded lactating females. To determine whether the development of diurnal feeding patterns in preweanling rats was influenced by the feeding habits of their mothers, offspring were weighed at various times during the day to estimate changes in their food intake. The body weight changes in neonatal rats (whether they had normal vision or were blinded) indicated that they ate more during the day than at night for the first 2.5 weeks of life if they were reared by dams with normal vision; in contrast, the offspring of blinded dams showed no clear diurnal feeding patterns. By the time of weaning (at approximately 18 days of age), blinded and sighted offspring reared by females with normal vision showed adult-like diurnal rhythms in food intake and ate the major portion of their food at night. Offspring reared by blinded mothers did not show mature patterns of food intake until much later; however, the maturation of this behavioral change was only delayed, not permanently arrested (418).

Early experience also produces changes in other aspects of feeding behavior. The presence of the dam or other adult rats strongly influences the type of diet selected by weanling rats and decreases the time it takes for the offspring to wean themselves completely onto solid food (224,226). Young rats offered solid food in the absence of adult rats do not eat it until they are approximately 25 days old, whereas solid food is eaten by 20-day-old offspring when it is presented in the presence of other adults (224,226). Lactating rats that have learned to avoid distinctly flavored foods previously paired with injections of lithium chloride transmit the learned taste aversion to their offspring, so that the littermates subsequently avoid the particular food even though it has not made them sick (223,225,227).

The nutritional experiences of young animals also appear to influence other aspects of their adult feeding behavior. Rats that were malnourished early in postnatal life and then subsequently rehabilitated with adequate diets may have permanently altered feeding habits as adults (111). Early malnutrition is associated with a variety of other, long-lasting physiological (150,675) and behavioral maladies (for a review, see Pollitt, *this volume*); however, it is unclear if all of these changes are related directly to the effects of the undernutrition or if the undernutrition alters the behavior of the mothers in caring for their young (130) and thus indirectly alters later behavior (564,565).

The quality of the diet consumed by nonprecocial mammals (e.g., the rat, cat, and human) may produce long-term changes in the numbers and sizes of various cells in peripheral tissues and the brain. In initial experiments Winick and his colleagues (206,790,791) showed that protein-calorie malnutrition experienced during the period of maximal cellular division produced a long-term reduction in the total number of cells in the brain and periphery; in contrast, protein-calorie malnutrition experienced at other times during the life span of animals produced an apparent reduction in cell size, with little effect on cell number. If undernutrition is experienced during the period of cell division (hyperplasia), the reduction in cell number appears to be permanent, inasmuch as subsequent nutritional rehabilitation has little restorative effect. On the other hand, the effects of undernutrition on cell size can be reversed with nutritional rehabilitation (790). These observations may have important ramifications for the effects of early nutritional experiences on subsequent eating behavior, since the changes in brain or adipose cell number (305,306) or size may alter peripheral or brain mechanisms that may be involved in the control of eating. Although it is unclear just how these early nutritional experiences might permanently alter eating behavior, these findings do point to a potentially interesting animal model that might prove useful in studies of early feeding experiences and subsequent behavior.

Other manipulations of early feeding history apparently have relatively little effect on later eating behavior. For example, in a recent report preweanling rats were totally deprived of maternal influence by being fed intragastrically from the time of birth until weaning. These animals thus had no previous suckling experience nor any obvious experience in learning how to locate food in the environment. In addition, they had little opportunity to respond to peripheral changes associated with eating or fasting, or to display the motor responses usually associated with eating behavior because they were fed automatically at preprogrammed times throughout the day. In this initial experiment the animals were allowed access to solid food for the first time at age 19 days and then were tested briefly for their relative ability to control eating behavior. The intragastrically fed pups appeared to have no difficulty in identifying or eating food the first time it was presented; in addition, they responded normally by increasing food intake after a period of fast and decreasing the intake of food adulterated with quinine (269).

### E. Other Environmental Stimuli Important to Feeding Behavior

The majority of most mammals' food consumption occurs during that portion of the day-night cycle when the animal is normally awake (236,410, 432,594,598,827). The rat's normal nocturnal feeding pattern can be reversed if it is exposed to artificial lighting schedules that are out of phase with the normal environmental light-dark cycles; retraining to the new lighting schedule usually takes several days to stabilize, but these animals continue to consume most of their food during the dark portion of the cycle, even though it is shifted as much as 180° out of phase with the original cycle (586). When rats are exposed to conditions of constant light or constant dark (598), or to 2-hr light-dark cycles (91), the feeding rhythm "free runs," but most of their food is still eaten during the time when darkness normally would have occurred. The mechanisms that mediate the diurnal patterns of food intake are unknown, although animals with lesions of the VMH nucleus no longer show rhythms in feeding behavior that are synchronized to the lighting schedule (60,412).

Other environmental changes (e.g., differences in ambient temperature) also influence feeding. Most mammals eat more food when placed in cold environments and eat less during exposure to hot temperatures (107). As is seen later, changes in food consumption resulting from differences in environmental temperatures have been offered as partial support for the hypothesis that one of the control factors important for feeding behavior involves thermostatic mechanisms (273).

Differences in environmental temperatures may also be important in the seasonal changes in food consumption observed in hibernating animals (136, 494,629). Again, it is not yet possible to specify the precise physiological mechanisms that mediate the effects of environmental temperature on feeding, although it is interesting to note that electrolyte imbalances observed in humans during a heat wave may have been due to temperature-induced changes in the type of food eaten (651).

Observations of human and animal eating behavior suggest that many subjects tend to increase food intake when they are emotionally upset, bored, or under stress (143,242,623). Apparently eating food during these times helps some individuals to be less disturbed by environmental stressors, and subjectively helps to attenuate the emotional responses to unpleasant stimuli (143). During times of stress human subjects tend to eat relatively greater quantities of palatable foods, whereas the consumption of bland foods does not seem to change (512,645,799). An animal model was recently described which shows that mild to moderate stress in rats (accomplished by pinching the tails of these animals) also induces hyperphagia and obesity, even in animals that appear satiated (28). Furthermore, preliminary evidence indicates that stress-induced changes in feeding behavior may be mediated by brain neurons known to participate in other aspects of eating (623).

Perhaps one of the most interesting research programs during the past few years involves the observations from several laboratories that obese or normal-weight human subjects may respond differently to various environmental stimuli associated with eating behavior (510,513,615,644,645). Stated simply, these observations suggest that obese people may be less responsive to internal cues that signal hunger and satiety, but may be more responsive to external stimuli associated with food. In support of this hypothesis it was found that obese humans eat more food than normal-weight individuals if they are led to believe that more time has elapsed since their last meal than in fact has, or that the normal time for a meal has been reached even though it has not (613,646). In addition, obese subjects eat more if the food is displayed prominently, whereas nonobese people do not change their food consumption in response to such visual cues (619). Finally, obese humans tend to eat more when the food is palatable but eat less than normal individuals if the food is slightly unpalatable (511,571). Some results do not support the contention that all obese humans are more responsive to external cues and less responsive to internal signals associated with eating (800). In an attempt to account for these discrepancies, Rodin (614,615) hypothesized that the responsiveness to external cues may influence body weight gain in the acute situation but may not be a strong influence on long-term weight regulation. Although these hypotheses need to be tested further, they do offer interesting preliminary support for the notion that various environmental factors may play a large role in the regulation of eating behavior and may somehow interact with various other mechanisms of weight regulation.

## F. Sociocultural Influences on Feeding Behavior

Detailed, cross-cultural comparisons of human eating behavior have appeared in the anthropological literature for quite some time; however, rigidly controlled investigations of the possible variables affecting human eating behavior are relatively sparse (572). Thus far the bulk of experiments conducted with humans suggest that the brain and peripheral mechanisms that appear to play a large role in the control of feeding behavior in animals are often secondary to environmental, and especially sociocultural, influences. It is impossible to discuss in detail here all of the socioeconomic factors thought important to human eating behavior, but several excellent reviews were recently published (168,510,562,614,615,721,789) summarizing various aspects of this area.

Most animals respond reflexively or instinctively to various aspects of the environment, whereas humans select from and modify their surroundings largely by using techniques, principles, rules, and symbols learned from other members of their society (168,763,789). Humans tend to adopt food habits which closely reflect those of other individuals within the society; although these food habits can be somewhat altered by individuals, societal values can influence the feeding patterns of the individual, even to the point where malnutrition results. For example, almost everyone is familiar with the recent problems associated with the introduction of new nutrient supplements into certain areas plagued by recurrent famine (419,610,672,673,763); these new foods are often rejected by the populace on the basis of social or religious taboos. In addition, many societies reject new foods on the basis of their unfamiliar tastes, smells, colors, or textures (610). Although human food habits can sometimes be altered as a result of changes in social, psychological, economic, or physiological needs, the degree of change is often related to various cultural biases or proclivities (672,673).

Besides these obvious effects, various cultural characteristics produce quite subtle influences on the feeding habits of individual members of the society. For example, the more a society relies on farming as a source of food, rather than on hunting or gathering wild foodstuffs, the less varied its diet becomes. The reliance on agriculture eliminates some wild food sources, and the time spent in cultivating fields decreases the time available for gathering wild foodstuffs and the need for travel across great distances for foods (210). In times of famine, however, some societies "rediscover" natural food sources and incorporate greater amounts of them into the diet.

In addition to cultural differences in food production, societal distinctions in food processing and preservation also influence human eating habits. For example, cultures that lack the technology for making fireproof utensils, or utensils for eating foods, tend to eat foodstuffs of different quality or consistency than do societies that have developed these accessories (210). Advances in food preservation and transportation within individual societies are also important since they tend to increase the number of available foodstuffs.

Cultural attitudes toward food and eating also influence food intake patterns. In some societies the urge to eat is tempered by religious ideologies: Some foods are sacred and are not gathered, processed, or eaten, but are used in religious ceremonies. In other societies some foods are grown or gathered to be used as barter, and in still other societies food preparation and eating are regarded as aesthetic expressions approaching an art form. Hence it appears that food habits play as large a role in the fabric of different societies as sociocultural factors play in altering food habits (610).

## IV. ORGANISMIC DETERMINANTS OF EATING BEHAVIOR

Any theory purporting to account for all of the control mechanisms thought to be important for eating behavior must include possible differences in the constitutional makeup of the individual organism. Differences in genetic history, age, sex, or hormonal state appear to be important for long-term energy and nutrient balance, and have been hypothesized to alter a "set point" around which body energy and nutrient levels are regulated. Many of these factors may also influence the short-term control of eating behavior by changing the extent to which food induces satiety, or lack of food produces hunger.

### A. Genetic Factors

Genetic factors strongly influence energy-nutrient metabolism, storage, and expenditure, as well as the precise ways in which animals acquire and eat food. The food-gathering habits of many species have been studied in some detail (789), and it seems safe to conclude that preprogrammed, genetically mediated eating responses are less influential, and experiential and environmental influences more so, in higher-order mammals (173,629,789). It is apparent, however, that factors such as the types of food selected (493) and energy-nutrient disposition are under some degree of genetic control in all animals, including humans (478). Unfortunately, little is known about the biochemical processes involved in the genetic translation and transmittance of food preference characteristics, basal metabolic rate, or energy-nutrient expenditure. The enormous differences in body size alone probably account for a great deal of the variance associated with species and individual feeding habits. However, genetic factors that influence eating behavior must also be considered in the context of their interactions with various other determinants of food intake. For example, "genetically" obese animals would not become overweight if they did not have access to adequate supplies of food (100,325).

Perhaps the most potent genetic influences on feeding behavior involve mechanisms that set the limits of normal weight and size for each animal (100).

Again, the genetic potential for body weight and size can be modified by various environmental factors: During a famine all animals lose body weight regardless of their particular genotype, although the rate of weight loss varies among species and individuals; when the famine has passed some animals retain their lean body mass, others regain normal body weight, and still others become obese.

If "normal" body weight is genetically determined, how might this be important for feeding behavior? Evidence gathered from experiments with animals having a genetic propensity toward obesity suggests that body composition may be related to genetically programmed differences in energy-nutrient metabolism, storage, and expenditure (100,325). Each genetically obese animal shares several characteristics not seen in its lean littermate counterpart: (a) In all cases where food intake has been measured, the obese animals have eaten more food than their lean control littermates, although the degree of hyperphagia varies considerably among the various strains. (b) In all of these animals, a high proportion of calories are stored as fat, suggesting that genetically obese animals have more efficient biochemical mechanisms for food absorption and energy storage. (c) Most genetically obese animals are hypoactive and thus expend few calories in exploratory and locomotor activity. (d) All genetically obese animals studied thus far show some degree of hyperglycemia associated with hyperinsulinemia (100). Even though these animals have rather high circulating insulin levels, they appear to be "insulin resistant;" they are insensitive to the hypoglycemic effects of exogenously administered insulin, and insulin-induced inhibition of amino acid release from skeletal muscle is impaired (100). Since many metabolic abnormalities in genetically obese rodents—as well as in obese human patients (320,325)—exist, many may be due to altered effects of insulin on glucose metabolism in the adipose tissue of the obese (73,320,638). This explanation, however, is clearly insufficient to account for all of the metabolic abnormalities associated with obesity. Another possibility is that the relative insulin resistance of obese animals limits the peripheral utilization of glucose and favors its metabolism into adipose tissue triglycerides; furthermore, the increased plasma insulin levels might promote carbohydrate and protein storage, decreasing adipose tissue lipolysis (73). Each of these factors would increase the tendency for obesity. Despite these explanations, it remains uncertain whether these metabolic abnormalities, presumably due to genetic influences, cause the obesity or are merely the response to hyperphagia. For example, the insulin resistance seen in the obese may be an adaptive mechanism for dealing with the additional nutrients and calories associated with excessive eating: The hyperglycemia, hyperinsulinemia, hypertriglyceridemia, and glucose intolerance in obese animals and humans disappear when food intake is decreased and weight loss occurs (785).

Studies of genetic obesity in animals show that the obesity can be transmitted via simple autosomal recessive or dominant traits or by polygenic inheritance involving several alleles at a number of different loci (100,325). There appear to be genetic bases for taste or food preferences as well, although the precise ways in which these traits are inherited remain to be determined. Since many of the genetic forms of obesity in animals do not become manifest unless the animals have access to an appropriate diet, it seems clear that even the genetic propensity toward hyperphagia is not always fixed but depends to some extent on the environment (100). Continuation of these studies may provide additional clues to the specific effects of genetic inheritance on eating behavior.

Although the evidence seems incontrovertible that genetic baselines for obesity or leanness help to determine the feeding responses to certain environmental circumstances, it still remains to be determined precisely how feeding behavior is influenced in this manner. Future experiments may establish if genetic factors directly alter behavioral response hierarchies so that some responses are emitted preferentially, or if behavior is altered indirectly via genetic influences on the various physiological changes associated with eating or fasting. However, since all animals—whether normal or over- or under-weight—appear to defend body weight once it has stabilized, it is necessary to understand the mechanisms underlying and influencing the genetically programmed set point before we can completely understand the factors controlling feeding behavior.

## B. Age-Related Factors

During the early stages of ontogenesis, feeding is determined in many nonprecocial mammals by the strength of the clinging, rooting, and suckling reflexes (5). As development proceeds, these reflexes gradually disappear and feeding becomes self-initiated and intertwined with regulatory mechanisms for temperature regulation, water balance, and other physiological homeostatic processes. The primitive clinging, rooting, and suckling reflexes present in the newborn may not disappear simply as the result of replacement by other, more mature feeding behavior. Interestingly, these reflexes may be inhibited by active brain mechanisms that become mature relatively later in development. The evidence for this inhibition is only indirect and is based on the fact that these reflexes have been observed in senile humans with arteriosclerosis, cortical trauma, or certain brain tumors (548).

A variety of evidence supports the notion that the mechanisms controlling eating behavior in immature animals differ somewhat from those important for the adult. During the preweanling period, many nonprecocial neonatal animals, including the rat and human, are greatly dependent on their mothers for the maintenance of homeostatic balance, as well as for survival. During the early developmental period, food intake relative to body weight is approximately similar to that of the adult, even though most of the energy and nutrients obtained from the food are used for growth (359); little energy and few nutrients are stored or expended on activities such as temperature regulation or locomotion, thus leaving relatively greater quantities of metabolites for cellular proliferation and enlargement (359,434).

Somewhat later many mammals progress through a stage in which food intake relative to body weight increases dramatically and is greater than at any other time. Growth at this time is critically dependent on the quality of the diet as well as on its amount; growth rates can be severely depressed if insufficient milk is available (790) or if the diet does not contain adequate protein (5). In some cases growth can be permanently altered, depending on the quality of the diet (5,790).

The weekly percentage of weight gain decreases around the time rats are weaned; survival can be threatened if weaning occurs too early, even if water and solid food are freely available (381). This decreased weight gain does not appear to result from changes in food intake, since the food intake/body weight ratio is still relatively high. Probably the slower weight gain reflects a change in energy expenditure; during the period between weaning and attainment of sexual maturation, the body weight of rats typically increases by approximately 300%, whereas the body surface area only doubles (358,359). Although heat loss and metabolic rate decrease somewhat (434,436), animals expend a great deal of energy because of the maturation of temperature control mechanisms and increased physical activity (436,482).

By the time they are sexually mature, many mammals have reached a stable body weight that is maintained at a fairly constant level throughout the rest of their lives. Exceptions to this general rule do exist, however: Whereas female rats have a relatively stable body weight, with slight fluctuations at particular times during the estrous cycle, male rats tend to increase body weight throughout their lives (albeit the increases normally occur at fairly stable rates).

Although relatively few studies have assessed possible ontogenetic changes in the control mechanisms for eating behavior, it seems clear that maturation of feeding behavior is a gradual process. For example, although preweanling rats can increase their food intake following food deprivation (322,323,438) and decrease it if they receive premeal intragastric loads of milk or the nonnutritive substance kaolin (190,215,322), they do not increase food intake as adult rats do when they are injected with insulin (131,438,737,738,742) or with 2-deoxy-D-glucose (2-DG) (322), a drug that decreases cellular glucose utilization (115). Similarly, adult animals, including humans, can compensate under some conditions for changes in the caloric density of diet by altering the amount of food eaten (123,354,696); human neonates also increase total food consumption when offered a calorically dilute diet, although the extent to which they compensate is insufficient to maintain normal weight gain (209). In the latter study it may have been that the neonates fed the calorically dilute diet could not ingest any more of the food because the volume capacity of the stomach was approached, preventing further intake. On the basis of these and other results, some investigators hypothesize that gastric fill and the rate of gastric emptying may be important satiety mechanisms in immature mammals, whereas other factors (e.g., changes in cellular glucose utilization) may become mature relatively late in development (86,190,215).

It is currently impossible to specify with any precision all of the developmental changes underlying the mechanisms that control feeding behavior; at least two interesting possibilities have been suggested, however. First, the qualities of diets consumed by young and mature animals are quite different, as are the ultimate metabolic uses of the energy and nutrients obtained. Both of these factors may play important roles in determining the control mechanisms for eating behavior. The milk ingested by many nonprecocial neonates constitutes a high-fat, low-carbohydrate diet; after weaning, the normal diet changes to one with relatively lower fat and higher carbohydrate levels (267). Although the hypothesis has thus far not been tested directly, it is possible that the preweanling rat may respond to lipostatic changes rather than to glucostatic cues for hunger and satiety. In contrast, carbohydrate levels or other cues may become more important for older animals.

Along similar lines, preliminary evidence (H. Anderson, *personal communication*) indicates that the food intake of immature animals is highly correlated with diet-induced changes in plasma amino acid patterns, whereas the food intake of older rats is not. Since growth during the early postnatal period depends largely on the protein content of the diet, it is possible that aminostatic cues influence food intake more during early development than during later life. Similarly, the high food intake/body weight ratio observed during the early postnatal period may be necessary to support normal growth; the higher the ratio the greater is the possibility for growth, and therefore young animals may regulate food intake simply on the basis of gastric filling or emptying, or the rates at which nutrients are absorbed from the GI tract (115,190). Later in development, as feeding behavior becomes more mature, other factors (e.g., learned changes in food habits or alterations in preferences or aversions based on taste) may become more important. Hence ontogenetic changes in the control of eating may be a direct function of age-related alterations in the type of diet consumed as well as in the metabolic utilization of foods. In this conception control mechanisms for feeding behavior are mature at birth, but as physiological requirements change with age, certain mechanisms play a greater role than others.

A second hypothesis accounting for the age-related differences in feeding behavior is that many of the peripheral and central control mechanisms important for eating may mature at different rates and possibly in fixed, genetically determined sequence (434,438,738,742). There is indirect support for this theory; the eating responses of differently aged rats were measured following developmental retardation induced by thyroidectomy or by partial starvation shortly after birth (131,742). Animals that were severely growth-retarded by these manipulations were completely aphagic and adipsic when they were offered wet, palatable food or ordinary laboratory chow and water at the time when normally developing rats were weaned. Animals less severely retarded ingested some of the wet palatable diet but did not eat enough to maintain body weight. Still other weanling rats, even less retarded by the experimental manipulations, gained body weight and were able to control their food intake if offered a liquid diet; however, even these animals were more finicky (ate less food than control animals if it was adulterated with quinine) and failed to increase their food intake in response to hypoglycemia induced by insulin injection (738,742). It was assumed that the deficits in the normal control of feeding behavior observed in the thyroidectomized or semistarved animals resulted from the arrested maturation of brain or peripheral mechanisms that participate in the control of eating behavior in mature animals; however, the precise mechanisms influenced by the experimental manipulations are unknown. There is enough evidence to demonstrate that young animals do not normally control feeding behavior to the same extent as mature animals: They do not respond to glucostatic challenges (86,437,738, 742); do appear to be prandial drinkers (they drink water only in association with the consumption of food) (369,738); do not respond normally to challenges to osmotic balance (215); and do not respond to anorexic drugs that decrease the food intake of mature animals (438). Finally, lesions in the VMH nuclei that produce hyperphagia and obesity in adult rats do not alter the food intake of weanling rats (218,356).

In each of these age-related differences, it has been assumed that the lack of mature responses is related to the relative functional immaturity of various peripheral or brain mechanisms that mediate these responses in adult animals; however, the maturational processes that underlie the ontogenetic changes in feeding behavior are currently unknown, and it seems clear that not all control mechanisms involved in eating are immature at birth. For example, lesions in the lateral hypothalamic area that produce long-term, permanent disruptions of feeding and drinking responses of adult rats also produce comparable changes in rats lesioned at a time when feeding behavior is still immature (10,433). Along similar lines, injection of insulin or 2-DG produces hyper- and hypoclycemia, respectively, in both young and adult animals (190,665); young animals do not increase food intake following treatment with these compounds, however, whereas adult animals do (131,322,438,742). Although a greater understanding of the ontogenetic changes in eating behavior may prove useful for treating early-onset disorders in these responses in humans, more descriptive studies cataloging feeding ontogenesis are necessary to clarify these developmental processes before clinical usefulness can be achieved.

## C. Hormonal Factors

Various hormones secreted from peripheral endocrine glands produce striking changes in many behavioral responses, including feeding behavior. The GI hormones (secretin, gastrin, enterogastrin, and cholecystokinin) and the pancreatic hormones (glucagon and insulin) appear to be essential for feeding behavior inasmuch as they are intimately involved in the digestion, absorption, utilization, and expenditure of nutrients. Other hormones—secreted from the pituitary, thyroid, adrenal, or pineal glands, or from the gonads— also influence nutrient digestion and metabolism and appear to be more important as determinants of long-term weight regulation and nutrient-energy balance. In addition, these hormones may mediate some of the age- and sex-related differences in feeding behavior previously described.

## *1. Pituitary Hormones*

Hypophysectomized animals (animals whose pituitary glands have been removed) show a particular syndrome of dysfunctions that may be important for feeding behavior. Their growth is retarded; total daily food consumption is reduced (297,363,689); and there is a general atrophy of the genitals and the thyroid and adrenal glands. Furthermore, hypophysectomy prevents the increase in body weight gain normally seen in animals made obese by a variety of genetic (291), surgical (153,297,814), or pharmacological (423,583) methods. Hence it is possible that the pituitary gland, or a hormone secreted by it, may be a factor in some nutritional and endocrine abnormalities associated with experimental and clinical obesity. Additionally, the normal, functioning pituitary gland may be a necessary mechanism for feeding behavior. Many studies have examined the possible roles played by two pituitary hormones—GH and prolactin—in these various effects.

GH is a protein secreted by the anterior pituitary gland. Its rate of secretion varies as a function of changes in plasma levels of glucose and amino acids (326,580,797), and its release can also be influenced by nonnutritive manipulations (620). GH levels in plasma are highest after animals have been fasted for a length of time sufficient to decrease blood glucose concentrations, and are lowest immediately after plasma glucose concentrations are elevated by a meal (620). Hence GH secretion varies as a function of eating or fasting, and its level in plasma is generally inversely related to the blood sugar level. *In vitro* and *in vivo* studies with animals and humans suggest that GH also influences the metabolism and utilization of nutrients: The hormone promotes bone, connective tissue, skin, and general growth in immature animals, and increases lipolysis in adipose tissue and amino acid incorporation into protein in various peripheral tissues (812). It also may participate in normal energy balance by decreasing cellular glucose utilization and increasing gluconeogenesis; in this respect its actions are antagonistic to those of insulin (536).

Hypophysectomy may inhibit feeding via interference with the secretion of GH since the reduction in food intake following hypophysectomy can be reversed by replacement doses of GH (556). Interestingly, GH treatment appears to be more effective in male than female rats (566). The extent to which GH may control normal food intake remains unclear: Although injection of the hormone increases food intake and growth in hypophysectomized male rats (814), the same treatment may depress food intake/body weight ratios in normal rats (255). It should be noted, however, that the plasma GH level is highest in normal weanling rats at the time when they are hyperphagic and eat the most food relative to body weight (247,363). It has been hypothesized that GH secretion during this time may increase food intake by inhibiting so-called "satiety" cells located in the VMH nuclei (360,363), although the evidence for this effect is indirect. Lesions of the VMH area produce hyperphagia and obesity if they are made in mature rats but have no immediate effect on the feeding behavior of weanlings (247,360). Furthermore, lesions of the VMH nuclei in young animals partially reverse hypophysectomy-induced reductions in food intake and block the ability of replacement doses of GH to restore the food intake reduced by hypophysectomy (247). However, GH treatment produces opposite effects in adult animals; it increases the food intake of hypophysectomized rats but decreases food intake in hypophysectomized animals that also have lesions of the VMH area (814). Some investigators tried to account for these ontogenetic differences by suggesting that the *ratio* of GH to insulin levels in the plasma, rather than the *absolute levels* of GH, may determine the hormone's possible role in the control of eating behavior (797); others have criticized this hypothesis (537). It may ultimately be shown that GH plays an important role in the control of eating behavior, especially in the developing animal, but current evidence is inconclusive. Thus far only a few assays are sensitive or reliable enough to measure GH in infraprimate mammals; future developments may greatly enhance our understanding of its role in feeding behavior.

One study, examining the possible effects of prolactin injection on the feeding behavior of hypophysectomized animals, showed that prolactin increases food intake to a greater extent in female rats than in males (556), but the roles of this and other pituitary hormones in eating behavior are unclear.

## 2. Thyroid Hormones

Thyroxine, a major hormone secreted from the thyroid gland, promotes gluconeogenesis by increasing the catabolism of fats, proteins, and glycogen; hence treatment with the hormone increases oxygen consumption and heat production in almost all tissues, except the brain and heart (536). Destruction of the thyroid gland early in development results in irreversibly retarded growth (cretinism) unless thyroxine replacement therapy is employed (99, 254). Relatively normal growth rates are maintained in adult thyroidectomized rats, even though food intake is often slightly decreased after the operation (255) owing to a decrease in the basal metabolic rate. Chronic treatment with thyroxine in adult thyroidectomized rats produces a large decrease in body weight, probably as a direct result of the action of the hormone on nutrient catabolism (99). Replacement doses of thyroxine in these animals produce larger weight losses in male than in female rats, although it is not clear if this is a sex-related difference in the direct effects of the hormone, or if the greater percentage of weight loss merely reflects the fact that adult male rats continue to grow throughout their lives whereas female rats show relatively less change after sexual maturity is reached (255). Normal intact animals treated with thyroxine show a rather large increase in total daily food consumption (692); whether these hormone-induced changes in feeding behavior are direct effects of the hormone or result indirectly from the nutrient imbalances created by the catabolic effects of thyroxine remains to be determined.

### 3. Adrenal Hormones

Glucocorticoids (corticosterone, cortisol) are steroid hormones secreted from cells in the adrenal cortex in response to the release of adrenocorticotropic hormone (ACTH) from the pituitary gland. These hormones alter intermediary metabolism by promoting the catabolism of fats and muscle proteins, stimulating the uptake and conversion of amino acids into glucose in liver cells, and inhibiting the uptake and oxidation of glucose in almost all tissues except the brain (536).

Animals with complete adrenalectomy show an immediate reduction in food intake accompanied by weight loss (255); injection of a relatively low dose of glucocorticoids increases food intake and weight gain in both adrenalectomized and intact animals (255,288,317). On the other hand, injection of a larger dose of the glucocorticoids decreases food intake and increases body weight loss (536,710). In rats the release of adrenal corticosterone is highest during the dark portion of the day-night cycle, when food consumption is greatest (228); similarly, animals allowed only restricted access to food show increased corticosterone secretion immediately prior to the scheduled feeding period (341). Furthermore, adrenal gland weight is greatly increased in obese rodents (100); however, the increased release of the glucocorticoids is not always correlated with the occurrence of hyperphagia and the development of obesity, inasmuch as rats with VMH lesions still become hyperphagic and obese even though they have been adrenalectomized (814).

Another major hormone, epinephrine, is secreted from the chromaffin cells of the adrenal medulla in response to increased activity of preganglionic sympathetic nerves that innervate the gland (802). High circulating levels of epinephrine usually increase the plasma glucose levels by stimulating the catabolism of liver glycogen and blocking glucose uptake into peripheral tissues; epinephrine also increases lipolysis in adipose tissue (636).

Injection of epinephrine usually decreases the food intake of normal animals (469,635,636) and those with VMH lesions (93). Because of its chemical structure, the epinephrine molecule does not penetrate the blood-brain barrier and so does not gain access to brain synapses when injected into the periphery

(782,802); thus the changes in feeding behavior seen after systemic injection of epinephrine are probably mediated by the effects of the hormone on peripheral mechanisms. However, the reduction in food intake following treatment with epinephrine is probably not related to its effect on energy metabolism since systemic injection of norepinephrine (the precursor of epinephrine in the adrenal gland) produces increases in body temperature and oxygen consumption comparable to the changes induced by epinephrine, even though treatment with norepinephrine does not alter food consumption (636). The mechanisms mediating the effects of peripheral injection of epinephrine on feeding behavior are still unknown.

### 4. Pineal Hormones

The pineal gland is a light-sensitive organ that secretes the hormone melatonin (473). The synthesis and release of melatonin changes in rats as a function of the diurnal lighting schedule, with peak concentrations of melatonin usually occurring during the dark portion of the day-night cycle (806). Because the pineal gland is light-sensitive, it is tempting to speculate that the diurnal rhythmic changes seen in food intake and other behavioral responses (i.e., locomotor activity, sexual behavior) depend on the integrity of the pineal gland. Thus far, no studies support this hypothesis; pinealectomized rats still show normal diurnal changes in the patterns of food and water intake and locomotor activity (432), and these behaviors can be retrained to new lighting schedules in adult animals with their pineal glands removed (55,432,575). Immature pinealectomized rats, however, show a slight increase in total daily food intake, and melatonin injection in normal or pinealectomized rats produces a small but insignificant decrease in food consumption (505). Additional studies are needed to clarify the possible role of the pineal gland in eating behavior, if indeed it plays any role at all.

### 5. Gonadal Hormones

Many aspects of feeding behavior differ among males and females of a variety of species. For example, male and female rats show marked differences in taste preference; normal female rats have a greater preference (or less aversion) to concentrated saccharin or glucose solutions than do males (768, 827). These sex-related differences in taste preference can be abolished if female rats are ovariectomized (768,769,771) or if they are treated with masculinizing doses of testosterone propionate during the early postnatal period (769). Similarly, ovariectomized, pregnant, or pseudopregnant female rats consume smaller amounts of concentrated saccharin or quinine solutions than do intact females (768,769,771). These sex-related taste preferences and aversions are apparently due to the high circulating levels of the gonadal hormones estradiol and progesterone, inasmuch as combined replacement therapy with these hormones restores the preference or aversion curve for saccharin or quinine to normal in ovariectomized females (771,826).

Male rats appear to be more sensitive than females to changes in the taste of the diet; they increase or decrease total daily food intake to a greater degree than female rats in response to dietary palatability (504). Similarly, male rats require a longer time to reach stable taste preferences than do females when they are allowed to choose between two solutions with different glucose concentrations (504). When intact or ovariectomized female rats or normal intact male rats are offered a choice of a protein-free or a high-protein diet, males and ovariectomized females choose to eat larger amounts of the high-protein diet than do the normal females (758); in addition, normal intact female weanlings and pregnant animals eat greater amounts of daily protein when offered a choice than do intact adult female rats (415). It is not at all clear whether these sex-related differences in taste preference, apparently due to differences in the secretion of the gonadal female sex hormones, result from the effects of the hormones on brain mechanisms underlying taste sensitivity or from direct hormonal effects on peripheral taste receptor mechanisms.

The body weights of most male mammals usually exceed that of their female counterparts, even if the males and females of a particular species are pair-fed equal amounts of an identical diet (395). There are comparable sex differences in total daily food intake: Beginning at puberty male animals generally eat more than females, and these differences become more pronounced with age (357,365). Even when male and female rats have comparable body weights, the males have more fat relative to lean body mass than do females (360). Sex-related differences in food intake and weight gain may depend on secretion of the gonadal sex hormones; injection of the female sex hormone estradiol in adult male or female rats decreases food intake and weight gain, whereas similar treatment in weanling rats has no effect on food intake (61,765,770). These age-related differences in the effects of estradiol may result from an interaction between it and ontogenetic changes in the synthesis and release of pituitary GH. Estradiol decreases food intake in hypophysectomized weanlings unless they are treated with replacement doses of GH (766). Although the mechanisms for these hormonal interactions have not been identified, the available data suggest that the relatively high circulating level of GH suppresses the action of estradiol in weanling rats; in contrast, estradiol might be active in adult animals because they have relatively low concentrations of GH.

Additional support for the possible involvement of gonadal hormones in the control of eating behavior is based on the observations that food intake, body weight, and energy expenditure change with phases of the estrous cycle (110,731,747,765). The plasma estradiol concentration is highest during proestrus and lowest during diestrus and metaestrus (110,731,747); food consumption is lowest during proestrus and estrus and is highest during diestrus (765). Ovariectomy abolishes these changes in food intake and results in a sharp increase in total daily food intake and long-term body weight gain (347,601). An ovariectomy-induced increase in food consumption can be reversed by daily systemic replacement doses of estradiol (731) or by injection of the hormone directly into the VMH nuclei (334,772). Although these data provide partial support for the notion that estradiol may normally decrease food intake by affecting hypothalamic mechanisms, animals with VMH lesions treated with estradiol still show a normal reduction in food intake, suggesting that the hormone probably affects other control mechanisms for feeding behavior besides the hypothalamus (591,707). One site for estrogen-induced changes in feeding behavior may be in the adrenal gland; ovariectomized, adrenalecto- mized rats do not increase food intake or body weight (266,481), and estradiol injection does not reduce their food consumption (584) unless they have been made slightly overweight by dietary manipulations (584,765).

Female rats eat smaller but slightly more frequent daily meals during proestrus than during other phases of the estrous cycle (75). Ovariectomized females increase meal size but decrease the number of meals per day (75). After the initial period of hyperphagia and weight gain following ovariectomy, body weight eventually levels off and is maintained at levels approximately 15–20% higher than the preoperative body weight (75). During this static period ovariectomized females still eat larger-than-normal meals, and the total number of daily meals is increased (75).

The mechanisms by which estradiol alters feeding behavior are unknown, although some evidence supports the hypothesis that it may change the functioning of brain catecholamine-containing neurons thought to mediate various aspects of feeding normally (178,179,207,669).

The effects of the other major female sex hormone, progesterone, on feeding behavior are less clear. Progesterone injections increase food con- sumption and body weight gain in intact, lean female rats but not in obese females or normal males (296,708). These effects are not blocked by ovariec- tomy or adrenalectomy, or by a combination of the two operations (607). It has been suggested that progesterone increases feeding behavior by antago- nizing the effects of estrogen, and some indirect support for this hypothesis has been gathered (767). If it is true, it may account for the observation that pregnant and lactating females, who have high progesterone levels, eat rather large amounts of food despite relatively high circulating levels of estrogen (767).

Even less information exists regarding the precise role played by the male sex hormone testosterone in the control of feeding behavior. Male or female rats injected with testosterone early in development eat and weigh more than castrated males or normal intact females when tested as adults (59,61,732). Mature female rats injected with testosterone also show an increase in weight gain (61). Gonadectomized rats treated with small doses of testosterone increase food intake and body weight gain, whereas treatment with larger doses of the hormone actually decreases feeding and body weight (233); in explanation, some investigators propose that large doses of testosterone are aromatized to form estrogens, which then suppress eating (233). The finding that treatment with the nonaromatizable testosterone analog dihydrotestosterone also stimulates food intake when given in small doses, but does not depress feeding in large doses, is compatible with this hypothesis (233). Similar but still indirect evidence is the observation that combined treatment with progesterone and large doses of testosterone does not decrease food consumption, suggesting that progesterone antagonizes the food-suppressing effects of the estrogen molecules formed from the aromatization of testosterone (233). However, these results may not be related to the aromatization of testosterone but may merely reflect the antagonistic effects of two drugs: progesterone (which increases food intake) and testosterone (which suppresses it).

As a whole, the evidence indicates that gonadal sex hormones not only play a role in altering taste preference, daily meal patterning, and total food consumption, but that they may also figure in the long-term control of body weight. Until more experiments are conducted, however, and more data derived from different techniques are presented, the possible involvement of any particular endocrine gland or hormone in the control of eating behavior must be considered with a certain amount of caution. Assumptions regarding the particular role of various hormones are based largely on studies using animals in which endocrine organs have been extirpated, or those that have been injected with doses of a hormone in concentrations several times those normally found in intact animals. Tissue extirpation results in many more changes than a reduction in the target hormones, and any one of these "other side effects" may actually be the critical variable producing the behavioral change. Similarly, injected hormones may have totally different fates from endogenous ones and may produce changes in eating behavior that do not normally result *in vivo*. Although the data gathered thus far point to an interesting interaction between various hormones and eating behavior, more experiments are needed to clarify these roles.

## V. PHYSIOLOGICAL DETERMINANTS OF EATING BEHAVIOR

As we have seen, eating behavior can be affected by environmental conditions and by the age, hormonal status, and genetic makeup of the organism. The physiological changes associated with eating or fasting also generate "hunger" and "satiety" signals from which the animal is able to determine when and how much food must be eaten to maintain survival (132). In the final analysis, whether animals eat or whether they gain weight depends on their ability to sense and respond to their metabolic needs.

It has been hypothesized that blood or cerebrospinal fluid (CSF) contains hunger and satiety factors (possibly hormones or certain nutrients or their metabolites) that influence feeding behavior and long-term body weight regulation (294,295). In an early study that has since been criticized (158), Luck-hardt and Carlson (431) transfused the blood taken from a hungry dog into a satiated dog and found that the number of stomach contractions increased in the sated animal. Sera taken from satiated dogs and injected into hungry ones inhibited the stomach contractions. Injection of blood from satiated rats into starved rats decreased the starved rats' food intakes by approximately 50% (158,159); it is not yet known if the food intake of satiated animals increases after injection with blood from starved rats.

Additional support for the existence of hunger or satiety factors in blood is based largely on feeding changes in parabiotic rats. In these experiments two rats were united surgically so they shared a common blood supply (approximately 2% of the total volume of blood crossed from one rat to the other per minute) (208,294). One member of the parabiotic pair, with electrolytic lesions in the VMH, became hyperphagic, rapidly gained weight, and become obese. At the same time, the other (unlesioned) member of the pair became ema-ciated, even though it was given equal access to the same diet consumed by the animal with the brain lesion (294). When one member of a parabiotic pair was allowed to eat for 2 hr prior to the time the second member of the pair was given food, the food consumption of the late-starting rat was significantly reduced (208). When less than 2 hr elapsed between the two rats' meals, there was no significant reduction in food consumption in the late-starting animal (208). Similarly, satiated monkeys injected with CSF obtained from starved donor monkeys began to eat within minutes after the injection (496). Although the nature of these possible hunger and satiety factors remains to be clarified and not all aspects of these studies have been replicated (208,279), several compounds have been proposed (454,497).

Two major questions guided the research efforts of scientists and clinicians interested in the physiological mechanisms that control eating behavior. What is the nature of the possible hunger or satiety signal(s) that tell the animal when to eat and when not to? How are these signals sensed, and what are the mechanisms that integrate them so the animal ingests enough nutrients for the maintenance of bodily functions?

## A. Peripheral Signals for Hunger and Satiety

### 1. Oropharyngeal Sensations

When animals chew food, receptors in the tongue and oral mucosa sensitive to sweet, salty, bitter, or sour taste stimuli relay gustatory information to the brain via the lingual, chorda tympani, and glossopharyngeal nerves (270). Gustatory information is also sent to the brain by way of the vagus nerve from receptors located in the pharynx and larynx (270).

Sensations resulting from the ingestion, chewing, or swallowing of food, although not absolutely essential, normally participate in many aspects of eating behavior. For example, when the nonnutritive sweetener saccharin or other palatable constituents are added to the diet overall food consumption increases, whereas the addition of bitter-tasting quinine decreases net food intake (272,332,355). Oropharyngeal sensations other than taste may be important satiety signals. For example, hunger seems to be satisfied in animals allowed to chew and swallow food regardless of whether the food enters the stomach. Animals whose esophagi have been severed to prevent food from entering the stomach still terminate eating, although the length of their individual meals is increased (339). In these experiments, however, factors other than satiety signals (e.g., fatigue) may contribute to meal termination.

Salivary secretion is also important to normal eating behavior. Salivary gland extirpation or salivary gland duct ligation decreases the food consumption of rats not allowed access to water (366,759). Rats prevented from salivating are prandial drinkers; when offered dry food and water, they eat small amounts of food, then drink small amounts of water, eat again, and so on (366,371). Normal rats eat rather large amounts of food in a single meal, then drink water (366).

Gustatory signals are relayed to the midbrain, in the nuclei of the solitary tract, and are transmitted to other brain areas including the ventral thalamus and cortex (514–516). The electrical activity of brain cells in these pathways responds to mechanical, electrical, or chemical stimulation of the tongue and oral cavity. Lesions that destroy the peripheral nerves linking the oral cavity and the brain, or that destroy brain regions such as the solitary nuclei, disrupt coordinated chewing movements and alter preferences for or aversions to flavored solutions (62,76,270,520,558).

Although taste and palatability do not appear necessary for the long-term regulation of food intake and body weight gain, they seem to contribute information that influences meal length and satiety. Furthermore, learned associations between the taste of a food and its other physicochemical characteristics may alter an animal's response to it.

## 2. Gastrointestinal Factors

Interest in GI factors as possible determinants of feeding behavior can be traced to the early experiments of Carlson (126) and Cannon and Washburn (124)—although, of course, people have always associated hunger or satiety with the sensations of an empty or a full stomach. It was once thought that changes in the rate of stomach contractions might be the critical peripheral signals for hunger or satiety. Recent experiments, however, provide evidence that other GI signals might be more important.

Animals that feed themselves by pressing a bar to deliver food directly to the stomach via a gastric tube consume a normal amount of food and maintain a relatively constant body weight even though they are deprived of oropharyngeal sensations normally associated with eating (192,345,690). Animals feeding themselves via this route are able to increase total food intake following periods of starvation, adjust total food consumption to compensate for changes in the caloric level of the diet, and show normal diurnal patterns of food intake during the day-night cycle (188). Although many aspects of feeding behavior appear to be normal in animals that feed themselves intragastrically, others are not. For example, these animals do not show normal food preferences and aversions, and are unable to select diets on the basis of taste (188).

*Gastric contractions.*

Cannon and Washburn (124) and Carlson (126) first proposed that the sensations of hunger were due chiefly to the contractions of the empty stomach; this theory dominated thinking about peripheral control mechanisms for eating behavior for approximately the next quarter of a century. In their original experiments Cannon and Washburn (124) found that strong gastric contractions inevitably preceded sensations of hunger in humans; furthermore, the contractions appeared to become stronger and more frequent as the length of time without food was increased (159). Experimental results compatible with this view include the observations that insulin injection, which increases feelings of hunger (and food intake in sated animals), increases the rate of gastric contractions (428,576), whereas injection of glucagon, which reduces food intake, also inhibits gastric contractions (290,726). Finally, electrical stimulation of cells in the VMH nuclei depresses food intake and GI motility, whereas electrical stimulation of the lateral hypothalamic area produces eating in sated animals and increases gastric contractions (386). These results suggest that brain mechanisms which integrate information important for feeding behavior also control gastric motility.

Although attractive and simple, the hypothesis that hunger sensations arise from changes in stomach contractions is not supported by the majority of contemporary experiments. Studies of eating behavior in humans (329) and rats (752) whose stomachs have been completely removed or denervated show that relatively normal sensations of hunger are still present, and that food consumption is almost normal. However, humans with their stomachs removed no longer localize sensations of hunger "pangs" to the abdominal region (called epigastric hunger pangs) (256,336); furthermore, they tend to increase the daily number of meals and decrease the amount of food consumed at each meal (256).

Gastric contractions do not occur only when the stomach is empty; strong gastric motility is observed when the stomach is full, and it has been impossible thus far to distinguish experimentally the stomach contractions associated with an empty stomach from those seen when the stomach is filled (336).

Finally, gastric "hunger" contractions occur at normal rates, even in animals made aphagic and adipsic by lateral hypothalamic lesions, or in animals made hyperphagic and obese with electrolytic lesions of the VMH nuclei (723). Apparently gastric hunger contractions are sometimes associated with the perception of hunger, and at other times they are not; at best, they are dispensable as peripheral signals of hunger (723).

*Gastric distention.*

Dogs fitted with esophageal fistulas that prevent ingested food from reaching the stomach tend to eat longer-duration and more frequent meals than do normal animals (339); if food or a water-inflated balloon is placed in the stomach prior to feeding, the duration of the sham-feeding can be decreased (666). Similarly, normal meal length can be reinstated in dogs with esophageal fistulas if they receive premeal, intragastric loads of food that are greater than 50% of the volume of a normal-sized meal (339).

In studies examining the feeding behavior of rats equipped with chronic gastric fistulas, Smith and co-workers (235,245,682,819) found that when these fistulas were open (and ingested food was prevented from reaching the small intestine), the sham-fed animals tended to increase the length of individual meals somewhat, suggesting that signals associated with food passing through the upper GI tract might provide weak signals for satiety. These animals never showed the complete, normal syndrome of behavioral satiety, however (680). Since normal behavioral satiety could be elicited in rats with gastric fistulas if liquid food was infused into the small intestine via a duodenal catheter during sham-feeding, it appears that ingested food must reach the small intestine for satiety to occur if gastric distention factors are eliminated (680).

Stretch receptors sensitive to changes in intragastric food volume may mediate the satiety associated with gastric distention. Inflation of intragastric balloons in hungry rats inhibits food intake and decreases locomotor activity (86). Similarly, the duration and frequency of eating is related directly to the size of intragastric preloading (666). Since intragastric loads of inert, metabolically unuseful bulk are as effective as nutritionally utilizable foods in producing short-term reductions in feeding behavior, it seems likely that these effects result from changes in gastric distention rather than short-term metabolic factors (335).

Although this evidence indicates that gastric distention produces short-term satiety, this factor may be important only when extremely large volumes of food are ingested (336) since animals with complete denervation of the upper GI tract show relatively few changes in the pattern of food intake or in long-term regulation of body weight (336).

*Osmolarity.*

In almost all mammals, eating food is usually associated with drinking liquids; a reduction in the availability of one produces concomitant changes in the intake of the other (4,366,367,413,630). The total food consumption of some animals is such that they maintain constant food/water intake ratios in the stomach and small intestine regardless of the amount of water made available with a meal (709). Furthermore, intragastric preloads of hypertonic saline decrease food intake (685,813). GI cells sensitive to the osmolarity of food in the lumen of the digestive tract were studied with electrophysiological techniques (667), but it is not yet clear how neural changes associated with osmolarity are related to the control of eating. Some indirect evidence supports the notion that osmoreceptors mediate the rate of gastric emptying and thus change the rates at which various nutrients are absorbed from the duodenum into the bloodstream (685,687); hypertonic, intragastric loads of glucose or saline decrease the rate of gastric emptying and generally produce subsequent reductions in food intake (462).

However, the overall evidence that osmocontrol mechanisms are important to feeding behavior is relatively weak. Animals can usually compensate well for changes in the caloric density of the diet (by increasing or decreasing food intake) regardless of relative changes in dietary osmolarity (332).

Other changes in the lumen (e.g., alterations in chemistry or pH) are normally associated with food digestions, but it remains unclear how, or if, these changes are important in the control of eating behavior.

*Gastric or duodenal secretion of hormones.*

Of the major GI hormones (gastrin, secretin, and cholecystokinin) involved in food digestion and absorption, only cholecystokinin has been implicated in the short-term control of feeding (29,235,245,425,682,725,819). Based on the evidence that intraduodenal loads of food inhibit sham-feeding in rats with open intragastric fistulas, Smith and Gibbs (235,679) proposed that the nutrient-induced release of cholecystokinin from cells in the duodenum may produce short-term behavioral satiety. In rats or monkeys (819) with open gastric fistulas, intraperitoneal injections of cholecystokinin decrease food intake and produce other signs of behavioral satiety (increased grooming, decreased locomotor activity, and increased periods of resting and sleeping). The satiety effect of cholecystokinin can also be elicited by treating the animals with synthetic octapeptide derivatives of the naturally occurring hormone (235); in contrast, treatment with other GI hormones (pentogastrin, gastrin, or secretin) produces little or no change in feeding behavior (235,682). Previous research established that gastric loads of the amino acid L-phenylalanine, but not D-phenylalanine, stimulate release of cholecystokinin (440,468); as might be anticipated from these results, feeding is inhibited in monkeys injected with L-, but not D-phenylalanine (680). These results are significant inasmuch as they demonstrate that feeding behavior may be mediated by nonneural, hormonally mediated mechanisms that are relatively unaltered in animals that have complex denervation of the lower digestive tract. These findings should stimulate future experiments designed to investigate the possible roles of the other, more recently discovered GI hormones (582) in the control of feeding behavior.

### 3. Carbohydrate Metabolism and Feeding Behavior

Several metabolic considerations indicate the importance of glucose and other carbohydrate levels to the control of eating behavior: (a) Brain cells (except under conditions of prolonged starvation) are obligatory glucose users, and normal brain function depends on the availability of the sugar. (b) Carbohydrates are not stored to any appreciable degree by body tissues; hence a relatively small elevation in the rate at which cells use glucose causes a major shift to metabolic pathways that use other nutrients (fats, amino acids) for energy. (c) Changes in carbohydrate metabolism are influenced by many hormones that produce corresponding changes in feeding behavior. (d) Surgical, pharmacological, or other manipulations that alter feeding behavior also influence carbohydrate utilization and metabolism (42,96,167). Since carbohydrates are generally not stored in abundance (compared to the amounts of fats typically stored), and since glucose is so important for normal brain function, changes in carbohydrate metabolism might provide hunger and satiety signals for eating behavior. Evidence relating carbohydrate utilization and feeding behavior has been assembled into what is called the glucostatic hypothesis, a theory that has dominated thinking about feeding behavior for the past several years (455,456). This theory, as currently formulated, states that changes in peripheral (or brain) cellular glucose utilization, occurring over relatively short periods, are detected by brain cells that control feeding behavior (457). Hunger and the subsequent increase in eating are associated with a decrease in glucose utilization by cells; conversely, satiety (the termination of feeding) is correlated with increased cellular glucose utilization (762). The evidence used to support glucostatic control of feeding behavior is largely indirect, since the rate of change of cellular glucose utilization (or glucose uptake) usually cannot be measured simultaneously with feeding behavior. Moreover, there is some disagreement as to where in the body changes in glucose utilization are important for feeding behavior. The precise mechanisms that monitor changes in glucose utilization are also controversial.

*Changes in glucose utilization and feeding behavior.*
   It has long been known that changes in the *level* of blood sugar, sensations of hunger or satiety, and subsequent changes in feeding behavior are not always correlated, e.g., in the case of the human disease diabetes mellitus (340,661); hence it has been assumed that the *availability* of glucose to cells and its *utilization* provide the signal critical for feeding behavior (455,457). The rate of glucose utilization can be measured indirectly by calculating the arteriovenous differences in plasma glucose across various tissues including the brain (762); because these differences are difficult to measure, however, most studies have used rough changes in plasma glucose levels, rather than arteriovenous differences, as rough indicators of glucose utilization.
   Remember that nutrients absorbed into the bloodstream from the small

intestine stimulate the release of insulin from the $\beta$-cells of the pancreas. Increased plasma insulin levels stimulate the uptake of glucose, FFAs, and amino acids into most peripheral tissues (Fig. 2). Once taken up, carbohydrates are metabolized for energy or are stored in the form of glycogen; FFAs are converted to triglycerides and stored in adipose tissue; and amino acids are incorporated into protein in various cells or are used in other metabolic pathways (e.g., some are used for the synthesis of neurotransmitters and vitamins). When the circulating plasma glucose level falls as a result of the action of insulin, glucagon and epinephrine are released from the pancreas and adrenal gland, respectively; these hormones increase blood glucose levels by inhibiting cellular uptake of the sugar and by promoting its synthesis in various peripheral tissues. On the basis of these metabolic changes, it might be anticipated that brain or peripheral changes in cellular glucose utilization, induced by a variety of manipulations, would alter feeding behavior.

Some changes in blood glucose and insulin and the rate of cellular glucose utilization are indeed correlated with feeding behavior; glucose and insulin levels rise shortly after animals begin to eat and peak just after a meal is ended (197,699,701). Moreover, feeding behavior is sometimes (762) but not always (77,219,256,349,492,574,622) related to peripheral arteriovenous differences in plasma glucose or to changes in the blood sugar level. Furthermore, glucose injection into the general circulation does not usually reduce food intake in hungry animals (2,256,280,337,340,633,684).

Studies manipulating glucose availability by altering the amount of insulin or glucagon generally produce changes in feeding compatible with the predictions of the glucostatic theory. Injection of short-acting forms of insulin produces time-related changes in feeding behavior; immediately after the treatment, when it might be anticipated that the intracellular uptake and utilization of glucose by cells is maximal, animals decrease food intake (430). However, approximately 30 min after injection, when blood glucose levels are low (and presumably when intracellular energy production from glucose has declined), food intake increases dramatically (40,85,87,700). If glucose is administered simultaneously with the short-acting form of insulin, the increase in food consumption is blocked (87). Chronic treatment with longer-acting forms of insulin also produces hyperphagia and eventually obesity (53,313, 439,532,544). This hyperphagia is characterized by an increase in the total number of daily meals, rather than by an increase in meal size (532). Glucagon injection generally produces changes in feeding behavior opposite to those induced by insulin; glucagon produces increased sensations of satiety in humans and decreased food consumption in a variety of animals (338,552,640,650).

Since glucose and insulin are synthesized by the $\alpha$- and $\beta$-cells of the pancreas, respectively, it might be anticipated that a disruption in pancreatic function would produce changes in eating behavior. Such manipulations, however, produce inconsistent results. Rats made diabetic following pancrea-

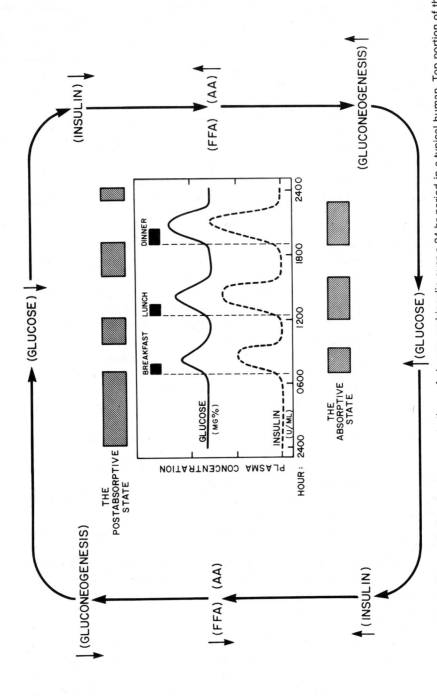

**FIG. 2.** Inner graph: Changes in the plasma concentrations of glucose and insulin over a 24-hr period in a typical human. Top portion of the diagram indicates the major metabolic changes in glucose availability during the postabsorptive state. The bottom portion indicates changes during the absorptive state. (Adapted from Cahill, ref. 121.)

tectomy (820) or after treatment with the pancreatic $\beta$-cell toxins alloxan or streptozotocin (214,384,814) overeat but usually do not gain weight because of the metabolic dysfunctions associated with inadequate insulin levels. The hyperphagia seen in animals with experimentally induced diabetes can be reduced by treating them chronically with insulin (820), thus lending support to the hypothesis that diabetic animals overeat, even though they are hypoglycemic, because cellular glucose uptake and utilization is impaired owing to decreased insulin secretion from the pancreas. However, the types of hyperphagia seen in diabetic animals vary, depending on the method used to induce the diabetic state. Alloxan-treated, diabetic rats are usually hypophagic for a few days following the treatment (384); thereafter they eat the same number of daily meals as normal animals, but they increase individual meal size by approximately 100% when they are offered highly palatable diets (543). Animals made diabetic by treatment with streptozotocin, on the other hand, usually decrease the size of individual meals but increase the number of meals eaten (83). These discrepancies may merely reflect differences in the relative palatability of the diets used in these two studies (543), but this possibility has not been directly tested. Although it is tempting to speculate that the hyperphagia associated with the various treatments might be related to a reduction in the circulating insulin level, studies using other techniques to produce transient reductions in insulin levels—i.e., treating animals with mannoheptulose (545) or anti-insulin serum (22)—do not produce an increase in total food consumption.

The results obtained from experiments using various glucose antimetabolites also lend support to the glucostatic theory. 2-DG, a structural analog of glucose, competitively inhibits the phosphohexoisomerase enzyme involved in glycolysis and inhibits the membrane transport system for glucose and mannose uptake by cells (115,116,592). It also stimulates the release of epinephrine from the adrenal gland (315,592,681), thereby increasing hepatic glycogenolysis; the net result of these effects is an increase in the circulating plasma glucose level, and a decrease in cellular glucose utilization (592). [The metabolic effects of 2-DG can be counteracted in animals pretreated with various doses of insulin (387).] There may be species differences in response to the effects of injected 2-DG; although rats and monkeys generally increase food consumption in response to the drug (82,250,322,324,519,545, 678,683,751), cats do not always do so (333). In cases where hyperphagia is associated with 2-DG treatment it does not seem to depend on the ability of the drug to release epinephrine, inasmuch as 2-DG-induced hyperphagia has been observed in adrenalectomized animals (751). In contrast, the increase in food intake after 2-DG is blocked in vagotomized animals (82,751); since insulin-induced hyperphagia can be blocked by adrenalectomy (82) but not by vagotomy, it has been proposed that the 2-DG-induced hyperphagia is probably mediated by mechanisms different from those associated with insulin (82). Animals treated with 2-DG begin eating sooner than when they are treated with comparable doses of insulin (678). This difference is thought to be related to the fact that 2-DG produces a rapid reduction in glucose utilization by decreasing the availability of glucose at specific glucose-sensitive transport sites, whereas insulin first *promotes* uptake of glucose into cells, eventually leading to a reduced plasma glucose level and decreased availability of the sugar for cellular utilization (678). Other glucose antimetabolites (e.g., 3-O-methyl glucose, 6-O-methyl glucose, or phlorizin) decrease glucose utilization to a lesser extent than 2-DG; these compounds also produce smaller increases in food intake than 2-DG, a finding compatible with the predictions of the glucostatic theory (82,239,692,751).

*Localization of glucoreceptor cells that mediate changes in feeding behavior.*

If changes in cellular glucose utilization are important signals for hunger or satiety, then it must be demonstrated that there are mechanisms for sensing changes in peripheral glucose utilization. Mayer and his colleagues (455,456,-458) originally postulated that glucose-sensitive cells might be located in the basomedial portion of the hypothalamus, an area of the brain known to be important for normal feeding behavior (300,528,535). The evidence that glucoreceptor cells in the VMH influence feeding behavior by mediating changes in cellular glucose utilization is summarized in Table 3 and is presented in detail elsewhere (458).

At first glance this impressive array of evidence seems to provide strong support for the theory that these cells play a critical role. However, the data accumulated in each of these studies have been criticized on theoretical and methodological grounds, and their adequacy as support for the glucostatic theory has been questioned (423,577,590). For example, the findings that changes in the electrical activity of cells in the VMH area correspond with changes in glucose utilization and feeding behavior do not provide direct evidence that these changes are unique to VMH cells (14,577) or that the altered electrical activity may result from some change not directly related to differences in glucose utilization (577); nor do they rule out the possibility that other regions of the brain or periphery might sense changes in glucose utilization and relay this information to VMH cells (14). Moreover, the changes in glucose utilization produced by glucose or insulin infusions in these studies were often out of the physiological ranges normally seen in animals during the fed and fasted states. Hence these studies do not establish if changes in cellular glucose utilization which normally occur during feeding or fasting are sensed uniquely and directly by VMH cells, or whether the electrical activity of these cells is influenced by glucoreceptors located elsewhere or by other changes associated with the experimental manipulations.

Although in a few studies glucose injection into brain reduced food intake, these changes were not immediate (531,540), nor have they been reproduced in other studies (2,256,280,337,340,684) using different injection routes for the sugar. It is also questionable that the delayed reduction in food intake seen

TABLE 3. *Evidence supporting the existence of glucose-sensitive cells important for control of feeding behavior*

| Location of cells | References |
| --- | --- |
| *Ventromedial hypothalamic area (VMH)* | |
| 1. Electrical activity of VMH cells increases after eating and decreases after food deprivation. | 18,20,307 |
| 2. Systemic glucose infusion increases electrical activity of VMH cells and causes satiety; injection of insulin or 2-DG decreases VMH electrical activity and induces eating. | 18,20,21,117,172,477, 508,524 |
| 3. Accumulation of radioactivity is greatest in the VMH region after intragastric infusion of $^{14}$C-D-glucose; uptake appears related to an insulin-sensitive transport mechanism. | 531,542,761 |
| 4. Rate of glucose turnover high in the VMH regions of hungry animals. | 13,20 |
| 5. Direct injection of glucose into the VMH area decreases VMH cellular electrical activity and causes satiety. | 324 |
| 6. Injection of gold thioglucose (GTG) destroys VMH cells and causes hyperphagia and obesity in mice. | 102,163,164,180,388,422, 423,451,452,780 |
| 7. Uptake of GTG into VMH region can be prevented by experimental induction of hyperglycemia, or can be blocked by insulin-induced hypoglycemia. | 161,162,165,166,239,426, 729 |
| 8. Degree of hyperphagia and obesity in animals with electrolytic lesions of the VMH is directly related to the occurrence of hyperinsulinemia. | 214,247,327,814,820 |
| *Lateral hypothalamic area (LH)* | |
| 1. Electrical activity of LH cells decreases after eating and increases after food deprivation. | 18,20,307 |
| 2. Systemic glucose infusion decreases electrical activity of LH cells and causes satiety; injection of insulin or 2-DG increases LH electrical activity and induces eating. | 18,20,21,47,80,117,172, 524 |
| 3. Glucose injection directly into the LH area attenuates insulin-induced eating; direct injection of 2-DG into this brain region causes eating. | 47,80 |
| 4. Systemic injection of GTG destroys cells in the LH region and causes obesity; direct injection of GTG into the LH area destroys cells and produces aphagia. | 423,676 |
| 5. Animals recovered from the initial effects of electrolytic lesions in the LH region do not increase food consumption following treatment with insulin or 2-DG. | 47,193,781 |
| *Liver or duodenum* | |
| 1. Glucose infusion into the hepatic portal vein reduces food consumption in hungry animals. | 82,122,517 |
| 2. Glucose infusion into the stomach or small intestine decreases food intake in animals that have free access to food. | 122,517,518, 761 |

TABLE 3.(*continued*)

| Location of cells | References |
|---|---|
| 3. 2-DG infusion into the hepatic portal vein causes increased food consumption in animals with free access to food. | 517,519,760 |
| 4. Vagotomized animals do not respond normally to hepatic portal glucose infusion, or to duodenal infusion of glucose or 2-DG. | 517,760 |
| 5. Insulin infusion into the hepatic portal vein causes increased food consumption in sated animals. | 517 |
| 6. A reduction in hepatic glucose concentration is correlated with eating. | 634 |
| 7. The electrical activity of the vagus nerve is inversely related to the hepatic glucose concentration; electrical stimulation of the vagus nerve causes eating in sated animals, whereas DC blockade of the nerve decreases eating in hungry animals. | 509,550,551 |
| 8. Hepatic-portal infusion of glucose alters VMH and LH cellular electrical activity; vagotomy blocks the hyperphagia and obesity associated with VMH electrolytic lesions, and the induced eating associated with LH electrical stimulation. | 569,570,649 |

after glucose injection into the VMH (535) reflects physiological changes since the injected doses greatly exceed normal brain concentration of the sugar. The delayed changes in feeding behavior after these injections may in fact indicate that the glucose had to diffuse to active sites geographically removed from the VMH nuclei before the behavioral changes could be initiated.

That VMH cells accumulate more radioactivity following intragastric injection of $^{14}$C-D-glucose (531,542) does not mean *ipso facto* that more glucose is taken up by this area than by other brain regions; no estimates of the concentration of radioactive *glucose,* as opposed to radioactive *metabolites* of the sugar, were reported (531). It is impressive that the accumulation of radioactivity was increased by pretreatment with insulin and slightly decreased in diabetic animals (531); however, other studies showed that glucose uptake by brain tissue does not appear to be insulin-dependent (237,303,546). Although it is possible that only cells localized in the VMH area have an insulin-dependent glucose-uptake system (161,676), other studies do not support this hypothesis. Insulin injection directly into this brain region does not alter feeding behavior, whereas a systemic injection does (536). In addition, lesions of the VMH area (which presumably destroy the hypothesized glucoreceptor cells) produce hyperphagia and obesity (534) but do not alter the hyperphagia seen after systemic injection of insulin (313) or 2-DG (477,508), whereas lateral hypothalamic lesions abolish the feeding effects of both of these compounds (193). Although it is possible that insulin-dependent, glucoreceptor cells may be localized specifically in the VMH area, these cells apparently do not mediate the effects of insulin or 2-DG on feeding.

The evidence from studies using gold thioglucose (GTG) has also been questioned (423,592). This toxic glucose analog is presumably taken up by glucoreceptor cells in the VMH; it then destroys them, producing hyperphagia and obesity. The destructiveness of this drug may not be due solely to the fact that it is a glucose analog; other substances (e.g., bipiperidyl mustard) that are structurally unrelated to the glucose molecule also destroy the VMH nuclei and produce hyperphagia and obesity (637). Furthermore, GTG-induced brain lesions are not confined solely to the VMH area; rather, massive tissue damage has been observed in other brain regions of mice treated with the drug, including the area postrema, subfornical organ, supraoptic crest, fornix, anterior hypothalamus, and premammillary area (423,554). It remains unclear if and how much damage to these other brain regions underlies the effects of GTG on feeding behavior; these results do demonstrate, however, that brain cells besides those located in the VMH area have the capacity to accumulate toxic levels of GTG (423). Some investigators suggest that the drug may not destroy glucoreceptor cells because it is actively and selectively taken up by these cells exclusively, but rather because it damages neural tissue as a result of nonspecific ischemia produced by the toxic effects of heavy metals on the vascular system (30,136,423,592). Even more suspect is the finding that GTG injections do not produce VMH damage, or hyperphagia or obesity, in any animals except the mouse (423). It has thus far been impossible to treat animals with a nonlethal dose of the drug that is still sufficient to induce changes in feeding behavior (423). If other animals have mechanisms similar to those of the mouse for the control of eating behavior, GTG would be expected to accumulate in, and destroy, their VMH cells as well. Finally, although some studies have shown that, following the induction of experimental diabetes, changes in blood glucose decrease the effects of GTG injection in mice, others using different methods for inducing blood sugar changes have not replicated these findings (182,183,555).

If glucoreceptor cells are not unique to the VMH area, or if they do not exist in this brain region at all, where else might they be found? Some experiments have provided indirect evidence that glucose-sensitive cells in various peripheral tissues, especially in the liver and duodenum, may detect changes in glucose utilization and relay this information to brain cells (and possibly to the VMH). All nutrients absorbed from the duodenum first pass through the hepatic portal blood supply before being distributed throughout the rest of the body by the general circulation. Russek and colleagues (631,632,634) were the first to report that reductions in hepatic glucose concentrations were associated with feeding behavior, and that increases in hepatic glucose levels were correlated with satiety. There were no similar correlations between food intake and changes in the glucose levels in adipose tissue, muscle, or plasma

(631). Novin and colleagues (517,519) extended these initial findings and found that infusion of a relatively small glucose dose into the hepatic-portal circulation decreased the food intake of starved animals but not of those that had access to food *ad libitum;* in contrast, gastric or duodenal infusion of a similar dose reduced the food intake of animals fed *ad libitum* but not of those that had been fasted for 24 hr. These preliminary findings suggest that glucoreceptor cells in the digestive tract may be maximally sensitive to changes in glucose levels (or perhaps to glucose utilization) only when animals are minimally hungry; hepatic-portal glucoreceptors, in contrast, may be maximally active when the need for glucose is more urgent (as during food deprivation) (517). Lower doses of 2-DG are needed to increase food intake when the drug is placed in the hepatic-portal circulation than when it is injected into the general peripheral circulatory system (519,634); this fact is also compatible with the existence of liver glucoreceptors, although alternative explanations are possible.

If glucoreceptor cells sensitive to changes in cellular glucose utilization do indeed reside outside the CNS, how does the information they receive reach the brain? Preliminary evidence suggesting that this information is carried via peripheral nerves from the lower GI tract or from the liver is summarized in Table 3. This evidence supports the notion that glucoreceptor cells located in the GI tract or the liver sense a change in the absolute glucose level in the lumen or the hepatic-portal circulation, and relay this information to brain mechanisms (possibly to cells located in the VMH nucleus). In turn, the latter cells might feed back, via the parasympathetic and sympathetic nervous systems as well as the vagal nerve, information to peripheral tissues that ultimately alters feeding behavior and the digestion, absorption, and metabolism of nutrients. Much more data are needed, however, to substantiate this hypothesis.

It was once thought that the metabolic consequences of feeding, especially as a result of changes in glucose utilization, probably occurred too slowly to be much of a factor in satiety. However, with the recent suggestion that glucoreceptors might be located in the digestive tract or liver, it seems possible that information regarding glucose utilization may well be important for both meal initiation and termination. Although glucostatic mechanisms may determine short-term feeding behavior, it is difficult to understand how changes in factors such as cellular glucose utilization or blood sugar levels might account for the long-term regulation of food intake and body weight. Other mechanisms, possibly based on changes in body fat stores, may fulfill this functional role.

### 4. Fat Metabolism and Feeding Behavior

Quite some time ago Kennedy proposed that mammals control long-term food intake and energy balance by monitoring fat stores and maintaining them as a constant proportion of total body weight (355). On the basis of this proposal, some investigators classified feeding behavior into two basic types: "caloric" feeding, which maintains daily energy requirements to fulfill metabolic needs, and "regulatory" feeding, which maintains the body fat/lean body mass ratio (534). With this view, regulatory feeding dominates when the body fat/body weight ratio changes. If the ratio is low, animals increase food consumption; if it is high, they eat less food per day until the normal ratio is restored. Although the precise mechanisms underlying regulatory feeding remain a matter of conjecture, it is known that most animals that have been force-fed (140) or made obese by chronic injection of long-acting forms of insulin (53,313,439,532) subsequently decrease food intake until they regain their normal pretreatment body weight. Similarly, animals that have been deprived of food overeat after the deprivation period until they attain their prestarvation body weight (113).

On the basis of these and other (353) results, it appears that mammals actively defend a set point around which they maintain a constant body fat/lean body mass ratio. The body weight set point hypothesis predicts that an animal will actively defend its body weight—be it overweight (obese), normal, or underweight (lean)—by altering food intake whenever its weight differs from the set point (353). This concept makes it easy to understand why it is so difficult for chronically overweight humans to maintain lower body weights reached after periods of rigorous dieting or using other methods for losing weight.

Certain questions have emerged from the set point hypothesis for long-term regulation of feeding behavior and body weight. What factors determine the set point level? What mechanisms enable animals to compare body weight with the set point? Finally, what is the evidence that changes in fat metabolism and storage do indeed influence long-term food intake and body weight?

It is always difficult if not impossible to isolate and assign relative importance to genetic and environmental influences. Both factors appear to be potent determinants of the set point around which feeding behavior and body weight are controlled. Fuller (221) recently reviewed the evidence that certain genetic manipulations produce profound changes in the eating behavior and body weight of some strains of rodents. It appears likely that many forms of obesity, in animals and in humans, are strongly influenced by genetic factors which are clearly separate from environmental influences (95). A possible genetic basis for leanness remains to be determined, although its existence certainly seems likely. It does appear that there are critical periods during which undernutrition results in permanent changes in the total number of cells in various peripheral tissues and the brains of animals (790) and humans (791). If it can be assumed that the set point monitors cell number, cell size, or both, then there seems to be good evidence that both genetic history and early experiences influence the value around which the set point is fixed. Once determined, the set point does not change except when the organism is subjected to severe environmental insult or radical physiological intervention. For example, when one fat organ in adult rats is removed surgically, remaining adipose tissue showed a compensatory hypertrophy so that total body fat was held constant (424). However, the mechanisms underlying these changes remain to be determined.

The set point for long-term body weight regulation may be mediated by hypothalamic mechanisms; bilateral electrolytic lesions of the VMH nuclei produce hyperphagia and obesity (300), whereas bilateral lesioning of the lateral hypothalamic area is associated with hypophagia and chronically reduced body weight (16,741). Once the new body weight stabilizes after these operations, both types of animal adjust their food intake to maintain the new body weight. For example, a previously starved animal with a VMH lesion overeats until its new body weight is reached if its weight is still reduced to preoperative levels; similarly, the animal decreases food intake if it is made more obese by force-feeding or with chronic insulin treatment (113,208). Results with lateral hypothalamus-lesioned rats are comparable (92,352,568). If a rat with a VMH lesion was made obese prior to the operation, less postoperative time is required to achieve its new body weight (313); in a similar manner, the lateral hypothalamus-lesioned rat starved prior to the operation recovers from the effects of the operation and resumes eating and drinking sooner than the rat that was not starved (647). Despite the attractive evidence that hypothalamic cells participate in the set point regulation of body weight and feeding, it is also possible that similar mechanisms reside in peripheral tissues or in other areas of the brain; no data yet exist regarding this point, however.

The nature of the signal by which animals detect the adipose tissue/lean body mass ratio is unknown. It seems relatively unlikely, however, that the brain contains liporeceptor cells similar to the glucoreceptor cells thought to monitor changes in carbohydrate metabolism, since brain cells normally are unable to use energy derived from fat rapidly and efficiently. Since all other peripheral tissues normally utilize the energy derived from fat, some investigators (697) suggest that cells sensitive to changes in fat metabolites might mediate a lipostatic control mechanism, but such cells have not been identified (295,774). Fat metabolism changes as a function of whether the animal has recently eaten or fasted. During the absorptive state lipid synthesis in the liver increases dramatically (412); in contrast, during the postabsorptive state hepatic lipogenesis decreases and lipolysis increases, raising plasma concentrations of fatty acids and glycerol (73,412). Pharmacological manipulation of lipogenesis or lipolysis produced corresponding changes in food intake (412, 727), suggesting that the reduction in the amount of energy derived from the breakdown of fat, or possibly changes in the circulating levels of fat metabolites, might be the critical "lipostatic" signal controlling food intake (409,412). The indirect observations that the basal release of glycerol and FFAs into the circulation is directly related to the size of the adipose tissue mass (74) and that plasma levels in these compounds increase during short periods of fasting (121,412,821) are compatible with this hypothesis.

The class of compounds called prostaglandins are also being considered as possible lipostatic signals. Prostaglandins are biologically active compounds synthesized from essential unsaturated fatty acids and released during adipose cell lipolysis (321). One compound in the prostaglandin series, prostaglandin $E_2$, increases or decreases the food intake of sheep, depending on the exact injection site in various hypothalamic areas (34,37,453,786). Since prostaglandin concentrations in plasma vary as a function of the adipose tissue mass and the fed or fasted state of the animal, it is possible that these compounds might be the link between lipostatic mechanisms and feeding behavior. However, they generally have short biological half-lives, a fact which casts doubt on their possible role in the long-term control of eating and body weight regulation.

Release of GH from the pituitary gland has also been proposed as the lipostatic signal (360). Its release is intimately related to changes in fat metabolism: High circulating GH levels increase lipolysis, and high concentrations of plasma FFAs decrease GH secretion (536,797). Since changes in GH also produce alterations in feeding behavior, it is possible that the hormone may be the critical link between changing adipose tissue size and eating behavior. Similar roles for other pituitary hormones—melanocyte-stimulating hormone, ACTH, or lipotropin—have also been proposed (350), although there is no firm evidence to establish the role of these hormones *in vivo*.

It is surprising that there is so little direct evidence to document the possible involvement of lipostatic mechanisms in the long-term control of eating behavior and body weight regulation; however, the hypothesis continues to enjoy popularity in current concepts of peripheral control mechanisms for the behavior.

## 5. Amino Acids and Feeding Behavior

Animals eat less food when they are offered diets that contain disproportionately low or high concentrations of protein (283); when their diets are deficient in, or devoid of, a single indispensable amino acid (282); or when the diet contains concentrations of amino acids that are far in excess of those normally needed (283). Animals also eat different amounts of two diets, depending on their amino acid concentrations (616). Hence it appears that some mechanisms exist whereby the amino acid or protein content of the diet can be detected. On the basis of these findings, several investigators (11,211, 416,463,464) proposed that feeding behavior may be at least partially controlled by diet-induced changes in the pattern of plasma amino acids.

Although some of the reductions in food consumption observed when animals are offered protein- or amino acid-imbalanced diets may result from decreased palatability of the diet, there are enough data to offer strong support for a possible "aminostatic" mechanism in the control of feeding behavior. Since adequate amounts of proteins and amino acids are absolutely essential for normal growth and health, it makes sense that bodily mechanisms should enable animals to alter the amount of food eaten when the quality of the diet changes. It now seems clear that brain mechanisms mediate changes in feeding behavior when animals are offered protein- or amino acid-imbalanced diets. The precise role played by these mechanisms remains to be determined. For example, rats decrease their food intake when offered a diet deficient in the amino acid threonine (416). These food intake depressions were abolished when threonine was infused into the carotid artery but not when the amino acid was injected into the jugular vein (416). These data suggest that brain cells which control feeding are sensitive to plasma amino acid concentrations and therefore to changes in the dietary concentrations of indispensable amino acids. If the limiting dietary amino acid is pharmacologically restored in the blood supply to the brain, food intake returns to normal levels, even though the diet is still amino acid-imbalanced. The brain regions containing aminostats are still poorly defined, but recent evidence suggests that certain brain areas may influence feeding behavior in response to some but not all amino acid-imbalanced diets. For example, rats with bilateral electrolytic lesions of the VMH nuclei do not decrease food intake as normal animals do when offered a diet deficient or imbalanced in isoleucine or histidine concentrations (416). However, these animals show normal food intake depression when presented with a leucine or threonine imbalance or with a diet that contains an excessively high protein level (416,647). Some but not all aminostatic control mechanisms are also disrupted in rats with medial septal lesions (616,647). Similarly, rats with anterior prepyriform cortical lesions do not decrease food intake when offered an amino acid-imbalanced diet or one missing a single indispensable amino acid; however, they do reduce food intake when offered a diet that contains an excessively high concentration of leucine or protein (417). Finally, balanced amino acid solutions injected directly into the lateral hypothalamic area inhibit food intake in hungry rats (539); unfortunately few studies have tested the effects produced by injecting single amino acids on feeding, so it is not yet possible to determine if some of these results are due to a nonspecific behavioral depression resulting from the treatment, or if they represent selective effects on eating behavior. On the basis of these initial results, however, it appears that specific brain regions contain aminostatic control mechanisms for feeding that are sensitive to some but not all diet-induced changes in plasma amino acid patterns. Of the brain regions examined thus far, however, no single area appears to have the capability of mediating all aminostatic responses.

It should be noted that the depressed food intake observed in animals offered diets containing an excessively low or high concentration of proteins or amino acids is not always permanent and apparently can be overridden by other metabolic needs (282). For example, although food consumption decreases when animals are first offered a high-protein diet, the daily food intake and growth rate return to near-normal levels within a few days (23). The compensatory ability of animals that adjust to these dietary imbalances appears to correlate in time with several biochemical adaptive changes. Animals offered a diet containing excess protein or amino acid(s) have increased activity of several amino acid degradative enzymes and an increased rate at which the excess amino acids are cleared; hence after a fairly short time these animals achieve a reasonably stable balance between nutrient intake and catabolism (282). Along similar lines, rats fed low-protein diets initially decrease total food consumption but then rapidly increase eating so that they eventually balance the nutrient intake and expenditure (281). Furthermore, the initial reduction in food intake following the first presentation of a low-protein diet is absent if other metabolic challenges arise, i.c., if animals have been maintained in a cold environment or are forced to exercise, or if the low-protein diet is also diluted with inert material (281,282). On the basis of these latter observations, Harper (282) proposed that food intake is normally controlled by mechanisms other than those arising from a change in the plasma amino acid pattern or amino acid metabolism. Since most adult animals usually have sufficient access to a diet that contains balanced mixtures of proteins and amino acids, aminostatic mechanisms would become dominant only when the experimental animal is restricted to protein- or amino acid-imbalanced diets.

Other results challenge this view. It is possible that diet-induced changes in plasma amino acids may directly alter the functional activity of brain neurons that mediate feeding behavior; although the evidence is still largely speculative, Fernstrom, Wurtman, and their colleagues (137,200,203,804,805) showed that diet-induced changes in plasma amino acids alter the concentrations of putative brain neurotransmitters. For example, synthesis of the brain neurotransmitter serotonin depends on an adequate concentration of its precursor amino acid, tryptophan. Mammals are unable to synthesize tryptophan *de novo;* hence the body concentrations of this amino acid depend ultimately on the presence of an adequate dietary concentration of tryptophan: (a) Animals chronically fed artificial or natural diets that contain inadequate amounts of tryptophan have reduced plasma and brain concentrations of the amino acid, and decreased brain concentrations of serotonin (202,437); conversely, animals eating diets with large concentrations of tryptophan have increased levels of brain serotonin (252). (b) Animals fed a high-carbohydrate, protein-free meal (200) or that were injected with low doses of insulin (201) have increased plasma and brain concentrations of tryptophan and increased brain levels of serotonin. (c) Tryptophan and serotonin concentrations in brain increase or decrease in response to artificial amino acid diets that either increase or decrease the ratio of plasma tryptophan to the sum of the concentrations of other large neutral amino acids (tyrosine, valine, leucine, isoleucine, or phenylalanine) which compete with tryptophan for transport into the brain (203,

805). The synthesis rates of other putative brain and peripheral neurotransmitters can also be influenced at least in part by diets that alter plasma and brain concentrations of their precursor compounds: (a) The consumption of diets that contain different amounts of tyrosine affect the synthesis rates of catecholaminergic neurotransmitters (Gibson and Wurtman, *in preparation*); and (b) similarly, rats have brain acetylcholine levels that are directly related to the amount of choline in the diet (137). Note that the brain neurotransmitters which are altered in animals consuming these various diets have been implicated in other studies as possible mediators of feeding behavior.

The major question is: Are there any data to show that qualitative changes in the diet alter brain mechanisms which specifically control feeding behavior? In a recent study Ashley and Anderson (31,32) described an animal model that may show this relationship. Animals offered two diets of different protein concentrations for long periods ate relatively constant amounts of their daily calories as protein; moreover, there were consistent relationships between the amount of protein eaten daily and the pattern of plasma amino acids. The ratio of tryptophan to the concentrations of competing neutral amino acids in plasma predicted almost perfectly the total daily amount of protein consumed (31); interestingly, the brain serotonin level was also highly correlated with protein consumption (Anderson, *personal communication*). Although it is still too early to tell whether the daily protein intake was the cause or the result of diet-induced changes in the plasma amino acid pattern, preliminary evidence suggests the following interconnected series of events: The quality of the diet alters the plasma amino acid pattern, which then changes brain serotonin levels; the changes in brain serotoninergic neurons then feed back and influence subsequent feeding behavior. If these preliminary results are repeated in future experiments, an important control mechanism for food intake may be the amino acid and protein quality of the diet.

### 6. *Temperature Change and Feeding Behavior*

The idea that food intake and body temperature are interrelated is not new—this relationship was hypothesized by Galen during the first century AD (273,792). In a more contemporary statement, Brobeck (107) proposed that animals eat to keep warm and stop eating to reduce hyperthermia. A variety of evidence indirectly supports this hypothesis. In most homeothermic mammals (i.e., animals that can maintain constant body temperature across a wide range of ambient temperatures), food intake varies inversely with ambient temperature. Animals tend to eat more food when placed in a cold environment and less at a warm ambient temperature (792). There are limits to this relationship; if the environment is extremely cold, the energy needed to maintain a viable body temperature may exceed the rate at which animals can ingest energy and nutrients; in an extremely hot environment, the small amount of food ingested may be inadequate to maintain body weight but sufficient to drive body temperature into the lethal range (274). Within these constraints, animals adjust their food intake to match closely the conservation or dissipation of body heat, even though a balance between energy intake and expenditure may be reached only after several days of exposure to new ambient temperatures (271). Environmental temperature change can also produce a rather rapid change in food consumption, however. Rats exposed to a cold or neutral temperature for only a 20-min period daily increase their food consumption during the subsequent hour as an inverse function of the temperature to which they were exposed (784).

Exposure to different environmental temperatures alters not only food consumption but the metabolism and storage of nutrients as well. In Alaskan husky dogs, for example, food ingested during the Arctic winter is used primarily to maintain body heat, since little change in body weight and growth occurs during this period; during the summer, body weight and growth increase, even though these animals consume less food and are more active (181). Changes in ambient temperature also alter the survival time of terminally starved animals, apparently by influencing the metabolic rate; rats survive longer and lose less body weight when they are food-deprived and exposed to a 20°C ambient temperature than when they are exposed to 30°C (373). At a neutral ambient temperature, rats fed extremely low protein diets do not consume enough of the diet to maintain body weight and die relatively quickly. If they are fed the same diet but are exposed to a cold temperature, they increase their total consumption of the diet and are able to gain weight and survive (26).

Dietary preferences as well as total food consumption are affected by the environmental temperature. In a warm environment mice offered a choice between a high-fat, high-carbohydrate, or high-protein diet eat more of the high-fat diet; in a cold environment they prefer the high-carbohydrate diet; however, when they are stressed by exposure to an extremely cold environment, the high-fat diet is preferred over the high-carbohydrate diet (177).

On the basis of these and other observations, Brobeck extended the thermostatic theory of food intake to take into account differences in the specific dynamic action (SDA) of food (106,719). The SDA of food refers to the increase in metabolic rate observed during the digestion and assimilation of nutrients. The metabolic rate of animals and humans, as determined by changes in oxygen consumption or body temperature, increases somewhat when a meal has been eaten, and the magnitude of increase varies as a function of the types of nutrient consumed; the heat generated after the digestion, absorption, and hepatic processing of a diet high in proteins and amino acids is greater than the metabolic heat generated after consumption of a high-carbohydrate or high-fat diet. Based on differences in the SDA of foods, Brobeck hypothesized that since metabolic rate (and body temperature) increases more after consumption of a diet high in protein than after one high in carbohydrate or fat, animals would be expected to consume less of a high-protein than of a high-carbohydrate or high-fat diet (so that they would not become too warm too fast). Hence animals can adjust food intake on the basis of the SDA of food rather than on its caloric content. Although other explanations are possible (rats may consume less high-protein diet because it is less palatable), this hypothesis has received some support; in animals that ingest comparable amounts of a protein, carbohydrate, or fat diet, subsequent food intake is initially lower after the protein diet than after the other two (240,720). Rats also eat less immediately after they have received an intragastric protein load than after an isocaloric carbohydrate or fat load (529). However, the protein load could be more toxic than isocaloric loads of other nutrients. Despite these results, the thermostatic theory of feeding behavior based on the notion of SDAs of food has not been widely accepted and has even been severely criticized (1,3,120,273,547).

If animals do alter their feeding behavior on the basis of thermostatic mechanisms, then eating and fasting should produce consistent, measurable changes in body temperature and oxygen consumption. Furthermore, it should be possible to locate cells in the brain or periphery that mediate these putative temperature-induced changes in feeding. Booth and Strang (90) reported that skin temperature increased approximately 2°C in nonobese humans shortly after they ate a high-protein diet, whereas the skin temperature of obese people consuming the same diet increased only slightly and at a later time after the meal. Although similar results were obtained in other studies with humans (724) and rats (273), the magnitude of change in body temperature was much smaller than that reported by Booth and Strang, and the difference between obese and nonobese humans has not been repeated (724). The problem in most of these studies is the inability to determine the best place to measure temperature changes. Are temperature sensors involved in controlling eating behavior located in the skin, colon, brain, and/or some other peripheral tissue?

The answer to this question is still in doubt. Some investigators provided evidence that changes in the temperature of the blood bathing certain brain regions may be important for normal eating. Andersson and Larsson (24) were the first to show that thermosensitive cells in the anterior hypothalamic and anterior preoptic areas may mediate temperature-induced changes in eating. Artificial heating or cooling of the preoptic areas of goats made them decrease or increase food consumption, respectively (24,25). However, the results must be interpreted with some caution, since it is unlikely that the temperature of this brain area normally changes as much as it was altered in these experiments. When similar experiments were attempted in rats using more modest increases in temperature in the hypothalamus, feeding increased rather than decreased (276,694). These latter findings demonstrate the complexities involved in interpreting studies that experimentally manipulate brain temperature; an increase in hypothalamic temperature was associated with a reduction in skin temperature (276,694). Depending on which temperature change (in brain or skin) one believes should be monitored, the thermostatic theory can be either supported or disproved. Rats with lesions of the anterior preoptic area of the hypothalamus have impaired temperature regulation and do not respond normally to a hot or cold environment; in contrast to normal intact rats, lesioned rats overeat following exposure to a hot environment and undereat when placed in a cold environment (275). It was also reported that temperature in the preoptic areas of rats decreases slightly before the onset of a meal and then increases rapidly after the cessation of feeding (1). Similar increases in the temperature of the abdominal cavity and in oxygen consumption have been correlated with the onset of eating (273). In any case, the rapid fluxes in temperature and oxygen consumption associated with the initiation of the meal make it extremely unlikely that these increases result from metabolic changes associated with the digestion, absorption, or utilization of nutrients. It also seems unlikely that a change in metabolic rate is the critical factor in meal termination, since increases in temperature and oxygen consumption reach a plateau long before meal termination. Finally, some suggest that the local changes in brain temperature may be more a function of the motor activity involved in chewing and swallowing food, and less a function of changes in metabolic rate (1,581).

Variations in deep core body temperature are usually small throughout the day; moreover, the normal transient fluctuations in body temperature that do occur are usually slow to change. Similarly, although the metabolic rate varies widely during the day, the rate changes measured thus far do not correlate well with meal initiation or termination (107). Ambient-temperature-induced changes in metabolic rate may account for some of the changes in feeding behavior in animals chronically exposed to different environments, but it is difficult to understand how they can account for the rather rapid increase in food intake seen in animals first placed in the cold (377,784). If a change in body temperature does not account well for altered feeding behavior, and if the ambient-temperature-induced change in metabolic rate does not easily account for the short-term changes in the feeding behavior of animals first exposed to a cold environment, then what other possible mechanisms might account for these changes?

Kraly and Blass (377) recently observed that animals fed a liquid diet in a cold environment increase their total daily food consumption by increasing the frequency rather than the size of meals. Since the rate of gastric emptying is faster when rats are maintained in the cold (377,581), these authors suggested that the ambient temperature might decrease intermeal intervals by reducing the satiety effects of food. Presumably cold-induced changes in the rate of gastric clearance accelerate the process of digestion and absorption in the small intestine, thus decreasing the time spent in the more satiated, absorptive state. Animals placed in the cold also appear to be "hungrier," in the sense that they perform an operant response for food reinforcement and eat food that has been adulterated with quinine (377).

Much more research is needed before it will be possible to determine the precise effects of feeding on body temperature or the role that body temperature may play in eating behavior. Until better data are presented to the contrary, it seems clear that changes in body temperature normally play only a minor role in the control of eating behavior. Thermostatic factors may outweigh other determinants of feeding behavior, however, when challenges arise to thermoregulatory homeostasis. The ingestion of food must, after all, be integrated with temperature regulation, since heat conservation and dissipation represent one of the primary ways in which animals expend energy. Even relatively minor discrepancies in the constancy of body temperature ultimately threaten energy-nutrient balance and survival.

Peripheral changes associated with the digestion and metabolism of food or, in some cases, the oropharyngeal sensations that arise during the process of eating appear to be important determinants for satiety and meal termination, and relatively less important for meal initiation. In contrast, many of the changes that result from the metabolism, storage, and utilization of nutrients during the postabsorptive state may be more important for hunger and meal initiation. These factors may be less important for satiety, inasmuch as most of the changes occur at times other than the short periods associated with the actual process of eating.

## B. Brain Integrative Mechanisms

All behavioral feeding responses are ultimately determined by the combined products of external and internal stimuli that impinge on, and are integrated by, cells in the brain and peripheral nervous systems. Neurons in the brain monitor the biochemical, hormonal, muscular, and electrophysiological changes that occur in the periphery during the absorptive and postabsorptive states, and then integrate this information into motor commands that tell the organism when to begin, continue, and stop eating. The precise means by which neurons influence behavioral feeding responses are still unknown, but the functioning of specific neuroanatomical and neurochemical systems in the brain appear essential for normal eating behavior.

Around the turn of this century, the hypothalamic area of the brain was singled out as the possible essential site for the control of eating behavior. This interest stemmed from clinical observations that, in many cases of human obesity tumors or lesions were found in the basal diencephalon. These abnormalities often encroached on the pituitary gland as well as on brain tissue, however, so it was not possible to determine with any accuracy whether this type of human obesity was caused by damage to brain cells in the hypothalamus or to the hormone-secreting cells of the pituitary gland (42,709).

From a series of experiments on the hypothalamus and pituitary gland (16,299,300) it was determined that the ventromedial and lateral hypothalamic areas are responsible for the control of eating behavior—not the pituitary. The dominant hypothesis that guided most research on the control of eating behavior until only recently was relatively straightforward: Peripheral changes that occurred during the fed or fasted state directly or indirectly stimulated cells in the ventromedial or lateral areas of the hypothalamus; relative changes in the activity of these cells resulted in the initiation or termination of eating (12,14,702). The VMH nucleus contained cells important for satiety and suppressed eating by inhibiting the activity of cells in the lateral hypothalamic feeding center. Animals were motivated to eat when cells in the lateral hypothalamic area were activated (14). Hence the dual-center theory of appetite regulation proposed that two brain centers in the ventromedial or lateral hypothalamus mediated eating behavior by reciprocally inhibiting each other's activity. Although the dual-center concept still plays an important role in contemporary research in this area, newer evidence indicates that feeding behavior may be controlled by anatomical brain *systems* and not brain *centers*.

### 1. Hypothalamic Neuroanatomy

The hypothalamic area of the brain is one of the most intricate neuroanatomical structures in the CNS. It contains a number of morphologically and functionally distinct nuclei, or cell bodies. Defined anatomically, the hypothalamic area usually includes all tissue that lies ventral to the subthalamus and dorsal to the base of the brain, lateral from the medial internal capsule, posterior to the optic chiasm, and anterior from the mammillary bodies (289). In most species the suprachiasmatic, supraoptic, paraventricular, ventromedial, dorsomedial, and mammillary regions of the hypothalamus form discrete nuclei, although in some species the anterior hypothalamic, periventricular, arcuate, and premammillary nuclei are less discernible (289,490).

One of the brain areas important for feeding behavior, the lateral hypothalamus, is not well defined because cells in this region are not morphologically uniform. Although better defined as a concentrated area of cells, the VMH nucleus also lacks uniformity with regard to cell type, size, or neuropil compared to other hypothalamic nuclei (474,476,506). These two hypothalamic regions are veritable way stations located in the middle of many of the major fiber bundles that traverse the anterior-posterior, dorsal-ventral, and medial-lateral axes of the brain (169,222,264,289,474,475,488,489). Because of their location, these cells can receive information from many areas in the brain and can influence the activity of cells in other parts of the brain and periphery. Moreover, due to the relatively heavy vascularization of the hypothalamus, its cells appear capable of sensing and responding to many plasma hormones secreted by endocrine glands in the periphery, as well as to plasma nutrients derived from the diet. Some hypothalamic cells also provide direct connections between brain neurons and the pituitary gland, and thus are a potentially important influence on peripheral biochemistry. Hence various hypothalamic nuclei may receive afferent information from the periphery and other brain areas important for eating, and because of their efferent connections can exert a strong influence over various neuroanatomical and endocrinological systems that may be important for feeding.

## 2. VMH: The "Satiety Center"

During the past 70 years or so, several classic procedures have been developed to determine the extent to which given areas of the brain might figure in different types of behaviors. These techniques include behavioral measurements combined with the use of: (a) procedures that damage the brain region of interest (electrolytic or radiofrequency lesions, or knife cuts that literally disconnect a brain area from surrounding tissue); (b) procedures in which a brain region is stimulated electrically or chemically with various compounds; and (c) procedures that measure changes in whole or regional brain electrical activity, or in the electrical activity of single cells.

*VMH lesions.*

In their pioneering studies, Hetherington and Ranson (299,300) showed that direct-current, electrolytic lesions of the VMH nuclei in rats resulted in hyperphagia and marked obesity. Based on the results of studies examining the effects of lesions in various areas of the brain, especially in the hypothalamic region, they concluded that hyperphagia and obesity resulted only when the lesions were fairly symmetrical and bilateral, and occupied the medial hypothalamic area, especially the area immediately lateral to the ventromedial nuclei (297,298,301,302). Later experiments confirmed these results, and it now seems clear that the area lateral to the VMH, and not the VMH *per se,* is the critical area whose damage leads to hyperphagia and obesity (105,108, 245,346,527,549,653,656). For the purposes of this chapter, however, no distinction is drawn between the VMH and this more laterally located hypothalamic region.

Experiments conducted after those of Hetherington and Ranson examined in great detail the factors necessary for the development of hyperphagia and obesity in VMH-lesioned animals, as well as the possible role that cells in this brain region play in the normal control of various aspects of feeding behavior (42,244,245,261,264,310,459,490,494,528,530,533,534,577,590,653–655,709). To summarize: The obesity of animals with VMH lesions results from three primary changes in energy balance: (a) VMH-lesioned animals alter food intake so that they eat more food per day than do normal intact animals. (b) VMH-lesioned animals are hypoactive and thus expend less energy postoperatively even though they eat more. (c) The VMH lesions produce several biochemical and endocrinological abnormalities which alter energy and nutrient metabolism, storage, and utilization to promote the storage of fat rather than its utilization as energy.

When the feeding habits and growth curves of VMH-lesioned animals are analyzed, it becomes clear that the changes in eating and body weight gain are not uniform throughout the duration of the postoperative period. Rats eat voraciously as soon as they have recovered from anesthesia and the trauma of the operation (712); this preliminary phase of hyperphagia continues for as long as 4 months after the operation, depending on the lesion placement, size, and symmetry (41). Rats typically double their initial preoperative body weight during this period of overeating, called the "dynamic" phase of obesity (109). The obesity that develops during the dynamic phase does not appear to result directly from a disruption in intermediary metabolism, since VMH-lesioned animals offered restricted access to food comparable to that consumed by control rats do not gain weight (109). The dynamic hyperphagic stage is followed by the "static" phase in which lesioned rats gradually reduce their food intake to preoperative control levels and eventually maintain a constant elevated body weight, even though food intake is not very different from normal (105). A portion of the obesity observed during the static phase appears to be related to changes in intermediary metabolism, rather than to the recovery of animals from the effects of the lesions; static-phase, VMH-lesioned animals deprived of food until preoperative body weight is reached once again overeat until they attain the plateau weight seen during the original static phase (109,113,353). Furthermore, animals given limited access to food so that they are not allowed to gain weight after the operation become hyperphagic and obese if they are then offered *ad libitum* access to food beginning as late as 2 months after the operation (109). As VMH-lesioned animals become heavier during the dynamic phase, they become more quiescent, less active, and have reduced basal metabolic rates; hence energy balance is once again attained, although this balance is regulated around a much higher set point of body weight (112).

The hyperphagia following VMH lesions is characterized by large individual meals, although the number of meals eaten per day depends on the type of diet presented (44,60,534,749). Animals eating solid food increase meal frequency (60,749), whereas animals offered liquid diets eat the same number of daily meals as intact controls (739). During the static phase of obesity, animals with VMH lesions actually eat fewer and slightly smaller meals than normal rats when offered calorically dense food (109,739). The diurnal pattern of eating also changes following VMH lesions; normal animals eat approximately 70% of their total daily intake during the dark portion of the day-night cycle; in contrast, VMH-lesioned animals eat as much food during the day as they do at night (60,114,348). On the basis of these findings, it appears that VMH-lesioned animals during the dynamic phase of obesity have a defect in the satiety mechanism for meal termination (hence individual meals are larger). Additionally, ingested food in VMH-lesioned animals may lose a portion of its hunger-reducing effect, inasmuch as meal frequency is increased (and so intermeal intervals are decreased). Finally, the lesions also disrupt mechanisms mediating the diurnal pattern for feeding.

The primary eating disorders seen in animals with VMH lesions involve a temporary disruption in satiety mechanisms for short-term control of feeding behavior. Nonetheless, many of the control mechanisms necessary for normal eating behavior appear to be spared by the lesion. In fact, with only a few exceptions (84), once VMH-lesioned animals reach the static phase of obesity, they have normal or near-normal feeding responses to various glucostatic (93,193,534,736), aminostatic (616), or thermostatic (354,355) challenges. Probably one of the most obvious and permanent defects in feeding behavior involves these animals' responses to changes in the palatability of the diet (354,720,733). Even during the dynamic phase of hyperphagia, VMH-lesioned animals are not indiscriminating eaters, and the amount of food consumed is highly dependent on its palatability; they undereat and lose weight if offered a diet inferior in taste or texture (147,354,420,472,720). This finickiness is even more pronounced during the static phase of obesity, and it appears to be permanent (733). Hence the feeding behavior of VMH-lesioned rats resembles that of both the gourmet and the gourmand; however, the development of obesity is not simply a result of an exaggerated responsiveness to the sensory aspects of food, inasmuch as VMH-lesioned animals that obtain food only by pressing a bar for intragastric injections become obese even when deprived of the oropharyngeal sensations associated with eating (460).

Since VMH-lesioned animals display few long-term impairments in control mechanisms for short-term feeding behavior, yet appear to have long-term, permanent disruptions in energy balance, many investigators propose that cells in the VMH area must play a major role in long-term body weight regulation. It is somewhat surprising that VMH-lesioned animals that have reached the static phase of obesity often consume less food per day than do normal intact animals; similar observations have been made in many cases of human obesity (342,512,645,698). The primary cause of obesity produced by the lesions must therefore involve disruption of energy storage and expenditure (354).

Body fat accumulates in VMH-lesioned animals even if they are offered an amount of food comparable to that consumed by intact, nonobese animals (113,277,278,573,578). In VMH-lesioned rats that are allowed to overeat, more than 80% of the body weight gain can be accounted for by increased fat deposits (300,709). Although it seems clear that these increased fat stores are primarily the result of fat cell enlargement, rather than an increase in the total number of fat cells (343), it is not yet known whether the increased concentration of cellular fat is the result of increased lipogenesis or a decreased rate of lipolysis (343,706).

The type of obesity seen in VMH-lesioned, hyperphagic animals differs greatly from that observed in intact animals made obese by force-feeding (95); obesity in the former group is accompanied by hyperinsulinemia, increased fat accumulation, and increased or normal insulin sensitivity; force-fed rats show hyperinsulinemia and increased fat accumulation, but decreased insulin sensitivity (66,95,218,268,319,327,328,670). The hyperinsulinemia seen in obese, force-fed animals probably results from adaptive metabolic changes; in contrast, the hyperinsulinemia of brain-lesioned rats may result directly from the disruptive effects of the lesion on the brain's control of pancreatic function (66,362,797), since hyperinsulinemia has been observed even when these animals are prevented from being hyperphagic (247,730). The increase in food intake or weight gain in VMH-lesioned animals may not produce hyperinsulinemia; but is it possible that the lesion-induced hyperinsulinemia might be necessary for hyperphagia and obesity? This question has not been resolved satisfactorily. Although treatments that decrease circulating insulin levels—pancreatectomy or drug-induced diabetes (214,248,764,814,820)—generally prevent the hyperphagia and obesity normally seen in animals with VMH lesions, other investigators have challenged this hypothesis (536).

In addition to the metabolic abnormalities that promote the storage and synthesis of fat, VMH-lesioned animals may suffer other endocrinological dysfunctions that contribute to the permanent elevation in body weight. Thyroid function is changed postoperatively (113), but it is unclear how these changes might contribute to the lesion-induced obesity. Pituitary hormone changes may well be factors in the VMH syndrome (hyperphagia, obesity, and hypoactivity), however. Hypophysectomized, VMH-lesioned rats do not eat as much food per day, nor do they gain weight as rapidly as lesioned animals with intact pituitary glands (153,297,814); however, since VMH lesions decrease the plasma GH levels in rats (66), it has been hypothesized that the fat accumulation in lesioned animals may be due in part to a decrease in lipolysis associated with a reduced GH level (797). Injection of GH in hypophysectomized animals with VMH lesions reduces the food intake and weight gain—a fact compatible with this hypothesis (556,814), although apparent ontogenetic differences exist in this effect (255). Adrenal corticoids appear to be unnecessary for the development of hyperphagia and obesity after VMH lesions, since lesioned animals with adrenalectomies still become hyperphagic (814). However, there are interesting interactions between VMH lesions and possible differences in hyperphagia and obesity induced by gonadal sex hormones. When male and female rats are matched for age or weight, lesioned females usually show greater hyperphagia and weight gain than do males (154,756). Furthermore, female VMH-lesioned rats ovariectomized during the static phase of obesity show less food intake and body weight gain than do neurologically intact, ovariectomized females (58,756). Hence VMH lesions may attenuate the hyperphagia and obesity associated with female gonadectomy; injection of estrogen into VMH-lesioned animals still produces a normal decrease in food intake (591), however, suggesting that at least some aspects of sex-related feeding behavior remain intact in animals with damage to the VMH nucleus. It is interesting to note that the hyperphagia and obesity seen in VMH-damaged animals or humans (709,756) are often, but not always (709), associated with gonadal atrophy; in addition, VMH lesions in female rats often disrupt the vaginal estrous cycle, rendering the animals relatively infertile

(361). However, these coincidental effects on feeding behavior and reproductive function may be due merely to lesion damage extending to brain areas immediately adjacent to the VMH (778).

Controversy persists regarding male and female animals' responses to VMH lesions. Some investigators claim that males show little hyperphagia and obesity after the lesions (152), whereas others report that animals of both sexes are hyperphagic and obese (253,585), although females show greater postoperative changes than males (152,568). Still others find that males get just as fat and overeat just as much as lesioned females (243). These differences may result from methodological variations in the time that animals are monitored after the lesion, in lesion size or placement, or in the preoperative body weight of the rats (243). More carefully controlled studies must be carried out so these differences in experimental results can be resolved.

Some of the weight gain in VMH-lesioned animals may result from decreased energy expenditure. Static-phase, VMH-lesioned rats have lowered metabolic rates (105,277) and are hypoactive (112,238,302,734). Some of these changes appear to result directly from the brain damage and are not consequences of the lesion-induced obesity. VMH-lesioned animals can become active under certain conditions; food deprivation produces locomotor activity comparable to that of intact animals in the static but not the dynamic phase of obesity (734).

Along similar lines, VMH lesions markedly reduce the locomotor activity level before obesity becomes apparent (734), suggesting that the lesion may simultaneously destroy two or more neuronal systems, one mediating feeding behavior and the other locomotor activity. Interestingly, the lesions may also destroy mechanisms involved in anticipatory responses for feeding behavior. Normal animals offered food on a rigid schedule at the same time each day show an anticipatory increase in locomotor activity just prior to the feeding period; VMH-lesioned rats in the dynamic phase of obesity show only a small, transient increase in activity (807,808). It would be interesting to pursue these results to determine if animals with VMH lesions lack other anticipatory feeding responses, e.g., a rise in insulin level prior to feeding (40,796).

Although the precise nature of the VMH syndrome differs somewhat when other species (490,709) or other methods (293,490,709) for producing damage in the basomedial hypothalamus are used, a rather impressive amount of evidence implicates these cells as possibly playing a role in both short-term satiety and long-term energy balance. The results of still other experiments, however, provide data that are not compatible with the basic assumptions of this model. In studies where alternative methods of ablating the VMH were used—thermocoagulation (589,590) or aspiration (40)—relatively little postoperative changes in food intake and obesity were observed, even though tissue destruction appeared to be as great as that seen after electrolytic lesions or following injection with gold thioglucose (GTG). Reynolds (590) and others (155,577,579) suggested that a portion of the obesity and hyperphagia observed after electrolytic lesions of, or knife cuts adjacent to, the VMH might result from an irritative side effect of the lesioning technique and not from a specific loss of tissue in the VMH. Within this framework, Reynolds found that hyperphagia and obesity resulted only when electrolytic lesions were made with electrodes that left scar tissue and metal deposits at the site of the lesion; when radiofrequency lesions were used (which apparently do not irritate tissue adjacent to the lesion), no hyperphagia or obesity was observed (590). These results were repeated in other laboratories (577), and it was proposed that electrolytic VMH lesions cause animals to increase food intake not by removing a satiety brake on eating behavior but by stimulating "hunger" cells in the lateral hypothalamus (577,590). Although some evidence suggests that the lesion-induced changes in behavior following different lesion or ablation techniques may be due to differences in methodology (e.g., the sex of animals, the palatability of the diet offered), this controversy is still not resolved satisfactorily.

There is also controversy regarding whether some of the feeding disorders seen in these animals result from changes in "hunger motivation" (i.e., defined operationally as the willingness of animals to work for their food) (144,472,528,777), or from indirect effects of the lesion, nutrient metabolism, energy utilization, and obesity (364,447,567,590,671). It now seems clear that VMH-lesioned animals generally respond to most of the cues that elicit changes in short-term eating behavior, whereas long-term energy balance and weight gain seem permanently changed by the lesion. Without a greater understanding of how the lesion might change various metabolic, endocrinological, and physiological functions normally associated with eating and weight regulation, it is difficult to determine the precise aspects of short-term eating behavior and long-term weight regulation dependent on the integrity of cells in the VMH.

*Effects of VMH stimulation.*
Since most experiments show that damage to the VMH produces hyperphagia and obesity in animals, it might be expected that electrical stimulation of this area would produce decreased eating in hungry animals. Experiments conducted quite some time ago by Smith (688) confirmed this expectation, and these results have been repeated in other laboratories (17,485,810); the specificity of these findings is in doubt, however. The intensity of stimulation necessary to inhibit feeding in hungry animals is of a magnitude sufficient to disrupt other types of behavioral responses, and animals actually learn operant responses to avoid electrical VMH stimulation (378,577). It is therefore unclear whether animals stop eating in response to VMH stimulation of "satiety" cells, or because the stimulation is aversive and generally suppresses all behaviors. Reynolds (590) and others pointed out that animals also stop eating in response to foot shock, although most investigators would be reluctant to suggest on the basis of these results that the satiety center resides

in the soles of the feet. Although changes in feeding behavior after VMH stimulation remain in doubt, it is clear that electrical activity of cells in this brain region does produce various peripheral changes important for feeding: decreased gastric motility (386) and alterations in glucagon secretion, blood sugar, and plasma insulin (217).

To circumvent the theoretical problems associated with feeding changes produced by VMH electrical stimulation, some investigators have tried other ways of altering neuronal activity. In one experiment, for example, the anesthetic procaine was injected into the VMH (presumably to decrease its electrical activity) and transient but reversible increases in the food intake of satiated animals were found (186). Although at first glance these data are consistent with the bulk of information showing that permanent damage to the VMH results in hyperphagia, a clear interpretation of these results is not possible because it is not known if the anesthetic specifically decreased the electrical activity of cells confined to the VMH or if it altered the activity of cells in other brain regions (577,590) as well. The fact that it took a relatively long time for animals to begin eating after the injection is compatible with the latter hypothesis (577,590).

Many laboratories attempted to alter the activity of putative glucosensitive cells in the VMH by local injection of glucose or insulin, but these attempts were unsuccessful (186,261,773) with only one exception (535). Food intake can be reduced in hungry animals by injecting hypertonic saline into the VMH (186), but the meaningfulness of these results is still unclear. Finally, prolonged chilling of the VMH in goats increased hay consumption but did not affect water ingestion (25). Since the temperature changes induced in the VMH by this manipulation appear to be outside the normal range of temperature changes thought to occur in intact animals (709), the specificity of the results remains in question.

In general, then, studies using a number of techniques designed to increase or decrease transiently the electrical activity of cells in the VMH have not produced clear-cut, easily interpretable effects on feeding. Although many investigators hypothesize that this brain region contains various cells receptive to changes in peripheral metabolism or to temperature changes associated with eating, the results of direct injection experiments yielded largely negative data.

*Electrical changes in the activity of VMH cells.*

If neurons in the VMH nucleus are in fact involved in the control of eating behavior, it might be assumed that their electrical activity would change as a function of whether the animal was eating. The results of these experiments are summarized in Table 3. Although studies measuring changes in the electrical activity of neurons in the VMH show that these cells are sensitive to changes in eating behavior, and to changes in the various biochemical, endocrinological, and metabolic factors known to influence the behavior, it is difficult if not impossible to determine on the basis of these data alone just what function these cells might have in the control of eating behavior. If electrical activity increases, does it mean that a certain behavioral response is more or less likely to occur? Furthermore, it is never certain that changes in neuronal activity following dietary, pharmacological, or surgical manipulations reflect the cells' ability to sense directly peripheral changes associated with feeding (e.g., changes in glucose utilization) or if the electrical changes result because cells located in other parts of the brain or the periphery influence hypothalamic unit activity through single or multisynaptic connections. Furthermore, it is not clear that *all* cells in a given area respond in a similar fashion to any experimental manipulation; the results of many single-unit studies in various brain regions, including the hypothalamus, indicate that several cells must be sampled in a given area before fair statistical assessment of the global electrical activity of that region can be established. For example, injection of amphetamine—an anorexic compound that reduces appetite and decreases food intake in hungry animals and humans (142)—is correlated with an increase in the firing rate of VMH neurons (380). The results of this single experiment might be interpreted as providing evidence that amphetamine produces anorexia by stimulating (or turning on) satiety cells in the VMH which inhibit food consumption. The results of other experiments are not easily explained by this hypothesis, since the anorexic effects of amphetamine are still present and may even be enhanced in animals with bilateral lesions of the VMH nuclei (185,588,713). It should be noted that amphetamine injection also decreases the electrical activity of a few cells in the lateral hypothalamic area (380), and since brain lesions in this region attenuate the anorexic potency of the drug (125,433) it seems reasonable to assume that a portion of amphetamine's suppressant effects on feeding behavior might be mediated by cells in this brain region (142). These conclusions are also supported by the results of other pharmacological (397) and neuroanatomical studies (7,205).

Within the context of the dual-center theory of brain mechanisms controlling feeding, increases in VMH activity are thought to represent a dominance of satiety mechanisms and a disposition to stop eating; conversely, an increase in the electrical activity of cells in the lateral hypothalamus is thought to reflect the dominance of mechanisms that predispose the animal to eat. Indeed there is some evidence that the firing rates of cells in the ventromedial and lateral hypothalamic areas are inversely related (525); on this basis it is thought that cells in the lateral and ventromedial hypothalamus probably inhibit each other's activity (14). Other studies, however, show no reciprocal correlation of activity of cells in these two hypothalamic regions (577). Some failed to find a decrease in the activity of VMH cells following stimulation of lateral hypothalamic neurons, or to find that lateral hypothalamic stimulation decreases the electrical activity of VMH cells—except when high-intensity stimulation is used (thus increasing the possibility of greater current spread) or when the stimulating electrode is close to the border of the VMH nuclei (495).

If a reciprocal circuit between the VMH and the lateral hypothalamic area is postulated, the timing of changes in the unit activity of cells in these two brain regions becomes important. In one study the injection of glucose produced an increase in the multiunit activity of cells in the VMH and a decrease in lateral hypothalamic electrical activity (117). The depression of activity in the lateral hypothalamus was long-lasting and detectable for at least 5 hr, whereas the increase in VMH unit activity was extremely short and apparently not correlated temporally with the lateral hypothalamic depression (577). Finally, even though glucose injection increased VMH electrical activity (18,20,117), it did not consistently decrease food intake (2,186,256,261,280,337,340,684,773). Along similar lines, even though injection of 2-DG and insulin changes VMH electrical activity (14,172), these compounds still increase food intake in animals with VMH lesions (313,477,508). Although at first glance changes in the single-unit activity of VMH cells seem consistent with the dual-center theory of feeding, much more data are needed if the many findings that are inconsistent with the predictions of this theory are to be negated.

### 3. Lateral Hypothalamus: The "Feeding Center"

Despite the substantial disagreement regarding the precise role played by the cells in the VMH, less controversy exists about the involvement of cells in, or coursing through, the lateral hypothalamic area. Again, these studies employ the classic lesion and the stimulation and recording techniques described previously.

### Lateral hypothalamic lesions.

Anand and Brobeck (16) were the first to show that bilateral electrolytic lesions placed in the lateral hypothalamic area resulted in aphagia and adipsia in both rats and cats. Animals with large lateral hypothalamic lesions died of starvation, even though food and water were freely available (16). Furthermore, lateral hypothalamic lesion-induced changes in feeding behavior overrode those induced by VMH lesions. When lateral hypothalamic lesions were made in animals previously rendered hyperphagic by VMH lesions, these animals were aphagic and subsequently died from starvation (19).

The aphagia and adipsia associated with bilateral damage to the lateral hypothalamic area have been confirmed in many different species, including birds, rabbits, cats, and monkeys (490,709). One of the most complete studies detailing the changes in feeding behavior after these lesions was conducted on rats by Teitelbaum and Epstein (741). Their results greatly influenced the types of experiments conducted subsequently and still form the reference point for current studies attempting to assess the effects of these lesions on the control of eating behavior.

Teitelbaum and Epstein repeated the experiments of Anand and Brobeck, and found that animals with bilateral lesions of the lateral hypothalamic area rapidly starved to death, despite *ad libitum* access to food and water (735, 741). However, if the lesioned animals were kept alive long enough by intragastric force feeding, they partially recovered from the immediate effects of the lesions and eventually ate food and drank water on their own. The course of recovery from these lesions progressed through relatively clear-cut stages, with the amount of postlesion time spent in each stage dependent on the placement and size of the lesion. Immediately after the operation the rats were completely aphagic and adipsic; if food or water was placed directly in their mouths, they refused to swallow it. After a period of time (the length of time was longer in animals with larger lesions), the animals entered a second distinct phase characterized by anorexia (a decreased appetite for food) and adipsia. During this stage, lesioned rats ate only foods that were palatable, but they did not eat enough to maintain their body weight and did not survive unless the caloric intake was supplemented with force-feeding. Animals in this stage still refused less palatable, dry foods, and they would not drink water. The aversion to food and water gradually disappeared, and the animals eventually swallowed food and water placed directly in their mouths. During the third stage of recovery, characterized by adipsia with a secondary dehydration aphagia, the lesioned rats began to regulate their caloric intake of wet, palatable foods, even though they still refused to drink water or to eat a dry, relatively unpalatable diet. When offered a high-calorie liquid diet, animals in the third stage ingested enough to maintain body weight. Under some conditions they learned to perform operant responses to obtain a food reward. In the later portions of this stage, the rats ate dry food if they were gastrically intubated with water. During the fourth stage, misnamed the "recovery" stage, the lesioned animals drank water and ate dry food if it was offered *ad libitum*. During this final stage the animals ate and drank enough to maintain body weight, even though weight was well below preoperative levels.

Even in the final recovery stage, lateral hypothalamic lesioned rats have a variety of regulatory deficits in food and water intake that appear to be permanent (741). These animals are unable to respond normally to manipulations that alter water balance; they do not increase water intake following injection of hypertonic saline (741) or after hypovolemia induced by injection of ethylene glycol (714). Furthermore, the lesioned rats are "prandial drinkers" (369); they drink only in response to dryness of the mouth, which increases when dry food is eaten. The unique prandial drinking in lateral hypothalamic-lesioned rats is potentiated by removal of the salivary glands and can be abolished when water is injected into the mouth (but not the stomach) during a meal (371). Hence the prandial drinking associated with these lesions appears to be related primarily to changes in eating foods of different osmolarities, and not to normal thirst (188,189).

The lesioned animals fail to respond normally to several manipulations that alter the feeding behavior of intact animals. They fail to increase food intake after insulin-induced hypoglycemia and thus die if injected with large doses of the hormone (189,193,678,741); and they do not decrease food intake after a fast if they are injected with the anorexic drug amphetamine (125). They are finicky eaters (189) and do not eat food or drink water adulterated with normally insignificant doses of quinine (741); they also are unable to form learned taste aversions to foods whose tastes have been paired with drug-induced lithium poisoning (621) or with presentations of electric shock (621). Furthermore, they have intense food neophobias (189). Food intake patterns are also permanently altered in animals that reach the "recovery" stage after lateral hypothalamic lesions. Intact animals wait longer before beginning a new meal if a large meal was eaten previously—the postprandial relationship (410)—whereas this relationship is abolished in lesioned rats (368). Prepran-dial relationships (a positive correlation between the length of an intermeal interval and the amount of food ingested during the subsequent meal) are not found in normal animals (43,44,407,409,410,690,749) but do occur for a brief period in lateral hypothalamus-lesioned rats (128). The feeding patterns of lateral hypothalamus-lesioned animals are extremely difficult to define because their eating is constantly interrupted by prandial drinking (371). Depending on the criterion used to define a meal, lesioned animals have been reported to eat a large number of small daily meals (if one uses a short intermeal criterion to define a meal operationally) or a small number of large meals each day (if the meal criterion involves longer times between bouts of eating) (368). One obvious difference in the meal patterns of recovered lateral hypothalamic-lesioned rats involves an exaggerated diurnal pattern of eating, with virtually all eating occurring during the dark portion of the day-night cycle (348,503). Compared with control animals, all of these animals show a large reduction in body weight and in food and water intake during the light but not the dark portion of the cycle (348,503). Some investigators (503,690) concluded from these studies that damage to the lateral hypothalamus inter-feres with an animal's ability to initiate eating and allows mechanisms involved in the termination of feeding to dominate eating behavior.

The lesioned animals also show an impaired ability to learn to approach food when hungry, to avoid electric shock (176,189,490,652,809), or to learn a bar-pressing response for food reward (49,617). In addition, rats with lateral hypothalamic damage have severely impaired ability to orient to many sensory stimuli (448–450,795). When lesions are made on only one side of the brain in the lateral hypothalamic area, these sensory deficits occur on the side contralateral to the lesion (448). Bilateral damage causes bilateral sensorimotor impairment which may correlate with the disruption of feeding and drinking seen during the early postoperative stages (448). Although the possible role of these sensorimotor deficits in the disruption of eating behavior is unclear, it has been suggested that failure to eat after these lesions is the result of a deficit in motor coordination (38,491). Although some motor disabilities in the lesioned animals have been reported, the degree of motor impairment appears to be unrelated to the degree of aphagia caused by the lesion (48,189,612).

Not all mechanisms shown to be important to controlling eating behavior in normal intact animals are disrupted by lateral hypothalamic lesions. Recovered lateral hypothalamus-lesioned animals respond normally by changing their food intake as a function of different environmental temperatures (741), by increasing food consumption when offered calorically dilute diets (741) or when deprived of food for various lengths of time (741), and by decreasing food intake when offered amino acid-imbalanced diets or diets that contain excessively high levels of protein (616).

Although the body weight of animals with lateral hypothalamic lesions never returns to postoperative levels, maintenance of the reduced body weight of animals recovered from this lesion appears to be as precise as weight regulation in normal animals. When the caloric density of the diet offered these animals is increased, body weights are maintained at the same percent change from control levels as are the body weights of lesioned animals fed normal diets (353); if the diet is adulterated with nonnutritive bulk or with a relatively large concentration of quinine, the body weights of intact and lesioned animals are reduced in a parallel fashion (353). Powley and Keesey (568) hypothesized that animals with lateral hypothalamic lesions may have a lowered control level, or set point, for body weight. The results of several studies support this notion; animals whose body weights were reduced prior to lesioning of the lateral hypothalamus show greatly attenuated or absent postoperative periods of aphagia and anorexia (46,568). In contrast, animals made overweight by force-feeding prior to the lesion, or those that were stomach-loaded for a period of time after the lesion show an extended postoperative period of aphagia and anorexia (46,568). Similar effects were observed in VMH-lesioned animals whose pre- or postoperative body weights were manipulated (199,353). Together, then, these data suggest that one of the primary deficits after lesions in the lateral or ventromedial areas of the hypothalamus involves disruption in the long-term set point for body weight regulation.

The permanently decreased body weight of animals with lateral hypothalamic lesions is probably the direct result of changes in energy expenditure, inasmuch as the daily food intake of these animals varies little from that of control animals matched for age. For example, locomotor activity levels undergo major changes after damage to the lateral hypothalamus. Shortly after the operation the animals were continuously hyperactive for a brief period, but during most of the early stages of recovery the animals are hypoactive and almost immobile. By the time of the third stage, when they regain the ability to initiate some feeding on their own, the animals again become hyperactive so that their activity level is higher than that of the controls during both the light and dark portions of the day-night cycle. During the "recovery" stage these bouts of hyperactivity eventually become confined to the dark portion of the lighting schedule, and the rats spend almost the entire night eating, drinking prandially, and moving around their cages (48,189,491,711).

The increase in locomotor activity induced by the lesion is accompanied by an immediate and permanent increase in basal metabolic rate (711). Analysis of the carcasses of these animals shows that the body weight loss can be accounted for almost entirely by a reduction in whole-body fat stores (353, 709). Indirect evidence that these lesions directly alter the processes of nutrient digestion, metabolism, and storage is convincing (490), but the precise nature of the changes remains to be defined. Some of these changes may be due to interactions between cells in the lateral hypothalamus and the peripheral tissues; animals with combined brain lesion and vagotomy tend to maintain body weight at a level even lower than that of animals with a lateral hypothalamic lesion alone or vagotomy alone (570).

Although it is unknown if any of the hormone-induced changes in feeding behavior are mediated by cells in the lateral hypothalamic area, the evidence seems convincing that these cells are intimately involved in glucostasis but probably have little to do with gonadal hormone-induced changes in eating (678,741). Animals recovered from the initial effects of the lesions fail to increase food intake following injection of insulin (741) or 2-DG (678); conversely, injection of 2-DG directly into the lateral hypothalamic area increases food intake in previously satiated, intact animals (47). Furthermore, direct glucose injection into this brain area blocks the normal hyperphagia of animals injected systemically with insulin (80). Direct, lateral hypothalamic injection of gold thioglucose (GTG) also produces aphagia, and this effect can be blocked by pretreating animals with 2-DG (676). Hence some investigators (47,189,534,678) suggested that this brain region contains glucosensitive cells that may normally mediate changes in feeding behavior associated with altered carbohydrate metabolism; at any rate, the evidence accumulated thus far for lateral hypothalamic glucoreceptors is more consistent that it is for the occurrence of these cells in the VMH. Manipulations involving feeding changes associated with the gonadal sex hormones (93,504), on the other hand, are indirect and do not suggest an involvement of lateral hypothalamic cells.

It is still unclear if all of the behavioral and metabolic abnormalities seen in animals with lesions in the lateral hypothalamus are the direct result of damage to neurons whose cell bodies are confined to this region, or if they represent the combined effects of local damage and the destruction of neurons whose axons or terminals course through this area. This question has long been the source of rather heated debate, inasmuch as the lateral hypothalamus contains many major fiber bundles that ascend or descend to other brain regions (265,488,490,801). In early studies aimed at answering this question, selective, small lesions located in the midlateral hypothalamic area produced little change in food intake but did decrease water consumption (479). These studies also suggested that the greatest reductions in food and water intake were associated with lesions that damaged the far-lateral aspects of this region (479). These initial findings were repeated in other laboratories: Animals with lesions predominantly in the midlateral area often spontaneously recovered some aspects of food and water intake regulation without being force-fed; animals with lesions confined primarily to the far-lateral area died, despite force-feeding (484,486). Morgane and co-workers (490) found that animals with bilateral damage to the far-lateral hypothalamic area (that also included damage to the medial aspects of the internal capsule) showed greater weight losses and higher mortality rates than did animals with midlateral damage; few if any animals with far-lateral damage recovered. These results led many investigators to postulate that the lesion did not destroy a functional "center" for food and water intake control; rather, the feeding disruption occurred because the lesion severed fibers (axons) passing through this area (487,488). Once techniques were developed that accurately described the neuroanatomy of brain cells containing specific types of neurotransmitter compounds, it became clear that many aspects of the lateral hypothalamic feeding dysfunctions induced by lesions probably resulted from damage to ascending neurotransmitter systems whose cell bodies lie in the midbrain but whose axons ascend in the medial forebrain bundle and medial internal capsule (523,753). The results of these studies redefined our thinking regarding the possible role of the lateral hypothalamic area in controlling eating behavior (and are considered in greater detail later).

Animals with lesions in either the lateral or ventromedial hypothalamus show striking changes in food and water intake as well as body weight regulation immediately after lesioning. Although many of these impairments appear permanent, some aspects of feeding behavior recover, even though histological or neurochemical analyses of the damaged brain area confirm that the cells and/or fiber tracts damaged by the lesion are still injured.

The changes underlying the partial recovery of behavioral function are unknown, although several mechanisms have been proposed (189,715,717, 738,776,824): (a) Cells not totally destroyed by the lesion might regenerate, replacing portions of the damaged neuron with healthy ones. (b) Particular groups of cells that normally mediate a given behavior may be only temporarily impaired by the trauma associated with the lesion, and their functioning may recover with time. (c) Cells not destroyed by the lesion may hyperfunction and be capable of supporting at least some of the original behavior. (d) Other cells in the brain, not normally involved in the behavior, may take over the function of the original core group of neurons.

Although each of these hypotheses has stimulated some research interest, only indirect evidence has thus far emerged. For example, recovered, lateral hypothalamic-lesioned animals can be made temporily aphagic and adipsic once again by induction of "cortical spreading depression" via local application of potassium chloride (KCl) to their cerebral cortices (740). These data suggest that cortical cells may somehow mediate a portion of the central control of eating behavior in the absence of lateral hypothalamic cells; however, KCl-induced spreading depression is a rather nonspecific procedure, and it is possible that other brain cells were also affected by the treatment. In another study the rate at which rats recovered from the effects of lateral hypothalamic lesions was found to be enhanced in animals that received daily electrical stimulation of this area (284). Although these data tentatively suggest that the cells remaining in this area after the lesion might be involved in the recovery process, additional experiments are needed to support this hypothesis. The possibility that behavioral recovery may be mediated at least in part by the regeneration of damaged cells is partially supported by the observation that behavioral recovery is enhanced by treating animals with nerve growth factor, a compound known to speed the growth of developing or injured neurons in the peripheral nervous system (64). Finally, the notion that remaining neurons not originally damaged by the lesion might hyperfunction enough to support some aspects of feeding behavior has received some support from the observation that various drugs, known to interfere with the functioning of neurons that contain catecholaminergic neurotransmitters, produce aphagia and adipsia when injected in lateral hypothalamus-lesioned animals during the recovery stage (823). In contrast, injection of similar doses of these drugs in intact animals produces little observable change in feeding behavior.

*Effects of lateral hypothalamic stimulation.*

It has long been known that stimulation of the lateral hypothalamic area with relatively low intensities of electrical current produces voracious eating in cats, fish, rats, goats, doves, and monkeys (12,14,170,309,310,490,709, 793,807). Although the particular type of feeding behavior and hyperphagia associated with electrical stimulation of the lateral hypothalamus has been called "stimulation-bound" eating (793), it is not always time-locked to the periods of the stimulation. Eating does not always begin synchronously with the stimulation; it may not always continue even though the electrical current is left on; and it does not always stop when the stimulation is terminated (793). Hence it is probably more correct to infer that changes in eating behavior are facilitated by, rather than bound to, the electrical stimulation.

The particular motor movements facilitated by stimulation of the lateral hypothalamus are not reflexive or stereotyped, but resemble in many ways the behavior of normally feeding animals (608,677). Moreover, animals learn to perform an operant task to obtain electrical stimulation in the lateral hypothalamus (465) just as they learn to perform a new behavioral response for food reinforcement. In fact, some evidence suggests that the sensations associated with the electrical stimulation may possess similar reinforcing properties not easily distinguishable from those of eating food. Animals trained to make a variety of operant responses for a food reward when they are hungry perform these same responses when stimulation of the lateral hypothalamus is substituted for food; conversely, responses learned with brain stimulation as the reward are performed by food-deprived animals for food reward (145). The effects of electrical brain stimulation and food reward also appear to be additive; rats electrically stimulated in the lateral hypothalamus ingest more of a quinine-adulterated solution or a previously preferred solution than do animals who are not stimulated (743).

Treatments that alter normal eating behavior of rats also influence stimulation-induced feeding. Animals previously satiated eat more food if they receive electrical stimulation of the lateral hypothalamic area; however, as the stimulated animal continues eating, a point of supersatiety is reached. As would be anticipated, the amount of current necessary to produce eating increases slowly during the process of supersatiation; in contrast, the current threshold necessary to induce drinking behavior does not change during the same time period (174). The electrical current threshold to elicit drinking can be altered similarly in rats that have drunk an excessive amount of water (174). Gastric intubation of food or water prior to stimulation specifically decreases stimulation-induced eating or drinking, respectively (145,174). Conversely, food deprivation reduces the current intensity necessary to elicit eating but not drinking, whereas prior water deprivation decreases the current threshold for drinking but not eating (174,249). Finally, if animals learn to avoid a previously preferred diet that has been poisoned with lithium chloride, they continue to avoid this food when they receive electrical stimulation in the lateral hypothalamus (743).

The lateral hypothalamic area apparently contains cells involved in the control of behavioral responses other than feeding. Hence it is not surprising that electrical stimulation of this brain region induces changes in sexual behavior (109,705), food hoarding (292), locomotor activity (618), and attack behavior (51), in addition to the changes in eating and drinking. Moreover, stimulated animals also drink, if only water is available, and gnaw, if only wood is available (755,757). If animals are stimulated when food, water, and wood are available, the animals can be trained to switch their stimulation-induced behavior from eating to drinking to gnawing (755). It therefore seems possible that electrical stimulation in this area can affect different populations of neurons that normally mediate these different behavioral responses (793). However, the lack of behavioral specificity associated with electrical stimulation of the lateral hypothalamus may also result from the spread of current into other, adjacent brain sites; in animals with brains larger than those of rats (e.g., cats or opossums), more specific behavioral responses can be elicited with electrical brain stimulation (609). Hence the multiple behaviors induced by brain stimulation in rats may result from the close anatomical proximity of various brain structures and fiber bundles as well as the possible current spread associated with electrical brain stimulation (793).

Animals perform an operant response (bar pressing) to obtain short pulses of electrical stimulation to the lateral hypothalamus (445,522,787). The rates at which animals bar press can be influenced by a variety of manipulations known to alter eating behavior (309). In some situations the same amount of stimulation that produces a high response rate in normal animals becomes aversive (animals perform an operant response to turn off the stimulation) when these animals are made obese by overeating (308,312,314). These results support the hypothesis that self-stimulation in the lateral hypothalamus bears a specific relationship to feeding, so that when stimulation of this brain area is rewarding animals become hyperphagic. Conversely, when stimulation of the lateral hypothalamus is less rewarding, anorexia results (309). However, the rate of self-stimulation for lateral hypothalamic reward is not always perfectly correlated with the level of feeding or anorexia; amphetamine injection decreases food intake in hungry animals (anorexia) but increases the rate of bar pressing for lateral hypothalamic stimulation (309,697). Similarly, female rats eat less during vaginal estrus but increase their rate of lever pressing for electrical stimulation (309).

Relatively few studies examined physiological changes resulting from lateral hypothalamic stimulation. Such stimulation produces a relatively prolonged hyperglycemia, a response that is blocked in bilaterally adrenalectomized rats (88) or in those with subdiaphragmatic vagotomy (568). Immediately after stimulation in the lateral hypothalamus is terminated, hypoglycemia appears (88). Lateral hypothalamic stimulation also increases GI motility; again, these effects can be blocked by vagotomy (568). Since changes in blood glucose produced by other manipulations also alter GI motility, it is unclear whether lateral hypothalamic stimulation or a stimulation-induced change in blood sugar is the prime stimulus for this alteration (709). Moreover, the stimulation-induced change in blood sugar may also result from an indirect change in intermediary metabolism, inasmuch as stimulation increases the glycogen content of the liver, possibly by activating the enzyme glycogen synthetase (50). The hypoglycemia seen after termination of lateral hypothalamic stimulation may therefore be due to enhanced glycogen synthesis. Few studies thus far have examined other changes that lateral hypothalamic stimulation might produce in peripheral mechanisms, which in turn control hunger or satiety.

Injection of a variety of compounds into this brain area also alters eating behavior. The effects of intrahypothalamic injection of neurotransmitters and drugs on eating behavior are reviewed below. Bilateral injection of isotonic glucose (but not saline) into the lateral hypothalamus blocks subsequent eating behavior induced by food deprivation or insulin (80); however, these injections also produce sedation and general drowsiness, so the changes in feeding behavior may not be specific (80). Local injection of amino acids rapidly suppresses feeding in hungry animals (539), although the mechanisms that underlie this effect are not understood, especially in light of the fact that animals with lateral hypothalamic lesions still reduce food intake when presented with amino acid-imbalanced or low-protein diets (616).

*Electrical changes in the activity of lateral hypothalamic cells.*

The electrical activities of cells in the VMH and lateral hypothalamus are sometimes inversely related (14). Some cells in the lateral hypothalamus increase their firing rates when animals see food. Interestingly, these cells are not activated when food is smelled, reached for, or eaten in the dark (617). Other cells in the lateral hypothalamus change electrical activity only when food is tasted, whereas some cells respond both to the sight and taste of food (617). Most of these cells appear to change firing rate only when the animal is hungry, not when food is presented after the animal has eaten (617). Hence brain regional activity important for eating behavior is altered only when it is physiologically appropriate (the "appetitive state"). Although cells in the VMH may provide this "gating" function, no direct evidence has yet been marshaled to support this hypothesis. Changes in the periphery associated with eating alter hypothalamic electrical activity. Hence glucose injection decreases the activity of some but not all lateral hypothalamic cells, and insulin injection reverses these effects (18,20). Changes in plasma FFA levels or iontophoretic application of some amino acids in the lateral hypothalamic area also change the electrical activity of these cells (15). Unfortunately there are no data to permit interpretation of the functional significance of these changes.

## 4. Other Brain Mechanisms

On the basis of the previous review, it can be seen that various hypothalamic nuclei appear to play a strategic role in the normal control of eating behavior; however, cells in these brain areas do not integrate, or participate in the control of, all aspects of feeding behavior. Although it seems quite likely that other brain regions share some control over aspects of eating, we know much less about their possible contributions; contemporary and future research should fill in some of these gaps.

The evidence implicating the involvement of brain regions other than the hypothalamus is reviewed in detail elsewhere (42,261,262,264,489,490). Thus far few other brain regions appear to have consistent roles in feeding. It has not yet been possible to discover how or to what extent the changes in eating behavior associated with manipulation of these brain regions are the direct result of functions idiosyncratic to cells in a particular area, or reflect changes that result from alterations in neural cells whose axons or terminals course through the area (263,488,489). Hence it is no longer considered useful to lesion the amygdala, for example, and look for specific changes in eating behavior without a greater understanding of how various nuclei in this brain area are related (by their efferent and afferent connections) to other brain regions. These types of analysis will ultimately depend on recently developed neuroanatomical "mapping" procedures that should allow for more precise descriptions of the input-output interconnections of cells in the brain.

## C. Brain Neurotransmitter Systems and Feeding Behavior

Mammalian organs utilize two types of chemical signal—hormones or neurotransmitters—to communicate with one another. Most neurotransmitters involved in feeding behavior are low-molecular-weight, water-soluble amines or amino acids. They are distributed only to the very few cells with which the neurons that synthesize them make synaptic contact, although potential receptors for some appear to be common to many types of cells. Neurotransmitters are the essential links for neural communication among cells and appear to influence feeding behavior by altering the actual integrative and control mechanisms involved. Hormones, on the other hand, have dissimilar physicochemical properties; they are for the most part ubiquitously distributed throughout the body following their release from specific sites; and their specificity of communication resides in their ability to interact with tissue-specific receptors on plasma membranes or in the cytoplasm (133). We already reviewed evidence that certain hormones—especially the pancreatic, GI, and gonadal hormones—normally participate in the control of food intake by affecting the metabolic fate of nutrients and by either providing signals to the brain regarding the relevant states of hunger or satiety, or directly altering peripheral or brain cells involved in feeding.

Of the neurotransmitter compounds currently known, most are released from the terminal areas of neurons into small gaps, called synapses, following electrical depolarization of the cell (33). Once released into a synapse, these molecules are believed to interact with receptors on postsynaptic cells to produce biological responses. Although it is not known precisely how these compounds effect changes in the postsynaptic cell, it appears that if enough neurotransmitter molecules are released by the presynaptic cell, the postsynaptic cell's electrical activity changes (if the postsynaptic cell is another neuron), releases a hormone (if the cell is part of the endocrine system), or contracts (if the cell is a muscle fiber). Synapses in the brain and peripheral nervous system can be classified into two functional types. One type is excitatory, because the release of sufficient amounts of neurotransmitter from the presynaptic nerve terminals causes the postsynaptic neural cell to depolarize and to propagate an electrical impulse down its axon toward the terminal regions. The other type is inhibitory; here the release of the presynaptic neurotransmitter makes it less likely that an electrical potential will be propagated in the postsynaptic neural cell.

It appears that only one kind of neurotransmitter is released from the terminals of any given neuron. Hence each neuron of the brain or peripheral nervous system can be characterized by the type of neurotransmitter it employs. With the advent of new neuroanatomical and biochemical techniques for locating cells that contain specific types of neurotransmitter, it has been possible to identify with some precision the brain and peripheral regions that contain the cell bodies, axons, and terminals of these cells. Although not all neurotransmitters have yet been identified, a formal set of criteria has been established to determine if a given chemical compound qualifies as a neurotransmitter: (a) The compound must be localized within nerve endings. (b) It must be released when the nerves that store it are stimulated. (c) The physiological effect of applying the compound to postsynaptic effector cells must be identical with that observed when the neuron thought to contain it is stimulated. (d) Drugs that either enhance or interfere with its synthesis, storage, release, inactivation, or effects on receptors must cause predictable changes in inactivation or transmission across the synapses where it is located (435). Most of these criteria have been satisfied in the identification of many neurotransmitters in the peripheral nervous system, but the difficulties in examining single CNS neurons or synapses in isolation preclude the definitive demonstration that any given compound functions as a central neurotransmitter. Nonetheless, good evidence indicates that several compounds— acetylcholine, aspartate, the catecholamines (dopamine, norepinephrine, epinephrine), γ-aminobutyric acid, glutamate, glycine, histamine, serotonin, and substance P—function as brain neurotransmitters. Since these compounds are essential for neurotransmission, it is not surprising that manipulations known to alter their synthesis, storage, release, receptor interaction, or inactivation also produce striking changes in eating behavior. The results of studies of this type dramatically changed our conception of how and which brain cells participate in the control of feeding behavior and led to the discovery of new procedures that hold some promise for the treatment of some human eating disorders.

## 1. Fate of a Typical Neurotransmitter

Even though particular neurotransmitters appear to play different functional roles in various regions of the brain and periphery, all share similar metabolic fates. Each is synthesized from precursor compounds (usually an amino acid or amino acid derivative) through the action of a rate-limiting enzyme, stored within distinct intracellular functional pools (which may be associated with subcellular organelles), released after nerve stimulation into synapses, complexed with pre- or postsynaptic receptors (which causes modification in ionic fluxes), and inactivated (usually but not always by reuptake into its neuron of origin).

Brain and peripheral neurons appear to contain all of the precursors, enzymes, and cofactors needed for the biosynthesis of their particular neurotransmitters. Most of the essential precursors for these compounds must be derived from the diet (e.g., tryptophan for the synthesis of serotonin, choline for the synthesis of acetylcholine) (804,805). The enzymes involved in synthesizing neurotransmitters are made in the cell body of the neuron and are then transported in the axon to the terminal nerve endings, where most of the synthesis occurs. Many factors can influence the rate of neurotransmitter synthesis (160,695,748), and some may be directly influenced by the diet (803).

Once synthesized, neurotransmitters are usually stored in at least two distinct intracellular pools, defined functionally but not morphologically. When the neuron is depolarized by presynaptic inputs or stimulated electrically, or when calcium enters its terminals, neurotransmitter molecules are released (478). It is believed that the amount released in response to physiological or electrical depolarizations per unit time is related to the number of action potentials the neuron generates and the number of molecules released per action potential.

If a sufficient number of neurotransmitter molecules are released from one or more presynaptic "excitatory" neurons per unit time, the postsynaptic effector cell depolarizes and generates an action potential. The precise ways in which neurotransmitters interact with the postsynaptic effector cell to produce depolarization (or in the case of "inhibitory" neurons, hyperpolarization) are poorly understood. It seems likely, though, that this process often involves specific receptors, which when stimulated modify the inward or outward fluxes of particular ions and which act to cause longer-term functional changes (e.g., in the synthesis of enzyme proteins). The sensitivity of postsynaptic receptors in intrasynaptic neurotransmitter molecules may depend on the extent to which the receptors are already occupied, the availability of hormones, and the effects of other compounds released into the synapses along with the neurotransmitters (adenine derivatives, storage proteins and peptides, etc.).

Once neurotransmitter molecules are released into synapses, they are rapidly inactivated by enzymes or are taken up again within the neuron of origin. Neurotransmitters released into peripheral synapses may also be inactivated by being "washed out" into the circulation.

On the basis of this brief review, it is clear that specific neurotransmitter-containing cell systems in the brain or periphery can be manipulated in relatively specific ways with a variety of dietary, surgical, or pharmacological techniques, and their relative contributions to feeding behavior can be assessed.

## 2. Catecholamine Neurotransmission and Feeding

*Metabolism and anatomical localization of catecholamine neurotransmitters.*

Dopamine, norepinephrine, and epinephrine are members of the class of neurotransmitters called catecholamines. These compounds have in common a chemical structure that consists of a ring of six carbon atoms to which are attached adjacent hydroxyl groups (the catechol nucleus) and an ethylamine side chain. The catecholamine neurotransmitters are synthesized from an amino acid, tyrosine, in a multienzyme pathway (Fig. 3). Recent histochemi-

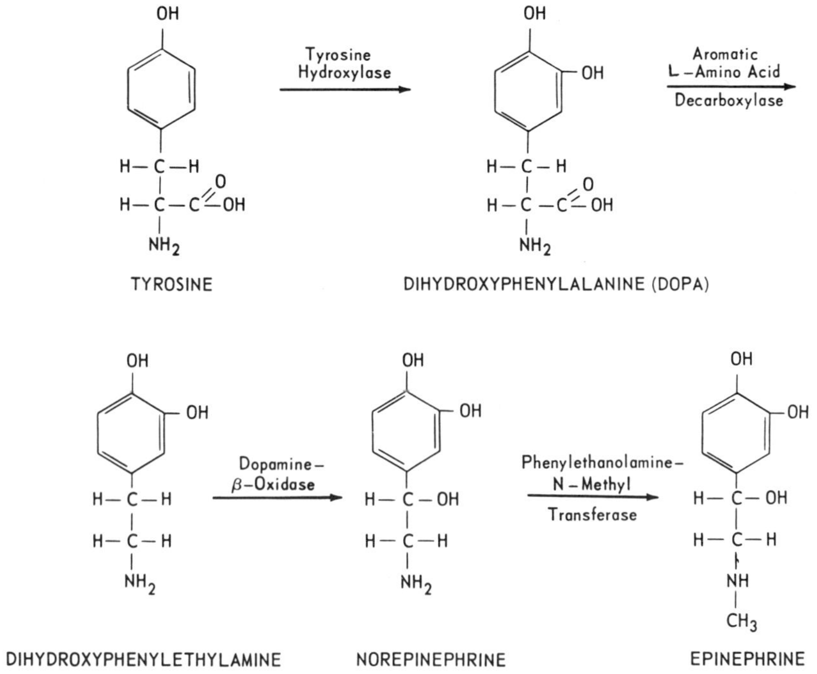

**FIG. 3.** Synthesis and metabolism of the catecholamine neurotransmitters dopamine, norepinephrine, and epinephrine.

cal and immunochemical fluorescence methods permit visualization and "mapping" of catecholaminergic neurotransmitters within specific cell bodies and neuronal tracts in the brain and peripheral nervous systems (72,127,156, 728). On the basis of this evidence, dopamine does not appear to be a neurotransmitter in its own right in the peripheral nervous system, with the possible exception of interneurons in the superior cervical ganglia (253). On the other hand, norepinephrine is the neurotransmitter released by the post-ganglionic neurons of the sympathetic nervous system. Epinephrine is localized in the chromaffin cells of the adrenal medulla and appears to act like a hormone rather than a neurotransmitter (802).

Using the fluorescence histochemical technique, dopamine was found to be concentrated within several major groups of brain neurons: the nigrostriatal, mesolimbic, tuberoinfundibular, and incertohypothalamic dopamine systems (754). The nigrostriatal bundle has cell bodies located in the midbrain ventral tegmentum; these cells send axons into cell masses deep in the forebrain, with prominent terminal projections in the neostriatum. The mesolimbic system also has cell bodies located in the midbrain, but it sends projections to selected forebrain areas, including the nucleus accumbens and the olfactory tubercles. The tuberoinfundibular system has cell bodies in the nuclei of the hypothalamus, and these neurons may provide one of the direct connections between the hypothalamus and the pituitary gland (the hypothalamic-hypophyseal portal system). The incertohypothalamic dopamine system was described only recently (427); it appears to have cell bodies located in the caudal thalamus and hypothalamus, as well as in the medial aspects of the zona incerta and dorsal anterior hypothalamus.

Several pharmacological and neuroanatomical techniques can produce relatively specific changes in catecholamine transmission in the brain and peripheral nervous systems. Certain drugs appear to alter specific aspects of catecholamine biosynthesis and metabolism, and thus neurotransmission: (a) administration of precursor compounds (e.g., tyrosine or L-DOPA) can increase the stores of releasable neurotransmitter and presumably increase the total number of molecules that might interact with postsynaptic cells. (b) Compounds such as $\alpha$-methyl-$p$-tyrosine block the synthesis of neurotransmitter molecules by inhibiting enzymes in this pathway and thus decrease the probability of neurotransmission. (c) Some drugs (e.g., amphetamine) promote the release of neurotransmitter molecules or block their reuptake by the presynaptic neuron (e.g., desmethylimipramine), thus increasing their intrasynaptic concentrations and the probability of receptor interaction. (d) Drugs such as reserpine block the storage of neurotransmitters in vesicles and interfere with neurocommunication by producing a net reduction in releasable and storage pools of the neurotransmitters. (e) Still other compounds (e.g., pargyline and tranylcypromine) block enzymes involved in the degradation of the catecholamines and thus increase the stores of biologically active compound available for release from the presynaptic neuron into the synapse. (f) Finally, drugs such as phenoxybenzamine or propranolol block adrenergic receptors and decrease catecholamine neurotransmission; other drugs (e.g., phenylephrine or isoproterenol) stimulate postsynaptic neuronal receptors and enhance neurocommunication (241,478). These drugs are injected into various brain regions or are administered systemically to determine the extent to which they produce predictable changes in eating behavior. In other studies, electrical or chemical lesions or stimulations are used to alter specific populations of neurotransmitter cells in the brain or peripheral nervous systems in order to determine their role in feeding behavior.

*Drug manipulation of catecholaminergic neurotransmitters: effect on feeding.*

In studies to determine the extent to which peripheral or brain catecholamine-containing neurons normally participate in the control of feeding behavior, the neurotransmitters themselves—or drugs known to alter the synthesis, storage, release, inactivation, or receptors for the catecholamines—are injected into food-deprived or satiated animals, and subsequent changes in eating are monitored. Sufficient experimental data have accumulated to show that a number of independent variables—including injection site, dose, species of animal tested, type of diet offered the animal—may influence the final results of these types of studies, and many of the present discrepancies in the results obtained in different laboratories may be due to differences in these parameters. Until recently most of the interest in the brain neurotransmitters that may be important for feeding behavior were directed at the involvement of catecholaminergic neurotransmitters; relatively less attention was paid to the contributions of other peripheral or brain transmitter candidates, although this deficiency should be remedied within the next few years.

It has long been known that injection of norepinephrine or epinephrine into the periphery generally produces anorexia in food-deprived animals (469,635, 636). Although it is possible that these generalized depressions in food intake are related to the effects of these compounds on peripheral neural control mechanisms for feeding behavior, the doses necessary to alter food intake also produce generalized behavioral depression, as well as a number of other biochemical, endocrinological, and metabolic changes that lead one to question whether these are specific neurotransmitter-mediated effects involving a control mechanism for eating (648). Since the chemical structures of the catecholamines do not allow them to cross the blood-brain barrier readily when injected into the periphery, it does not seem likely that the changes in feeding behavior result directly from their effects on brain neurons (782). These compounds do produce striking physiological changes in the periphery, however, and it is possible that alterations in feeding behavior following norepinephrine or epinephrine injection might indirectly influence the activity of brain control mechanisms important for the behavior.

In order to determine if a change in brain catecholamines influences feeding, in most studies these compounds were injected into the brain ventricles or into various brain regions in order to circumvent the problems associated with their peripheral effects, as well as to bypass the blood-brain barrier. Using these methods, Grossman (257) showed that noradrenergic and adrenergic brain systems may be important for feeding behavior. He found that the injection of relatively large concentrations of norepinephrine or epinephrine into the perifornical hypothalamic region (the area of the hypothalamus just lateral to the ventromedial region and slightly medial to the lateral hypothalamic area) increased food intake in previously satiated rats. In contrast, local application of another neurotransmitter, acetylcholine, or the cholinomimetic drug carbachol into these same injection sites increased water intake, with relatively little effect on feeding. The catecholamine-induced eating occurred 5–10 min after the injection and persisted for approximately 30–60 min; during this time animals ingested up to 25% of their total daily intake of a dry food laboratory diet. Animals injected daily with these compounds for 8 weeks increased their body weight significantly over that of vehicle-injected animals (258,259). The drug-induced changes in feeding or drinking were altered by other manipulations that influence normal food or water consumption: Prior food deprivation potentiated the catecholamine-induced increases in eating but not the carbachol-induced changes in drinking; in contrast, water-deprived animals drank more water when injected with carbachol but did not eat more food after injection with norepinephrine. Hence the drug treatment effects on eating and drinking behaviors were specifically related to the particular physiological need state of the animal.

Recent experiments extended the initial results of Grossman by providing a more detailed pharmacological analysis of the catecholaminergic control of eating behavior. Although it was initially reported that perifornical hypothalamic injection of dopamine induced eating only slightly in sated animals (81,258,674), and with a slower onset of action than that observed after injection of the other catecholamine neurotransmitters, other investigators (35,399,606) generally failed to replicate these results. Injection of desmethylimipramine, a drug that blocks the reuptake of norepinephrine and thus increases the intrasynaptic concentrations of the neurotransmitter (80,674), potentiated norepinephrine-induced increases in food intake; similarly, injection of the monoamine oxidase inhibitor nialamide prior to administration of the reserpinelike drug tetrabenazine also increased food intake (674). However, the reverse combination of drugs (injection of tetrabenazine prior to nialamide) did not alter feeding behavior (674), presumably because there were fewer releasable molecules of norepinephrine in the presynaptic neuron.

In the peripheral nervous system the catecholaminergic neurotransmitters may produce different, and sometimes opposite, physiological effects, depending on the tissue innervated and the receptors stimulated (6). For example, some catecholamine-containing nerves that innervate blood vessels cause them to dilate when the nerves depolarize, whereas others cause vasoconstriction when they are electrically active. Pharmacological evidence indicates that these two effects are mediated by different receptors activated by norepinephrine. The receptors mediating vasoconstriction can be blocked by the drugs phentolamine or phenoxybenzamine but not by the drug propranolol. Moreover, these receptors, called $\alpha$-noradrenergic receptors, are more sensitive (produce greater constriction) to the receptor stimulant drugs phenylephrine or norepinephrine and less sensitive to treatment with isoproterenol or epinephrine. In contrast, $\beta$-noradrenergic receptors (the ones producing vasodilation) are more sensitive to isoproterenol or epinephrine, and are less affected by phenylephrine or norepinephrine; propranolol is the drug most effective in blocking the effects of the receptor agonists, whereas phentolamine or phenoxybenzamine are least effective. The pharmacological distinctions between $\alpha$- and $\beta$-receptors are not always perfect, nor do these receptors always mediate physiological effects that are opposite one another. However, in a contemporary neuropharmacological restatement of the dual-center theory for the control of eating behavior, Leibowitz (392–394, 396,399, 400) and others (34–36,442,443,605,606,674) showed that distinct receptor systems at brain adrenergic or noradrenergic brain synapses may be important as control mechanisms for eating behavior.

Local injection of epinephrine or norepinephrine in brain will either stimulate or inhibit food consumption, depending on the site of injection. Using the pharmacological profiles described above, Leibowitz presented fairly convincing evidence that the medial hypothalamus (primarily the ventromedial nuclei) contains $\alpha$-receptors that, when stimulated, increase food consumption in animals fed *ad libitum;* in contrast, the lateral hypothalamic area (actually the anterolateral hypothalamus) contains $\beta$-receptors, so that when they are stimulated anorexia results in food-deprived animals (392,393,396). The perifornical hypothalamus contains both types of receptor, and some animals eat or stop eating after injection of catecholamines, depending on the amount administered (401). A low dose of norepinephrine or epinephrine into the perifornical hypothalamus produces eating, whereas a relatively high dose of epinephrine or isoproterenol suppresses food consumption by hungry animals. The increase in food intake seen in animals with a low dose of norepinephrine or epinephrine could be blocked by pretreating them with an $\alpha$-receptor blocking drug but not with a $\beta$-receptor antagonist. In contrast, the food intake depression seen in hungry animals treated with a high dose of epinephrine or isoproterenol injected into the perifornical hypothalamus could be blocked with propranolol but not with an $\alpha$-receptor antagonist drug. The lateral hypothalamic $\beta$-receptor *satiety* system and the VMH $\alpha$-adrenergic *hunger* systems appear to antagonize one another reciprocally: Increased eating following ventromedial $\alpha$-receptor excitation is presumably the result of ventromedial "satiety" cell inhibition; anorexia associated with lateral hypothalamic $\beta$-receptor activation results from the inhibition of lateral hypothalamic "feeding" cells (393). Evidence for the possible reciprocal antagonism between these two receptor systems is largely indirect but suggestive: Combined injection of a $\beta$-receptor agonist and an $\alpha$-receptor antagonist into the perifornical hypothalamic area potentiates the anorexic effects of the $\beta$-receptor agonist (393). Injection of an $\alpha$-receptor antagonist into the VMH but not the lateral hypothalamic area decreases eating in food-deprived rats, whereas injection of a $\beta$-receptor antagonist into the lateral hypothalamic area but not the VMH slightly increases the food intake of hungry rats (393).

Leibowitz (401) also examined the sensitivity of other brain regions to the feeding effects of locally applied catecholamine agonists and antagonists, and found that the paraventricular nucleus of the hypothalamus was the area most sensitive to these drugs: Injection of norepinephrine into this brain region elicited feeding in rats at the lowest dose and with the shortest latency after injection of any area. Interestingly, the feeding effects of noradrenergic stimulation of the paraventricular nucleus may be mediated by neuroendocrinological changes, inasmuch as the drug-induced changes in feeding were absent in hypophysectomized animals (401). Catecholamine-induced changes in feeding behavior have also been found in the anterior, posterior, and dorsal regions of the hypothalamus (79,257,258,401), as well as in the amygdala (260), thalamus (79), septum (79), hippocampus (251), and various portions of the diencephalon (811). However, the specificity and pharmacological profiles for these effects remain to be determined.

The Leibowitz model for VMH α-noradrenergic receptors for hunger and lateral hypothalamic β-noradrenergic receptors for satiety is controversial, and differs from the results of some other laboratories (442–444). For example, most of the data for the Leibowitz model were obtained from experiments with rats; injection of α- or β-receptor agonists in sheep or cattle *both* elicit feeding in satiated animals (34–36), whereas cats do not generally respond to this local drug injection (34). Furthermore, Margules (442,443) found that injection of α-receptor agonists into the perifornical hypothalamus suppresses eating when rats are fed a liquid milk diet, whereas β-receptor agonists decrease food intake only when these animals are fed unpalatable, quinine-adulterated milk solution. Although both Margules and Leibowitz agree that β-noradrenergic receptors probably mediate satiety, they do not agree about the precise role played by α-noradrenergic receptors. However, there are a number of methodological differences in the procedures used by these two investigators, and any or all of these differences may account for their respective results (395).

Other drugs known to alter noradrenergic neurotransmission in the peripheral nervous system also change feeding behavior when injected into the brain. Lateral hypothalamic injections of desmethylimipramine, a drug that blocks the reuptake of norepinephrine into the presynaptic neuron, increases feeding in food-deprived and water-satiated rats, and increases drinking behavior in animals that are food-satiated and water-deprived (480). Perifornical, intrahypothalamic injection of chlorpromazine increases food intake (395). Although chlorpromazine is usually thought to be an α-noradrenergic and dopaminergic receptor blocking drug (691), it may also release norepinephrine from the presynaptic neuron, since the drug-induced hyperphagia can be blocked in animals pretreated with drugs that deplete presynaptic stores of norepinephrine (402). Hence in these experiments chlorpromazine may increase feeding behavior by increasing the turnover and release of norepinephrine (395).

Both norepinephrine- and epinephrine-containing neurons have axons and terminals in the hypothalamic region; hence it is possible that both of these neurotransmitters normally participate in the control mechanisms for feeding behavior. In contrast, evidence for the third catecholamine neurotransmitter, dopamine, and its role in feeding behavior are not clear, at least on the basis of studies using local injection of the neurotransmitter directly into brain regions. In some experiments injection of dopamine into the lateral hypothalamus produces a small but delayed increase in food intake (81,258,674); in other experiments, however, dopamine injection appears to have no effect on eating behavior in satiated animals (35,399,606). In yet other experiments ventricular injection of dopamine somewhat decreases food intake in hungry animals (606); similarly, systemic injection of the dopamine receptor agonist apomorphine produces anorexia (382). These effects can be reversed by pretreating animals with systemic injection of the dopamine receptor antagonist pimozide

(382). However, perifornical hypothalamic injection of drugs that block the conversion of dopamine to norepinephrine, thus increasing brain dopamine and decreasing brain norepinephrine concentrations, potentiates food intake in hungry animals (213). Furthermore, injection of the catecholamine precursor amino acid L-DOPA also increases food intake, apparently by a dopaminergic mechanism (213).

The results obtained from studies using local application of various compounds into brain areas have provided interesting new information regarding the various neurotransmitters that may underlie feeding and drinking behavior; however, one must use caution in interpreting results based on these experiments. First, the doses of the neurotransmitters generally used to induce or suppress eating are usually 2–200 times greater than the entire whole brain concentrations of these substances in normal animals. For example, the total amount of norepinephrine in brains of normal rats usually varies between 0.5 and 1.5 $\mu$g; since the norepinephrine doses injected into the perifornical hypothalamus to elicit or inhibit feeding in most experiments are greater than 20 $\mu$g, it is difficult to know if these effects are related to the aphysiological concentration of the compound in brain regions, or if they are due to the stimulation of receptors that normally mediate changes in eating behavior. Second, it is surprising that in almost all instances feeding behavior does not appear to change for at least 5–10 min following local injection of the neurotransmitter (257,401). These temporal delays may reflect the time it takes the solution to diffuse away from the injection site into an active tissue site or to metabolize the large numbers of molecules typically injected before an effective dose is reached, and so forth. Regardless of the reason, one would expect an immediate drug-induced change in behavior if the drug is indeed stimulating receptors at the injection site. The results recently obtained by Leibowitz in which doses of norepinephrine as low as 16 ng reliably increased feeding and drinking behavior within 1 min after injection into the paraventricular hypothalamic nucleus (401) are promising in this regard. The dose and time response discrepancies obtained in these earlier studies might also depend on whether the animal is eating or has been fasted: Relatively small doses of norepinephrine increase meal size by approximately 200% when the injection occurs at the beginning of spontaneously initiated meals (605); in contrast, these same doses have no effect on eating when administered during intermeal intervals (605). The time during the light-dark cycle when the drug is injected might also influence its behavioral potency, although the results obtained thus far have been inconsistent (401,446). Finally, the type of diet offered drug-injected animals may also be important, depending on its relative palatability (395,441,443,490).

On the basis of the previous pharmacological results, one might expect that the concentration of catecholamine neurotransmitters in brain should change as a function of whether the animal was eating or fasting. Periods of food deprivation increase the concentration of hypothalamic dopamine but not norepinephrine (213), and the efflux of radioactively labeled dopamine and norepinephrine from the hypothalamus into the brain ventricles is increased when rats eat food or drink water, or when they perform operant responses for food reinforcement (498). However, not enough data have accumulated to understand the functional importance of these results. Furthermore, it is too early to tell if the various drug-induced changes in eating behavior described previously represent the direct effect of the drugs on brain control mechanisms for the behavior or if they occur indirectly as a result of drug-induced changes in peripheral mechanisms important for normal feeding. For example, chlorpromazine injection into the lateral ventricles of rats produces a rapid increase in blood sugar that may either cause or result from its effects on food consumption (220).

*Electrically or chemically induced lesions in catecholaminergic brain tracts: Effect on feeding.*

It has long been known that lesions of the lateral hypothalamic area, resulting in aphagia and adipsia, also produce long-term changes in brain catecholaminergic neurotransmitter levels (483). Somewhat surprisingly, the relationships between the neurochemical and behavioral effects of the lesions were not firmly established until recently (753). Histochemical fluorescence procedures for visualizing brain neurotransmitters show that the axons for brain dopamine-, norepinephrine-, epinephrine-, and serotonin-containing neurons course through the mid- and far-lateral hypothalamus, the areas most effective after lesioning for producing aphagia and adipsia (156,728,754). Ungerstedt (753) was the first to show that at least some of the lesion-induced changes in feeding behavior were probably the result of damage to the ascending nigrostriatal dopaminergic pathway. This neurotransmitter system has cell bodies in the pars compacta of the substantia nigra of the midbrain and sends axons through the far-lateral hypothalamus and the medial internal capsule (728). Since other neurotransmitter axons and terminals are also found in this region, electrolytic lesions nonspecifically destroy most of these other projection systems as well (483). To obtain relatively selective lesions of the catecholaminergic nerve tracts coursing through this area, Ungerstedt destroyed portions of the nigrostriatal bundle at various anteroposterior placements using local injection of 6-hydroxydopamine (6-OHDA) (753). 6-OHDA is a neurotoxic drug taken up quite selectively by neurons that contain only the catecholaminergic neurotransmitters; once the drug accumulates in these neurons, it releases the catecholamines and then destroys the axons and terminals of these neurons by an as yet poorly understood mechanism (344). Although there is some controversy regarding the specificity of its neurotoxic effects when the drug is injected directly into brain tissue (344) or into the ventricles surrounding the brain (344), Ungerstedt found that 6-OHDA lesions of the nigrostriatal dopamine system produced aphagia and adipsia in rats (753) that was strikingly similar to the syndrome of behavior described previously in rats with electrolytic lesions in the lateral hypothalamic area (741). These animals died from starvation unless appropriate postoperative thera- peutic measures were employed, i.e., feeding the animals a high-calorie liquid diet via stomach intubation. During the time the lesioned animals had to be tube-fed, they showed a pronounced hypoactivity that could be reversed by treating them with the dopamine-receptor stimulant apomorphine (753). Radiofrequency or 6-OHDA lesions along the entire anteroposterior extent of the nigrostriatal bundle (but not in other ascending catecholamine pathways) also produced aphagia and adipsia. Furthermore, the amount of weight loss associated with bilateral hypothalamic damage caused by electrolytic lesions is highly correlated with the lesion-induced decrease in striatal dopamine concentration and not with the lesion-induced changes in other monoamine neurotransmitters (523). This, then, further supports the notion that the lateral hypothalamic syndrome is related specifically to the effects of the lesion only on brain dopamine-containing neurons.

If damage to the nigrostriatal dopamine system were the critical variable for producing the long-term feeding and drinking behavior deficits associated with the lateral hypothalamic syndrome, it might be expected that these deficits are identical to those seen in animals with lesions of the substantia nigra. A detailed series of experiments in several laboratories (103,146,204,205,448, 449,500,715,716,718,822,824) indicates that damage to the nigrostriatal dopa- mine system reproduces almost all of the long-term food and water intake regulatory deficits seen in animals with lateral hypothalamic damage, with one possible exception: Lateral hypothalamus-lesioned animals decrease food or water intake when a small dose of quinine is added to the diet or water, whereas dopamine bundle-lesioned animals tolerate greater amounts of the bitter-tasting substance but are still more sensitive than normal intact animals (448).

In other experiments the feeding behavior of animals was assessed after intraventricular injection of 6-OHDA. Rats treated in this fashion showed a large reduction in brain norepinephrine concentration and a relatively smaller but still substantial decrease in brain dopamine; food intake in these animals was transiently decreased after the injection but returned to normal within 2–3 days (205,715,718,822,824), even though body weight appeared to be regulated at levels below those of vehicle-treated animals (716). Other groups of rats injected intraventricularly with the same dose of 6-OHDA, but this time after pretreatment with a monoamine oxidase inhibitor, showed a large reduction in brain dopamine but a decrease in norepinephrine similar to that in rats treated with 6-OHDA alone (205,714,718,822,824). Animals with a brain dopamine concentration reduced to less than 2% of the normal value are completely aphagic and adipsic (716), and appear never to recover from the effects of the lesion. These results parallel those described earlier with electro- lytic lesions in the far-lateral hypothalamus (486) and suggest that these lesions are more potent than those confined to the midlateral hypothalamic area because the far-lateral lesions damage almost all of the ascending, dopaminergic nigrostriatal axons (753).

When more than 2% of the dopamine concentration in the striatum remains after electrolytic or chemical lesions, animals show gradual recovery from the initial aphagia and adipsia associated with the treatment (716). Some evidence indicates that the catecholamine-containing neurons surviving the lesion may participate in the recovery: Animals with partial striatal dopamine depletion, injected during the recovery stage with the tyrosine hydroxylase inhibitor $\alpha$-methyltyrosine or with the $\alpha$-noradrenergic receptor blocking drug phentolamine (716), become aphagic and adipsic, even though the same doses of these drugs injected in neurologically intact animals have little apparent effect on feeding or drinking behavior. That a portion of the behavioral recovery might also be mediated by the ability of damaged neurons to repair themselves has been shown indirectly. Lateral hypothalamus-lesioned aphagic and adipsic animals recover faster if they are treated intravenously with nerve growth factor (64), a compound that stimulates the growth of immature (71) or injured catecholamine-containing neurons in the brain and periphery. These data suggest that feeding and drinking behavior after lateral hypothalamic lesions is at least partially supported by the hyperfunctioning of catecholamine neurons that have survived the lesion or that have regrown. Additionally, the behavioral recovery could be mediated by an increased synaptic concentration of neurotransmitter released from surviving or regenerated neurons coupled with changes in the sensitivity of postsynaptic effector cell receptors of the catecholamines (63,716).

The long-term feeding and drinking deficits that remain after the lateral hypothalamic, nigrostriatal lesions may be related to the animal's decreased ability to sense peripheral changes important for the control of feeding in normal, intact animals. Lateral hypothalamus-lesioned or 6-OHDA-treated animals that have reached the recovery stage do not eat when injected with single large doses of 2-DG or insulin (189,718,741). However, if these animals are made chronically hypoglycemic with repeated low doses of insulin (718), or if they are pretreated with drugs that increase postsynaptic catecholaminergic neurotransmission, they respond normally to decreases in cellular glucose utilization by increasing food intake (716). Even normal animals treated with the dopamine receptor-blocking drugs haloperidol or pimozide show feeding and drinking regulatory deficits similar to those of the lateral hypothalamic nigrostriatal syndrome (prandial drinking, failure to increase water intake following injection of hypertonic saline, lack of response to the anorexic effects of amphetamine or to the hypoglycemic effects of insulin, finicky eating and drinking) (825).

There are many parallels between ''natural'' feeding and feeding induced by lateral hypothalamic, electrical stimulation; hence it might be anticipated that manipulations of brain dopamine-containing neurons that alter normal feeding produce parallel changes in electrically induced eating behavior. This hypothesis has received partial support; treatment with haloperidol decreases the incidence of stimulation-induced feeding in rats (561), and injection of 6-OHDA into the ventral striatum produces hypophagia, hypodipsia, and a decrease in locomotor activity and operant responding for the reward of lateral hypothalamic electrical stimulation (507). Local injection of crystalline dopamine reverses the 6-OHDA-induced depression in self-stimulation rates (507). Despite these results, the relationships among changes in stimulation-induced feeding and natural feeding are not always perfectly correlated. Although injection of haloperidol decreases stimulation-bound eating, it does not decrease eating in food-deprived rats (825); similarly, local injection of dopamine increases self-stimulation behavior but does not always elicit normal feeding (35,399,606). Although both lateral hypothalamic electrolytic- and 6-OHDA-induced lesions produce complete aphagia and adipsia, these effects can be obtained with as little as 50–60% reductions in striatal dopamine following the electrolytic lesions, whereas only transient hypophagia and hypodipsia are observed in animals treated with 6-OHDA unless the extent of striatal dopamine depletion is greater than 95% (716,717). Furthermore, perifornical or midlateral hypothalamic lesions produce long-term feeding and drinking deficits, even though damage to the nigrostriatal dopamine system seems to be minimal (523,716). Hence it may be that several different subsystems coursing through the lateral hypothalamic area are involved in feeding and drinking, and that lesions or stimulation might alter some of these systems but not others.

Lesions that damage specific aspects of brain norepinephrine-containing nerves also alter feeding behavior. The major cell bodies for norepinephrine-containing neurons are localized in the brainstem. The axons from these cell bodies ascend in two distinct fiber bundles (the anterior and dorsal noradrenergic bundles) to innervate rostral brain structures, including the hypothalamus, septum, and cerebral cortices (754). It is unclear what role, if any, neurons in the dorsal noradrenergic pathway play in feeding behavior, although recent evidence suggests that neurons in the ventral noradrenergic pathway may be involved in a satiety control mechanism much like that described previously for cells in the VMH nucleus. Injection of 6-OHDA directly into the ventral noradrenergic pathway (at a site posterior to the substantia nigra) produces long-lasting hyperphagia and weight gain in rats (7,8). These behavioral changes appear to be directly related to the effects of 6-OHDA on this specific fiber bundle inasmuch as injection of the drug into the dorsal noradrenergic pathway or into the ventral bundle following pretreatment with desmethylimipramine (a drug that blocks 6-OHDA uptake and prevents neurotoxicity in norepinephrine-containing neurons), produces no significant change in food intake or body weight gain (8). A portion of the nerve terminals of the ventral noradrenergic pathway innervate cells immediately lateral to the ventromedial nucleus (754), and lesions in this area produce hyperphagia and obesity, as well as small but significant reductions in the forebrain norepinephrine concentration (148). Since norepinephrine injection into this brain region also influences eating behavior, it is tempting to speculate that the functions previously ascribed to the VMH nucleus may actually reflect changes in a ventral noradrenergic bundle satiety system. The results of several experiments argue against this possibility however: (a) Lesions of the ventral noradrenergic bundle attenuate amphetamine anorexia, whereas VMH lesions do not. (b) Hypophysectomy blocks the hyperphagia and obesity seen after VMH lesions but not that seen after ventral noradrenergic pathway lesions. (c) Animals with VMH lesions are finicky eaters and drinkers, whereas rats with ventral noradrenergic bundle lesions show normal sensitivity to changes in dietary palatability. (d) Rats with ventral noradrenergic lesions overeat primarily during the dark portion of the day-night light cycle, whereas VMH-lesioned animals overeat primarily during the day. (e) Animals with combined lesions of the ventral noradrenergic pathway and the VMH eat more and gain weight faster than animals with lesions of either the VMH or the noradrenergic ventral bundle alone (9,311). Furthermore, the hyperphagia and obesity associated with lesions of the ventral noradrenergic pathway are never as great as those typically seen after VMH damage (although it is not possible to equate the extent of tissue damage in these two brain regions) (9,311). Hence there may be at least two distinct brain systems mediating satiety; the possible extent to which these systems interact to control eating behavior remains to be determined.

### 3. Indoleamine Neurotransmission and Feeding

*Metabolism and anatomical localization of serotonin neurotransmitters.*

Serotonin is the only known indoleamine in brain that is also likely to be a neurotransmitter. Brain neurons appear to contain all of the precursors and enzymes necessary to synthesize and catabolize the neurotransmitter; this pathway is outlined in Fig. 4.

A significant concentration of serotonin is found in various peripheral tissues, including the enterochromaffin cells of the GI tract, the parenchymal cells of the pineal gland (where serotonin appears to be a precursor for the synthesis of melatonin), blood platelets, nerve endings of sympathetic neurons innervating the pineal gland, and in mast cells of some species (435,804,806). It seems clear that serotonin probably does not function as a neurotransmitter in most of these peripheral tissues. Serotonin-containing neurons are also found

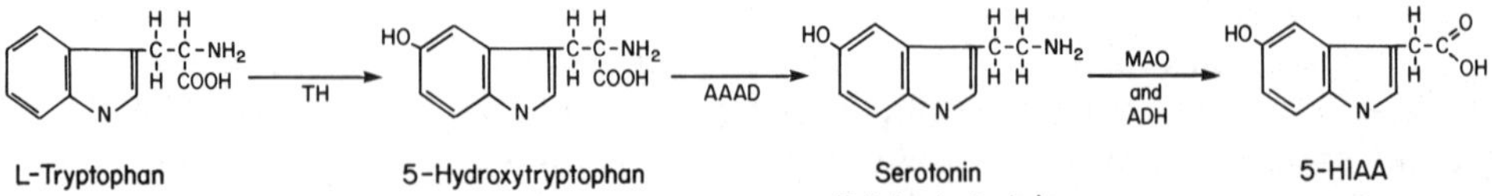

FIG. 4.  Synthesis and metabolism of the neurotransmitter serotonin.

in the CNS; and although they are not visualized well by the fluorescence histochemical method, sufficient data indicate that virtually all of the serotonin cell bodies in brain are confined to the midline raphe nuclei of the medulla and pons (72). Fibers from these cell bodies give rise to large numbers of collaterals that descend in the spinal cord to innervate gray matter and ascend in the medial forebrain bundle (which courses through the lateral hypothalamic area) to innervate most of the telencephalon and diencephalon (754).

*Drug manipulation of serotonin neurotransmission: Effect on feeding.*
Several experimental drugs have relatively specific effects on the functioning of serotoninergic neurons, although there are fewer of these compounds than those available for manipulating catecholaminergic neurotransmission. Furthermore, although pharmacological manipulation of brain serotoninergic neurotransmission indicates that these cells probably participate in the normal control of eating behavior, the evidence accumulated thus far is not as consistent as the evidence implicating the catecholaminergic transmitters.

Peripheral injection of serotonin decreases food intake in free-feeding rats (593) but may either increase or decrease the food intake of deprived animals (101,411,693); however, it is unclear if the effects are mediated solely by serotoninergic synapses. These feeding changes are probably not mediated by serotonin-containing neurons in brain, since serotonin does not readily cross the blood-brain barrier when it is injected into the periphery.

Injection of serotonin into the brain ventricles (501) or directly into the hypothalamic areas (674,773) generally fails to alter feeding in rats, although some (34) but not all (773) studies report a small reduction in food consumption following its injection into the VMH or perifornical hypothalamic areas (246). There may be species differences in response to local brain injection of serotonin, however, inasmuch as relatively large doses of the neurotransmitter injected into various diencephalic sites in monkeys (663) or into the ventromedial or anterior hypothalamic areas of sheep (67) produce a small, delayed increase in food intake.

Food intake is altered more successfully by systemic administration of drugs thought to influence serotoninergic neurotransmission. Injection of 5-hydroxytryptophan, the immediate amino acid precursor of brain serotonin, suppresses food intake in normal rats and in those with lateral hypothalamic lesions (78). Similarly, animals treated with fenfluramine or *p*-chloramphetamine, drugs thought to increase acutely the release of serotonin from presynaptic nerves, are also anorexic immediately after the injection (70,78,134,135, 212,414,641,642,668,798). However, the long-term reduction in brain serotonin concentration (286,287,467) seen in animals treated with these drugs suggests that they might also be neurotoxic to these neurons in a manner analogous to the catecholamine neurotoxicity seen after 6-OHDA.

Somewhat paradoxically, systemic injection of *p*-chlorophenylalanine, a drug that irreversibly inhibits tryptophan hydroxylase and reduces brain serotonin levels (374), generally produces transient anorexia and hypodipsia in rats (69,541). The meaning of these results is unclear, however, inasmuch as animals treated with p-chlorophenylalanine appear to be sick (541). Furthermore, the anorexia seen after drug treatment may not reflect specific drug effects on brain serotonin neurons, since p-chlorophenylalanine also reduces catecholaminergic neurotransmitter levels (374); it thus may produce anorexia by altering brain catecholaminergic control mechanisms for feeding rather than by inhibiting brain serotonin synthesis. That food intake patterns return to normal even though brain serotonin concentrations are still reduced (69) is compatible with this alternative hypothesis. Similarly, although injection of 5-hydroxytryptophan in animals pretreated with p-chlorophenylalanine restores brain serotonin concentrations to normal, it does not prevent the p-chloro-phenylalanine-induced reduction in food intake (107). Different results are obtained, however, when p-chlorophenylalanine is injected into the lateral ventricles of rats; with this route of administration the drug produces long-lasting hyperphagia and weight gain, paralleling the drug-induced reduction in brain serotonin concentration (104). Since the drug does not seem to alter the concentration of brain norepinephrine or dopamine when given intraventricularly, these data support the notion that a brain serotoninergic mechanism may normally inhibit food intake. Along similar lines, systemic injection of cyproheptadine, a drug believed to block serotonin receptors, also increases appetite and weight gain in humans (664), cats (129), and food-deprived rats (57,234).

*Electrically or chemically induced lesions in serotoninergic brain tracts: Effect on feeding.*

Electrolytic lesions of serotonin cell bodies in the raphe nuclei (429) or intraventricular or intracerebral injection of 5,6-dihydroxytryptamine, a neurotoxic drug that destroys neurons containing serotonin and norepinephrine (but not dopamine) (56), usually do not significantly influence food intake for more than 1–2 days (499). However, Saller and Stricker (639) showed that significant hyperphagia and obesity occur in animals pretreated with desmethylimipramine prior to intraventricular injection of another serotoninergic and noradrenergic neurotoxin, 5,7-dihydroxytryptamine. Apparently the dihydroxytryptamine-induced changes in feeding and weight gain occur only if the drug-induced brain noradrenergic neurotoxicity is blocked with desmethylimipramine, a drug that apparently eliminates the uptake of dihydroxytryptamine into these neurons and thus enchances its neurotoxic action on serotonin-containing neurons in brain. Many of the other pharmacological treatments aimed at determining if brain serotonin neurons participate in feeding may have produced no effects because they also changed the functioning of other neurotransmitter cells and thus counteracted the serotoninergic-mediated effects. This hypothesis must be tested directly.

Other evidence that brain serotonin-containing neurons participate in the regulation of food intake is largely indirect. Brain serotonin concentration varies rhythmically as a function of the diurnal lighting schedule and is lowest at the onset of darkness, the time when rats eat most of their daily food (201). Moreover, brain serotonin turnover rates are higher when rats have been deprived of food than when they have just eaten (553). Finally, the amount of daily calories consumed as protein is directly related to the ratio of plasma tryptophan relative to the concentration of other neutral amino acids that compete with tryptophan for uptake into brain (31); this observation deserves further study and suggests tentatively that the feeding habits of the animal alter brain neurotransmitters such that these changes might directly influence other behavioral responses, including eating behavior.

## 4. Other Neurotransmitter Mechanisms

Obviously there are many more putative neurotransmitters in the brain and periphery than the catecholamines and indoleamines. Unfortunately we know little about these other compounds and have fewer experimental tools (pharmacological, surgical, or nutritional) to manipulate them. Hence their possible functional roles in eating behavior remain to be determined. The little information available is reviewed in detail elsewhere (34).

Thus far, good neuroanatomical techniques exist only for the precise localization of brain dopamine, norepinephrine, epinephrine, and serotonin; until such techniques are developed to localize the other neurotransmitters, it is impossible to produce discrete and precise lesions, or to stimulate electrically cells that contain these compounds. Along similar lines, we know relatively little about the metabolic pathways involved in the synthesis and degradation of the other compounds (with the possible exception of acetylcholine and $\gamma$-aminobutyric acid) or about the enzymes involved in these pathways. Because of these gaps in our knowledge, few drugs exist (compared to those available for the catecholamine and indoleamine neurotransmitters) by which to attain relatively specific manipulations of these compounds.

Despite the fact that rather impressive evidence suggests that brain catecholamine and indoleamine neurotransmitters are essential components of the brain, it is often not immediately apparent how these neurochemical results relate to the neuroanatomical control mechanisms for the behavior. Whereas lesions of the nigrostriatal bundle suggest that dopamine-containing neurons in this tract are important for normal eating behavior, injection of dopamine into various diencephalic sites that should contain dopamine synapses has little if any effect on feeding behavior. Similarly, norepinephrine induces eating if it is injected into the VMH, and it causes a reduction in eating if injected into the lateral hypothalamic area; in contrast, electrical stimulation of cells in the VMH produces satiety, but electrical stimulation in the lateral hypothalamus induces eating. It is not immediately obvious why neurochemical stimulation produces one type of change in eating behavior and electrical stimulation in the same brain area the opposite effect. These discrepancies must be resolved before we can determine with any precision the functional role of cells in various brain regions in regard to eating behavior.

### D. Pharmacological Control of Eating Behavior

Since the late 1930s when it was first noticed that narcoleptic patients treated with amphetamine had decreased appetites associated with weight loss, a great deal of clinical interest has been focused on the usefulness of various pharmacological agents in the treatment of human eating disorders.

The appetite-suppressing effects of amphetamine made it the treatment of choice for human obesity during the past 20 years, and most of the anorexic drugs currently available share similarities to the chemical structure of the parent drug. Amphetamine produces many physiological and behavioral effects (149), most of which appear to be related to its action on brain and peripheral catecholamine-containing neurons (149,318). The drug alters catecholaminergic neurotransmission in at least two basic ways, both of which effectively increase the concentration of the catecholamines intrasynaptically: Administration of the drug stimulates the release of dopamine and norepinephrine from presynaptic nerve terminals and blocks their reuptake back into these cells by interfering with the neuronal transport mechanisms for these neurotransmitters (149,241). Hence the drug facilitates neurotransmission at adrenergic synapses in the brain and in the peripheral nervous system. Based on a variety of neuropharmacological observations, it appears likely that the drug produces anorexia by altering catecholamine neurotransmission in the brain (78,125,135,141,142,397,398,641,643) rather than by acting on peripheral control mechanisms for eating behavior (142). A rather massive literature has accumulated regarding the precise mechanisms by which amphetamine produces anorexia (142,398), and most of the evidence is consistent with the hypothesis that amphetamine-induced suppression in feeding behavior probably results from the release of dopamine or norepinephrine from lateral hypothalamic nerve endings such that dopaminergic and/or $\beta$-noradrenergic "satiety" receptors in this brain region are stimulated (379,397,398). However, alternative hypotheses regarding the mechanism of action of anorexic drugs also have some experimental support (141,142).

The use of amphetamine for treating obesity is currently in disfavor among most physicians due to its large potential for abuse (it is a psychomotor stimulant and produces euphoria); furthermore, tolerance eventually develops when amphetamine is used chronically for the control of appetite, such that the rate of weight reduction eventually reaches a plateau, unless increasingly greater doses of the drug are used. A number of congeners of amphetamine have been developed that appear effective as reducing aids. These drugs have the same basic chemical structure as the parent amphetamine molecule, with only slight modifications, but they have different neurochemical, physiological, and behavioral effects. For example, one of these compounds, fenflura-mine (N-ethyl-*m*-trifluoromethylamphetamine), is now widely used as an anorexic drug in Europe and the United States (668,798). Fenfluramine has equipotent anorexic activity compared with that of amphetamine but lacks the stimulant and cardiovascular side effects of the latter drug (212). Hence it does not have the drug abuse potential associated with the use of other amphetamine derivatives. Because the drug is halogenated on the benzene ring, many of its effects, including anorexia, appear to be mediated primarily by the action of the drug on brain serotoninergic, rather than on brain catecholamine-containing neurons (70,134,135,641,668). Recent evidence suggests that this drug may produce a neurotoxic-like effect on brain serotonin neurons in rats (286); although it is too early to tell if the drug produces similar effects on humans, however, future use of the drug for weight control may be in jeopardy.

The effectiveness of anorexic drugs currently used for treating human obesity depends in part on the definition of "effectiveness" (94). There seems to be little question that amphetamine congeners are effective agents for producing short-term reduction in body weight; however, the weight loss associated with the drug treatment is usually only temporary, and many patients rapidly regain weight to pretreatment levels following the termination of drug therapy (94). Although research scientists and pharmaceutical companies have solved many of the problems associated with the side effects and abuse potential of amphetamine-like drugs by chemically modifying the parent molecule (68,149), it remains to be determined if any effective long-term weight control drug can be developed whose primary action is related to its ability to decrease appetite and thus reduce the *amount* of food eaten. The reasons for this uncertainty are several. Many forms of human obesity appear to result from metabolic or endocrinological abnormalities in the storage and utilization of nutrients (772), rather than from an inability to control appetite. Even in cases of human obesity involving overeating, it is not clear that the overeating is always due to an alteration in physiological control mechanisms for feeding behavior (upon which amphetamine-like drugs are thought to act). Many factors—food palatability and accessibility, previous eating habits, sociocultural differences, to mention only a few—influence the amount of food eaten during a meal, and it is doubtful that anorexic drugs will ever be developed that completely suppress the effects of all of these other factors. The recent success claimed for alternative methods of treating weight regulation—which use behavior modification procedures for changing the psychological or sociological determinants of eating—hold promise as potentially effective means for appetite control (722).

It seems unlikely that drugs may become effective weight control agents by directly altering mechanisms that control when or how much food is eaten; however, drugs may someday be developed that have more utility for weight control if they can be made to change the storage or utilization of ingested nutrients after they are eaten. Some drug and hormone therapies currently available appear to be potentially useful in this regard, but their clinical effectiveness remains to be proved (94). Jejunoileal bypass surgery for the treatment of obesity is a radical operation with many untoward side effects (175) that has proved to be an effective means for reducing the body weight of extremely obese humans who fail to respond to other treatments. Drugs have not yet been developed that prevent the complete digestion of foodstuffs, block the absorption of nutrients from the GI tract into the bloodstream, interfere with the process of fat storage or the utilization of specific types of nutrients for energy, or enhance thermogenesis or energy expenditure without producing other undesirable side effects. The possibility that drugs of this type will someday be available depends in large part on increasing our understanding of the mechanisms that control energy and nutrient acquisition, utilization, and expenditure.

## VI. SUMMARY AND PROSPECTUS

Probably the most dramatic change in current conceptions regarding control mechanisms for eating behavior involves the understanding that behavioral responses are not determined exclusively by single mechanisms operating *in vacuo*. Eating behavior does not begin or stop simply because our blood sugar level changes, our fat cells are empty or full, our blood amino acid pattern varies, our stomachs are empty or full, or even because our body supply of metabolic fuel is high or low. Moreover, changes in our peripheral physiology are not sensed and integrated by a single brain mechanism that influences muscle physiology such that the likelihood of our searching for and finding food is increased; nor does a single brain mechanism increase the probability that we will eat the food once it is located. Similarly, there is no guarantee that we will always eat when we are "physiologically hungry" or when we are offered food that is essential for survival.

In the final analysis, whether we eat depends to some extent on *all* of the environmental, organismic, and physiological factors previously discussed, as well as on a number of other variables that have not yet been well studied. To incorporate all of the variables that seem to influence eating behavior into a single theory such that the theory has some predictive value is an imposing task, and many researchers have used the modern language of machine control theory in an attempt to grapple with these complexities.

Most machines have physical control systems that maintain a constant output over a substantial period of time; perturbations in the control system result in the implementation of feedback mechanisms to restore the output of the system to its original, preset level (98). Feedback control systems for machines usually consist of three major components: the controlled system, the controller, and the feedback elements. The controlled system is that part of the machine which generates the output. In the case of control systems designed to maintain constant room temperatures, for example, the controlled system is the actual temperature of the room and includes those elements that produce, distribute, and dispose of heat (heaters, fans, air conditioners, vents, etc.). The controller elements generate modifying signals that regulate the magnitude of response of the controlled system. Again, to use the analogy of room temperature control devices, the controller is the switch that turns a heater or an air conditioner on or off, depending on the signal generated from feedback elements. Feedback elements transform the output of the controlled system into a variety of signals that influence a reference input, or set point, that is applied to the controller to command a specific action of the controlled system. In the case of room temperature regulation, the feedback signal is the room temperature as measured by a thermometer, and the reference input is the desired room temperature as set on a thermostat. Changes in the room temperature above or below the reference point activate a switch (controller) that influences the control system to alter heat production. Each feedback control system has a certain amount of hysteresis, or delay, in influencing the regulatory capacity of the control system. Hence the actual temperature of a room oscillates at any given moment around the desired, or set point, temperature.

A number of investigators proposed that eating behavior is regulated by a control system in much the same manner as is room temperature (98). In this respect the output of the machine is concerned with maintaining a constant amount of calories, and the controlled system is concerned with the storage, distribution, and disposal of calories; the controller elements involve various brain regions and peripheral organs and endocrine glands; feedback elements include biochemical signals that change as a function of the quality or quantity of the diet consumed.

Although several gaps in our knowledge remain, we know a great deal more about the processes that influence the acquisition of energy and eating behavior; however, do we know enough about eating behavior to use control systems analysis? Although it is still too soon to answer this question completely, there are major differences in the basic nature of physical machines and biological machines that make this type of analogy suspect.

In most cases it is usually easy to specify the output, or controlled system, of most physical machines, because these systems are designed for well-defined purposes. However, the nature of the output, or the thing that is being regulated, is not always obvious in biological machines. With regard to eating behavior, it seems clear that mammals sometimes, but not always, regulate their amount of stored calories. However, it is not always certain if the storage of calories is *the* important endpoint, or if animals regulate other outputs that co-vary with, or are even not related to, calories. In any case, calories may be regulated on a long-term basis but not on a meal-by-meal basis (98,184).

In control systems for machines, the controller elements are usually sensory transducers that alter the response output; in biological systems these elements are not always passive sensors but may themselves be altered substantially by the output of the controlled system. For example, the ingested nutrients not only provide biochemical or physiological signals that are sensed or acted on by body tissues, they also change the response characteristics of the system itself. The quality and quantity of nutrients obtained from food ultimately provide the only precursor substances for the synthesis of various neurotransmitters, hormones, and enzymes that are essential components of the controlled system and the controller elements. Hence nutrients derived from food provide feedback signals important for eating behavior and change the basic nature of the biological machine itself.

The feedback elements for machines can be clearly specified and are dictated by the design inherent in the normal functioning of the machine. It is not always easy to specify the necessary and sufficient feedback elements operative in biological systems. Following the consumption of a meal, changes can be detected in a host of tissue and plasma chemicals (glucose, fatty acids, glycerol, amino acids, etc.); which if any of these signals provides biologically relevant information for the biological control system is still a matter of debate. The length of simple lists specifying all of the biochemical and physiological changes that occur following consumption of a meal is staggering; guessing which of these are the relevant feedback elements for eating behavior presents an imposing task that will continue to occupy the research efforts of scientists for years to come.

With machine control systems, the reference point (set point) is preset by the builder of the machine. It is often difficult if not impossible to discern the nature or level of the set point for biological control systems. In the case of eating behavior, if there is a set point for body weight regulation it appears to vary from species to species, from individual to individual, and within individuals as a function of time. For example, the caloric need for a single individual varies throughout life: Young animals ingest more food per unit body weight than do old animals; female animals ingest more or less food depending on the stage of the estrous cycle, whether they are pregnant, whether they are active, etc. Do these apparent changes in caloric "need" imply that the set point varies with time, or do they mean that the other feedback elements, predominant in furnishing information concerning the nutritional status of the organism, influence the level of the set point on a moment-by-moment basis?

It is evident from this brief description that it will be quite some time before machine systems analyses will have utility in helping us to understand the control mechanisms involved in feeding behavior. In the final analysis, the usefulness of this approach depends on future advancements in the "hard" and "soft" life sciences. Although we currently know a good deal about the control mechanisms for feeding behavior in rodents and other animals, we simply do not know very much about our own behavior. Certainly animal research has told us much about the delicate biological machinery that underlies various aspects of our own eating behavior, and we could not have this information without studying animals. However, we will never completely understand why we eat what we eat when we eat until we study ourselves with the same intensity and rigor that has characterized animal research.

## ACKNOWLEDGMENTS

The author is grateful to Louise Kittredge and Marjorie Lytle for their excellent assistance in the preparation of the manuscript. The work was supported in part by research grants from the National Institute of Mental Health, the Grant Foundation, and the National Foundation Basil O'Connor Research Starter Grant Program. The author holds a fellowship in neurosciences from the Alfred P. Sloan Foundation.

## REFERENCES

1. Abrams, R., and Hammel, H. (1964): Hypothalamic temperature in unanesthetized albino rats during feeding and sleep. *Am. J. Physiol.,* 206:641–646.
2. Adair, E. R., Miller, N. E., and Booth, D. A. (1968): Effects of continuous intravenous infusions of nutritive substances on consummatory behavior in rats. *Comm. Behav. Biol.,* 2:25–37.
3. Adams, T. (1963): Hypothalamic temperature in the cat during feeding and sleep. *Science,* 141:932–933.
4. Adolph, E. F. (1947): Urges to eat and drink in rats. *Am. J. Physiol.,* 151:110–125.
5. Adolph, E. F. (1957): Ontogeny of physiological regulations in the rat. *Q. Rev. Biol.,* 32:89–137.
6. Ahlquist, R. P. (1967): Development of the concept of alpha and beta adrenotropic receptors. *Ann. NY Acad. Sci.,* 139:549–558.
7. Ahlskog, J. E. (1974): Food intake and amphetamine anorexia after selective forebrain norepinephrine loss. *Brain Res.,* 82:211–240.
8. Ahlskog, J. E., and Hoebel, B. G. (1973): Overeating and obesity from damage to a noradrenergic system in the brain. *Science,* 182:166–168.
9. Ahlskog, J. E., Randall, P. K., and Hoebel, B. K. (1975): Hypothalamic hyperphagia: Dissociation from hyperphagia following destruction of noradrenergic neurons. *Science,* 190:399–401.
10. Almli, C. R., and Golden, G. T. (1974): Infant rats: Effects of lateral hypothalamic destruction. *Physiol. Behav.,* 13:81–90.
11. Almquist. H. J. (1954): Utilization of amino acids by chicks. *Arch. Biochem. Biophys.,* 52:197–202.
12. Anand, B. K. (1961): Nervous regulation of food intake. *Physiol. Rev.,* 41:677–708.
13. Anand, B. K. (1963): Functional importance of the limbic system of the brain. *Indian J. Med. Res.,* 51:175–222.
14. Anand, B. K. (1967): Central chemo-sensitive mechanisms related to feeding. In: *Handbook of Physiology,* Sect. 6, Vol. 1, edited by C. F. Code, pp. 249–263. American Physiological Society, Washington, D. C.
15. Anand, B. K. (1974): Neurological mechanisms regulating appetite. In: *Obesity Symposium,* edited by W. L. Burland, P. D. Samuel, and J. Yudkin, pp. 116–145. Churchill Livingstone, New York.
16. Anand, B. K., and Brobeck, J. R. (1951): Hypothalamic control of food intake. *Yale J. Biol. Med.,* 24:123–140.
17. Anand, B. K., and Dua, S. (1955): Feeding responses induced by electrical stimulation of the hypothalamus in cat. *Indian J. Med. Res.,* 43:113–122.
18. Anand, B. K., Chhina, G. S., Sharma, K. N., Dua, S., and Singh, B. (1964): Activity of single neurons in the hypothalamic feeding centers: Effect of glucose. *Am. J. Physiol.,* 207:1146–1154.

19. Anand, B. K., Dua, S., and Shoenberg, K. (1955): Hypothalamic control of food intake in cats and monkeys, *J. Physiol. (Lond.),* 127:143–152.
20. Anand, B. K., Dua, S., and Singh, B. (1961): Electrical activity of the hypothalamic "feeding centres" under effect of changes in blood chemistry. *Electroencephalogr. Clin. Neurophysiol.,* 13:54–59.
21. Anand, B. K., Subberwal, V., Manchanda, S. K., and Singh, B. (1961): Glucoreceptor mechanisms in the hypothalamic feeding centres. *Indian J. Med. Res.,* 49:717–724.
22. Anderson, J. W., Kilbourn, K. C., Robinson, J., and Wright, P. H. (1963): Diabetic acidosis in rats treated with anti-insulin serum. *Clin. Sci.,* 24:217–430.
23. Anderson, M. L., Benevenga, N. J., and Harper, A. E. (1968): Associations among food and protein intake, serine dehydratase, and plasma amino acids. *Am. J. Physiol.,* 214:1008–1013.
24. Andersson, B., and Larsson, B. (1961): Influence of local temperature changes in the pre-optic area and rostral hypothalamus on the regulation of food and water intake. *Acta Physiol. Scand.,* 52:75–89.
25. Andersson, B., Gale, C. C., and Sundsten, J. W. (1962): Effects of chronic central cooling on alimentation and thermoregulation. *Acta Physiol. Scand.,* 55:177–188.
26. Andik, I., Donhoffer, S., Farkas, M., and Schmidt, P. (1963): Ambient temperature and survival on a protein-deficient diet. *Br. J. Nutr.,* 17:257–261.
27. Anonymous (1944): Self-selection of diets. *Nutr. Rev.,* 2:199–203.
28. Antelman, S. M., Szechtman, H., Chin, P., and Fisher, A. E. (1975): Tail pinch-induced eating, gnawing and licking behavior in rats: Dependence on the nigrostriatal dopamine system. *Brain Res.,* 99:319–337.
29. Antin, J., Gibbs, J., Holt, J., Young, R. C., and Smith, G. P. (1975): Cholecystokinin elicits the complete behavioral sequence of satiety in rats. *J. Comp. Physiol. Psychol.,* 89:784–790.
30. Arees, E. A., Veltman, B. I., and Mayer, J. (1969): Hypothalamic blood flow following gold thioglucose-induced lesions. *Exp. Neurol.,* 25:410–415.
31. Ashley, D. V. M., and Anderson, G. H. (1975): Correlation between the plasma tryptophan to neutral amino acid ratio and protein intake in the self-selecting weanling rat. *J. Nutr.,* 105:1412–1421.
32. Ashley, D. V. M., and Anderson, G. H. (1975): Food intake regulation in the weanling rat: Effects of the most limiting essential amino acids of gluten, casein, and zein on the self-selection of protein and energy. *J. Nutr.,* 105:1405–1411.
33. Axelrod, J. (1974): Neurotransmitters. *Sci. Am.,* 230:58–71.
34. Baile, C. A. (1974): Putative neurotransmitters in the hypothalamus and feeding. *Fed. Proc.,* 33:1166–1175.
35. Baile, C. A., Krabill, L. F., and Simpson, C. W. (1973): Feeding elicited by $\alpha$ and $\beta$ adrenoceptor agonists in sheep and cattle. *Pharmacol. Biochem. Behav.,* 1:531–538.
36. Baile, C. A., Martin, F. H., Simpson, C. W., Forbes, J. M., and Beyea, J. S. (1974): Feeding elicted by $\alpha$ and $\beta$ adrenoceptor agonists injected intrahypothalamically in sheep. *J. Dairy Sci.,* 57:68–80.
37. Baile, C. A., Simpson, C. W., Bean, S. M., McLaughlin, C. L., and Jacobs, H. L. (1973): Prostaglandins and food intake of rats: A component of energy balance regulation? *Physiol. Behav.,* 10:1077–1085.
38. Baille, P., and Morrison, S. D. (1963): The nature of the suppression of food intake by lateral hypothalamic lesions in rats. *J. Physiol. (Lond.),* 165:227–245.
39. Baker, R. A. (1953): Aperiodic feeding behavior in the albino rat. *J. Comp. Physiol. Psychol.,* 46:422–426.
40. Balagura, S. (1968): Conditioned glycemic responses in the control of food intake. *J. Comp. Physiol. Psychol.,* 65:30–32.
41. Balagura, S. (1972); Neurophysiologic aspects: Hypothalamic factors in the control of eating behavior. *Adv. Psychosom. Med.,* 7:25–48.
42. Balagura, S. (1973): *Hunger: A Biopsychological Analysis.* Basic Books, New York.
43. Balagura, S., and Coscina, D. V. (1968): Periodicity of food intake in the rat as measured by an operant response. *Physiol. Behav.,* 3:641–643.
44. Balagura, S., and Devenport, L. (1970): Feeding patterns of normal and ventromedial hypothalamic lesioned male and female rats. *J. Comp. Physiol. Psychol.,* 71:357–364.

45. Balagura, S., and Harrell, L. E. (1974): Effect of size of food on food consumption: Some neurophysiological considerations. *J. Comp. Physiol. Psychol.,* 86:658–663.
46. Balagura, S., and Harrell, L. E. (1974): Lateral hypothalamic syndrome: Its modification by obesity and leanness. *Physiol. Behav.,* 13:345–347.
47. Balagura, S., and Kanner, M. (1971): Hypothalamic sensitivity to 2-deoxy-D-glucose and glucose: Effects on feeding behavior. *Physiol. Behav.,* 7:251–255.
48. Balagura, S., Wilcox, R. H., and Coscina, D. V. (1969): The effect of diencephalic lesions on food intake and motor activity. *Physiol. Behav.,* 4:629–633.
49. Balinska, H. (1968): The hypothalamic lesions: Effects on appetitive and aversive behavior in rats. *Acta Biol. Exp.,* 28:47–56.
50. Ban, T. (1975): Fiber connections in the hypothalamus and some autonomic functions. *Pharmacol. Biochem. Behav.,* 3:3–13.
51. Bandler, R., and Flynn, J. P. (1971): Visual patterned reflex present during hypothalamically elicited attack. *Science,* 171:817–818.
52. Bare, J. K. (1949): The specific hunger for NaCl in normal and adrenalectomized rats. *J. Comp. Physiol. Psychol.,* 42:242–253.
53. Barnes, B. O., and Keeton, R. W. (1940): Experimental obesity. *Am. J. Physiol.,* 129:305–306.
54. Barnett, S. A. (1956): Behaviour components in the feeding of wild and laboratory rats. *Behav. Neth.,* 9:24–44.
55. Baum, M. J. (1970): Light-synchronization of rat feeding rhythms following sympathectomy or pinealectomy. *Physiol. Behav.,* 5:325–329.
56. Baumgarten, H. G., Bjorklund, A., Lachenmayer, L., Nobin, A., and Stenevi, U. (1971): Long-lasting selective depletion of brain serotonin by 5,6-dihydroxytryptamine. *Acta Physiol. Scand. [Suppl.],* 373:1–16.
57. Baxter, M. G., Miller, A. A., and Soroko, F. E. (1970): The effect of cyproheptadine on food consumption in the fasted rat. *Br. J. Pharmacol.,* 39:229P–230P.
58. Beatty, W. W., O'Briant, D. A., and Vilberg, T. R. (1975): Effects of ovariectomy and estradiol injections on food intake and body weight in rats with ventromedial hypothalamic lesions. *Pharmacol. Biochem. Behav.,* 3:539–544.
59. Beatty, W. W., Powley, T. L., and Keesey, R. E. (1970): Effects of neonatal testosterone injection and hormone replacement in adulthood on body weight and fat in female rats. *Physiol. Behav.,* 5:1093–1098.
60. Becker, E. E., and Kissileff, H. R. (1974): Inhibitory controls of feeding by the ventromedial hypothalamus. *Am. J. Physiol.,* 226:383–396.
61. Bell, D. D., and Zucker, I. (1971): Sex differences in body weight and eating: Organization and activation by gonadal hormones in the rat. *Physiol. Behav.,* 7:27–34.
62. Benjamin, R. M. (1963): Some thalamic and cortical mechanisms of taste. In: *Olfaction and Taste,* edited by Y. Zotterman, pp. 309–329, Pergamon Press, New York.
63. Berger, B. D., Wise, C. D., and Stein, L. (1971): Norepinephrine: Reversal of anorexia in rats with lateral hypothalamic damage. *Science,* 172:281–284.
64. Berger, B. D., Wise, C. D., and Stein, L. (1973): Nerve growth factor: Enhanced recovery of feeding after hypothalamic damage. *Science,* 180:506–508.
65. Berkun, M. M., Kessen, M. L., and Miller, N. E. (1952): Hunger-reducing effects of food by stomach fistula versus food by mouth measured by a consummatory response. *J. Comp. Physiol. Psychol.,* 45:550–554.
66. Bernardis, L. L., and Frohman, L. A. (1970): Effect of lesion size in the ventromedial hypothalamus on growth hormone and insulin levels in weanling rats. *Neuroendocrinology,* 6:319–328.
67. Beyea, J. S., and Baile, C. A. (1973): 5-HT and dibutyryl cyclic-AMP injections in the hypothalamus of sheep, and feeding. *Fed. Proc.,* 32:304.
68. Biel, J. H. (1970): Structure-activity relationships of amphetamine and derivatives. In: *Amphetamines and Related Compounds,* edited by E. Costa and S. Garattini, pp. 3–19. Raven Press, New York.
69. Biggio, G., Mereu, G. P., Piccardi, M. P., Demontis, G., Caruso, P. L., Olianas, M., and Vargiu, L. (1973): Is brain serotonin involved in hunger and satiety? *Riv. Farmacol. Terap.,* 4:183–188.
70. Bizzi, A., Bonaccorsi, A., Jespersen, S., Jori, A., and Garattini, S. (1970): Pharmacological

studies on amphetamine and fenfluramine. In: *Amphetamines and Related Compounds,* edited by E. Costa and S. Garattini, pp. 577–595. Raven Press, New York.

71. Bjorklund, A., Bjerre, B., and Stenevi, U. (1974): Has nerve growth factor a role in the regeneration of central and peripheral catecholamine neurons? In: *Dynamics of Degeneration and Growth in Neurons,* edited by K. Fuxe, L. Olson, and Y. Zotterman, pp. 389–409. Pergamon Press, New York.

72. Bjorklund, A., Falck, B., and Owman, C. (1972): Fluorescence microscopic and microspectrofluorimetric techniques for the cellular localization and characterization of biogenic amines. In: *The Thyroid and Biogenic Amines,* edited by J. E. Rall and I. J. Kopin, pp. 318–368. North-Holland Publishing, Amsterdam.

73. Bjorntorp, P. (1972): Disturbances in the regulation of food intake. *Psychosom. Med.,* 7:116–147.

74. Bjorntorp, P., Bergman, H., Varnauskas, E., and Lindholm, B. (1969): Lipid metabolization in relation to body composition in man. *Metabolism,* 18:820–840.

75. Blaustein, J. D., and Wade, G. N. (1976): Ovarian influences on the meal patterns of female rats. *Physiol. Behav. (in press).*

76. Blomquist, A. J., and Antern, A. (1967): Gustatory deficits produced by medullary lesions in the white rat. *J. Comp. Physiol. Psychol.,* 63:439–443.

77. Bloom, R. A., and Fenton, P. F. (1956): Glucose tolerance in relation to obesity and food intake. *Am. J. Physiol.,* 184:438–440.

78. Blundell, J. E., and Leshem, M. B. (1974): Central action of anorexic agents: Effects of amphetamine and fenfluramine in rats with lateral hypothalamic lesions. *Eur. J. Pharmacol.,* 28:81–88.

79. Booth, D. A. (1967): Localization of the adrenergic feeding system in the rat diencephalon. *Science,* 158:515–517.

80. Booth, D. A. (1968): Effects of intrahypothalamic glucose injection on eating and drinking elicited by insulin. *J. Comp. Physiol. Psychol.,* 65:13–16.

81. Booth, D. A. (1968): Mechanism of action of norepinephrine in eliciting an eating response on injection into the rat hypothalamus. *J. Pharmacol. Exp. Ther.,* 160:336–348.

82. Booth, D. A. (1972): Modulation of the feeding response to peripheral insulin, 2-deoxy-glucose or 3-0-methyl glucose injection. *Physiol. Behav.,* 8:1069–1076.

83. Booth, D. A. (1972): Some characteristics of feeding during streptozotocin-induced diabetes in the rat. *J. Comp. Physiol. Psychol.,* 80:238–249.

84. Booth, D. A. (1976): Approaches to feeding control. In: *Dahlem Workshop on Appetite and Food Intake,* edited by T. Silverstone, pp. 417–478. Dahlem Konferenzen, Berlin.

85. Booth, D. A., and Brookover, T. (1968): Hunger elicited in the rat by a single injection of bovine crystalline insulin. *Physiol. Behav.,* 3:439–446.

86. Booth, D. A., and Jarman, S. P. (1975): Ontogeny and insulin-dependence of the satiation which follows carbohydrate absorption in the rat. *Behav. Biol.,* 15:159–172.

87. Booth, D. A., and Pitt, M. E. (1968): The role of glucose in insulin-induced feeding and drinking. *Physiol. Behav.,* 3:447–453.

88. Booth, D. A., Coons, E. E., and Miller, N. E. (1969): Blood glucose responses to electrical stimulation of the lateral hypothalamic feeding area. *Physiol. Behav.,* 4:991–1001.

89. Booth, D. A., Toates, F. M., and Platt, S. V. (1976): Control system for hunger and its implications in animals and man. In: *Hunger: Basic Mechanisms and Clinical Implications,* edited by D. Novin, W. Wyrwicka, and G. Bray, pp. 127–143. Raven Press, New York.

90. Booth, G., and Strang, J. M. (1936): Changes in temperature of the skin following ingestion of food. *Arch. Intern. Med.,* 57:533–543.

91. Borbely, A. A., and Huston, J. P. (1974): Effects of two-hour light-dark cycles on feeding, drinking and motor activity of the rat. *Physiol. Behav.,* 13:795–802.

92. Boyle, P. C., and Keesey, R. E. (1975): Chronically reduced levels of body weight in LH-lesioned rats maintained upon diets and drinking solutions of varying palatability. *J. Comp. Physiol. Psychol.,* 88:218–223.

93. Bray, G. A. (1974): Endocrine factors in the control of food intake. *Fed. Proc.,* 33:1140–1145.

94. Bray, G. A. (1974): Pharmacological approach to the treatment of obesity. In: *Treatment and Management of Obesity,* edited by G. A. Bray and J. E. Bethune, pp. 117–131. Harper & Row, Hagerstown, Md.

95. Bray, G. A. (1974): The varieties of obesity. In: *Treatment and Management of Obesity,* edited by G. A. Bray and J. E. Bethune, pp. 61–76. Harper & Row, Hagerstown, Md.

96. Bray, G. A. (1976): Peripheral metabolic factors in the regulation of feeding. In: *Dahlem Workshop on Appetite and Food Intake,* edited by T. Silverstone, pp. 141–176. Dahlem Konferenzen, Berlin.

97. Bray, G. A., and Bethune, J. E., editors (1974): *Treatment and Management of Obesity.* Harper & Row, Hagerstown, Md.

98. Bray, G. A., and Campfield, L. A. (1975): Metabolic factors in the control of energy stores. *Metabolism,* 24:99–117.

99. Bray, G. A., and Jacobs, H. S. (1974): Thyroid activity and other endocrine glands. In: *Handbook of Physiology,* Sect. 4, edited by E. Astwood and R. Greep, pp. 413–433. American Physiological Society, Washington, D. C.

100. Bray, G. A., and York, D. A. (1971): Genetically transmitted obesity in rodents. *Physiol. Rev.,* 51:598–646.

101. Bray, G. A., and York, D. A. (1972): Studies on food intake in genetically obese rats. *Am. J. Physiol.,* 223:176–179.

102. Breckcr, G., and Waxler, S. H. (1949): Obesity in albino mice due to single injections of gold thioglucose. *Proc. Soc. Exp. Biol. Med.,* 70:498–501.

103. Breese, G. R., Smith, R. D., Cooper, B. R., and Grant, L. D. (1973): Alterations in consummatory behavior following intracisternal injection of 6-hydroxydopamine. *Pharmacol. Biochem. Behav.,* 1:319–328.

104. Breisch, S. T., Zemlan, F. P., and Hoebel, B. G. (1976): Hyperphagia and obesity following serotonin depletion by intraventricular p-chlorophenylalanine. *Science,* 192:382–385.

105. Brobeck, J. R. (1946): Mechanisms of the development of obesity in animals with hypothalamic hyperphagia. *Physiol. Rev.,* 23:541–559.

106. Brobeck, J. R. (1948): Food intake as a mechanism of temperature regulation. *Yale J. Biol. Med.,* 20:545–552.

107. Brobeck, J. R. (1960): Food and temperature. In: *Recent Progress in Hormone Research,* edited by G. Pincus, pp. 439–466. Academic Press, New York.

108. Brobeck, J. R., Larsson, S., and Reyes, E. (1956): A study of the electrical activity of the hypothalamic feeding mechanism. *J. Physiol. (Lond.),* 132:358–364.

109. Brobeck, J. R., Tepperman, J., and Long, C. N. H. (1943): Experimental hypothalamic hyperphagia in the albino rat. *Yale J. Biol. Med.,* 15:831–853.

110. Brobeck, J. R., Wheatland, M., and Strominger, J. L. (1947): Variations in regulation of energy exchange associated with estrus, diestrus, and pseudo pregnancy in rats. *Endocrinology,* 40:65–72.

111. Bronfenbrenner, U. (1968): Early deprivation in mammals and man. In: *Early Experience and Behavior,* edited by G. Newton and S. Levine, pp. 627–764. Charles C Thomas, Springfield, Ill.

112. Brooks, C. McC. (1946): The relative importance of changes in activity in the development of experimentally produced obesity in the rat. *Am. J. Physiol.,* 147:708–716.

113. Brooks, C. McC., and Lambert, E. F. (1946): A study of the effect of limitations of food intake and the method of feeding on the rate of weight gain during hypothalamic obesity in the albino rat. *Am. J. Physiol.,* 147:695–707.

114. Brooks, C. McC., Lockwood, R. L., and Wiggins, M. L. (1946): A study of the effects of hypothalamic lesions on the eating habits of the albino rat. *Am. J. Physiol.,* 147:735–742.

115. Brown, J. (1962): Effects of 2-deoxyglucose on carbohydrate metabolism. *Metabolism,* 11:1098–1112.

116. Brown, J., and Bachrach, H. L. (1959): Effects of 2-deoxyglucose on blood glucose levels in the rat. *Proc. Soc. Exp. Biol. Med.,* 100:641–643.

117. Brown, K. A., and Melzack, R. (1969): Effects of glucose on multiunit activity in the hypothalamus. *Exp. Neurol.,* 24:363–373.

118. Brozek, J., and Vaes, G. (1961): Experimental investigations on the effects of dietary deficiencies on animals and human behavior. *Vitam. Horm.,* 19:43–94.

119. Bruch, H. (1976): The treatment of eating disorders. *Mayo Clin. Proc.,* 51:266–272.

120. Burton, A. C., and Murlin, J. R. (1935): Human calorimetry. III. Temperature distribution, blood flow, and heat storage in the body in basal conditions after injections of food. *J. Nutr.,* 9:281–300.

121. Cahill, G. F., Jr. (1974): Obesity and the control of fuel metabolism. In: *Treatment and Management of Obesity,* edited by G. A. Bray and J. E. Bethune, pp. 3–16. Harper & Row, Hagerstown, Md.

122. Campbell, C. S., and Davis, J. D. (1974): Licking rate of rats is reduced by intraduodenal and intraportal glucose infusion. *Physiol. Behav.,* 12:357–365.

123. Campbell, R. G., Hashim, S. A., and Van Itallie, T. B. (1971): Studies of food-intake regulation in man: Responses to variations in nutritive density in lean and obese subjects. *N. Engl. J. Med.,* 285:1402–1407.

124. Cannon, W. B., and Washburn, A. L. (1912): An explanation of hunger. *Am. J. Physiol.,* 29:441–454.

125. Carlisle, H. J. (1964): Differential effects of amphetamine on food and water intake in rats with lateral hypothalamic lesions. *J. Comp. Physiol. Psychol.,* 58:47–54.

126. Carlson, A. J. (1916): *The Control of Hunger in Health and Disease.* University of Chicago Press, Chicago.

127. Carlsson, A., Falck, B., and Hillarp, N-A. (1962): Cellular localization of brain monoamines. *Acta Physiol. Scand.,* 196:1–28.

128. Castro, J. M. de, and Balagura, S. (1975): Ontogeny of meal patterning in rats and its recapitulation during recovery from lateral hypothalamic lesions. *J. Comp. Physiol. Psychol.,* 89:791–802.

129. Chakrabarty, A. S., Pillai, R. V., Anand, B. K., and Singh, B. (1967): Effect of cyproheptadine on the electrical activity of the hypothalamic feeding centres. *Brain Res.,* 6:561–569.

130. Chavez, A., Martinez, C., and Yaschine, T. (1975): Nutrition, behavioral development, and mother-child interaction in young rural children. *Fed. Proc.,* 34:1574–1582.

131. Cheng, M-F., Rozin, P., and Teitelbaum, P. (1971): Starvation retards development of food and water regulations. *J. Comp. Physiol. Psychol.,* 76:206–218.

132. Chernigovsky, V. N. (1963): The significance of interoceptive signals in the food behavior of animals. In: *Brain and Behavior,* Vol. 2, pp. 319–348. American Institute of Biological Sciences, Washington, D. C.

133. Clark, J., Klee, W., Levitski, A., and Wolff, J. (1976): *Dahlem Workshop on Hormone and Antihormone Action at the Target Cell.* Dahlem Konferenzen, Berlin.

134. Clineschmidt, B. V. (1973): 5,6-Dihydroxytryptamine: Suppression of the anorexigenic action of fenfluramine. *Eur. J. Pharmacol.,* 24:405–409.

135. Clineschmidt, B. V., McGuffin, J. C., and Werner, A. B. (1974): Role of monoamines in the anorexigenic actions of fenfluramine, amphetamine and p-chloromethamphetamine. *Eur. J. Pharmacol.,* 27:313–323.

136. Coffyn, Z. E. Y. (1972): Early vascular changes in the brain of the mouse after injections of goldthioglucose and bipiperidyl mustard. *Physiol. Behav.,* 106:49–56.

137. Cohen, E. L., and Wurtman, R. J. (1976): Brain acetylcholine synthesis: Control by dietary choline. *Science,* 191:561–562.

138. Cohn, C. (1963): Feeding frequency and body composition. *Ann. NY Acad. Sci.,* 110:395–409.

139. Cohn, C., and Joseph, D. (1959): Changes in body composition attendant on force feeding. *Am. J. Physiol.,* 196:965–968.

140. Cohn, C., and Joseph, D. (1962): Influence of body weight and body fat on appetite of "normal," lean and obese rats. *Yale J. Biol. Med.,* 34:598–607.

141. Cole, S. O. (1973): Hypothalamic feeding mechanisms and amphetamine anorexia. *Psychol. Bull.,* 79:13–20.

142. Cole, S. O., and Gay, P. E. (1974): Brain mechanisms underlying the effects of amphetamine on feeding and non-feeding behaviors: Dissociation and overlap. *Physiol. Psychol.,* 2:80–88.

143. Conrad, E. H. (1970): Psychogenic obesity—effects of social rejection upon hunger, food craving, food consumption, and drive-reduction value of eating for obese versus normal individuals. *Psychosom. Med.,* 32:556.

144. Coons, E. E., and Quartermain, D. (1970): Motivational depression associated with norepinephrine-induced eating from the hypothalamus: Resemblance to the ventromedial hyperphagic syndrome. *Physiol. Behav.,* 5:687–692.

145. Coons, E. E., Levak, M., and Miller, N. E. (1965): Lateral hypothalamus: Learning of food-seeking response motivated by electrical stimulation. *Science,* 150:1320–1321.

146. Cooper, B. R., Howard, J. L., Grant, L. D., Smith, R. D., and Breese, G. R. (1974): Alteration of avoidance and ingestive behavior after destruction of central catecholamine pathways with 6-hydroxydopamine. *Pharmacol. Biochem. Behav.,* 2:639–649.
147. Corbit, J. D., and Stellar, E. (1964): Palatability, food intake, and obesity in normal and hyperphagic rats. *J. Comp. Physiol. Psychol.,* 58:63–67.
148. Coscina, D. V., Rosenblum-Blinick, C., Godse, D. D., and Stancer, H. C. (1973): Consummatory behaviors of hypothalamic hyperphagic rats after central injection of 6-hydroxydopamine. *Pharmacol. Biochem. Behav.,* 1:629–642.
149. Costa, E., and Garattini, S. (1970): *Amphetamines and Related Compounds.* Raven Press, New York.
150. Coursin, D. B. (1972): Nutrition and brain development in infants. *Merill-Palmer Q.,* 18:177–202.
151. Covian, M. R., and Antures-Rodrigues, J. (1963): Specific alterations in sodium chloride intake after hypothalamic lesions in the rat. *Am. J. Physiol.,* 205:922–926.
152. Cox, V. C., and Kakolewski, J. W. (1970): Sex differences in body weight regulation in rats following hypothalamic lesions. *Comm. Behav. Biol.,* 5:195–197.
153. Cox, V. C., Kakolewski, J. W., and Valenstein, E. S. (1968): Effects of ventromedial hypothalamic damage in hypophysectomized rats. *J. Comp. Physiol. Psychol.,* 65:145–148.
154. Cox, V. C., Kakolewski, J. W., and Valenstein, E. S. (1969): Ventromedial hypothalamic lesions and changes in body weight and food consumption in male and female rats. *J. Comp. Physiol. Psychol.,* 67:320–326.
155. Dahl, E., and Ursin, H. (1969): Obesity produced by iron and tissue destruction in the ventromedial hypothalamus. *Physiol. Behav.,* 4:315–317.
156. Dahlstrom, A., and Fuxe, K. (1964): Evidence for the existence of monoamine containing neurons in the central nervous system. I. Demonstration of monoamines in the cell bodies of brain stem neurons. *Acta Physiol. Scand.,* 62:1–55.
157. Davenport, H. W. (1971): *Physiology of the Digestive Tract.* Year Book Publishers, Chicago.
158. Davis, J. D., Gallagher, R. J., and Ladove, R. F. (1967): Food intake controlled by a blood factor. *Science,* 156:1247–1248.
159. Davis, J. D., Gallagher, R. J., Ladove, R. F., and Turausky, A. J. (1969): Inhibition of food intake by a humoral factor. *J. Comp. Physiol. Psychol.,* 67:407–414.
160. Davis, J. N., and Carlsson, A. (1973): Effect of hypoxia and tryptophan hydroxylation in unanesthetized rat brain. *J. Neurochem.,* 20:913–915.
161. Debons, A. F., Krimsky, I., and From, A. (1970): A direct action of insulin on the hypothalamic satiety center. *Am. J. Physiol.,* 219:938–943.
162. Debons, A. F., Krimsky, I., From, A., and Cloutier, R. J. (1969): Rapid effects of insulin on the hypothalamic satiety center. *Am. J. Physiol.,* 217:1114–1118.
163. Debons, A. F., Krimsky, I., From, A., and Cloutier, R. J. (1970): Goldthioglucose induction of obesity: Significance of focal gold deposits in hypothalamus. *Am. J. Physiol.,* 219:1403–1408.
164. Debons, A. F., Krimsky, I., From, A., and Cloutier, R. J. (1970): Site of action of goldthioglucose in the hypothalamic satiety center. *Am. J. Physiol.,* 219:1397–1402.
165. Debons, A. F., Krimsky, I., From, A., and Pattinian, H. (1974): Phlorizin inhibition of hypothalamic necrosis induced by gold thioglucose. *Am. J. Physiol.,* 226:574–578.
166. Debons, A. F., Krimsky, I., Likuski, H. J., From, A., and Cloutier, R. J. (1968): Gold thioglucose damage to the satiety center: Inhibition in diabetes. *Am. J. Physiol.,* 214:652–658.
167. Decke, E., and Vasselli, J. R. (1974): Metabolic hormones and regulation of body weight. *Psychol. Rev.,* 81:26–43.
168. DeGarine, I. (1972): The socio-cultural aspects of nutrition. *Ecol. Food Nutr.,* 1:143–163.
169. De Groot, J. (1967): Organization of hypothalamic feeding mechanisms. In: *Handbook of Physiology,* Sect. 6, Vol. 1, edited by C. F. Code, pp. 239–247. American Physiological Society, Washington, D. C.
170. Delgado, J. M. R., and Anand, B. K. (1953): Increase of food intake induced by electrical stimulation of the lateral hypothalamus. *Am. J. Physiol.,* 172:743–750.
171. Denton, D. A. (1967): Salt appetite. In: *Handbook of Physiology,* Sect. 6, Vol. 1, edited by C. F. Code, pp. 433–459. American Physiological Society, Washington, D. C.

172. Desiraju, T., Banerjee, M. G., and Anand, B. K. (1968): Activity of single neurons in the hypothalamic feeding centers: Effect of 2-deoxy-D-glucose. *Physiol. Behav.,* 3:757–760.
173. Dethier, V. G. (1967): Feeding and drinking behavior of invertebrates. In: *Handbook of Physiology,* Sect. 6, Vol. 1, edited by C. F. Code, pp. 79–96. American Physiological Society, Washington, C. C.
174. Devor, M. G., Wise, R. A., Milgram, N. W., and Hoebel, B. G. (1970): Physiological control of hypothalamically elicited feeding and drinking. *J. Comp. Physiol. Psychol.,* 73:226–232.
175. De Wind, L. (1974): Jejunoileal bypass surgery for obesity. In: *Treatment and Management of Obesity,* edited by G. A. Bray and J. E. Bethune, pp. 132–140. Harper & Row, Hagerstown, Md.
176. Di Cara, L. V., and Wolf, G. (1968): Bar pressing for food reinforcement after lesions of efferent pathways from lateral hypothalamus. *Exp. Neurol.,* 21:231–235.
177. Donhoffer, S., and Vonotsky, J. (1947): The effect of environmental temperature on food selection. *Am. J. Physiol.,* 150:329–333.
178. Donoso, A. O., and Cukier, J. (1968): Estrogen as depressor of noradrenaline concentration in the anterior hypothalamus. *Nature (Lond.),* 218:969–970.
179. Donoso, A. O., and Stefano, F. J. E. (1965): Sex hormones and the concentration of noradrenaline and dopamine in the anterior hypothalamus of castrated rats. *Experientia,* 23:665–666.
180. Drachman, R., and Tepperman, J. (1953): Aurothioglucose obesity in the mouse. *Yale J. Biol. Med.,* 26:394–401.
181. Durrer, J. L., and Hannon, J. P. (1962): Seasonal variations in caloric intake of dogs living in an arctic environment. *Am. J. Physiol.,* 202:375–378.
182. Edelman, P. M., Schwartz, I. L., Cronkite, E. P., and Livingston, L. (1965): Studies of the ventromedial hypothalamus with autoradiographic techniques. *Ann. NY Acad. Sci.,* 131:485–501.
183. Edelman, P. M., Schwartz, I. L., Cronkite, E. P., Brecher, G., and Livingston, L. (1965): The effect of hyperglycemia on hypothalamic gold uptake and hyperphagia in gold thioglucose-treated mice. *J. Exp. Med.,* 121:403–413.
184. Edholm, O. G., Adam, J. M., Healy, M. J. R., Wolff, H. S., Goldsmith, R., and Best, T. W. (1970): Food intake and energy expenditure of army recruits. *Br. J. Nutr.,* 24:1091–1107.
185. Epstein, A. N. (1959): Suppression of eating and drinking by amphetamine and other drugs in normal and hyperphagic rats. *J. Comp. Physiol. Psychol.,* 52:37–45.
186. Epstein, A. N. (1960): Reciprocal changes in feeding behavior produced by intrahypothalamic chemical injections. *Am. J. Physiol.,* 199:969–974.
187. Epstein, A. N. (1967): Feeding without oropharyngeal sensations. In: *The Chemical Senses and Nutrition,* edited by M. R. Kare and O. Maller, pp. 263–280. Johns Hopkins Press, Baltimore.
188. Epstein, A. N. (1967): Oropharyngeal factors in feeding and drinking. In: *Handbook of Physiology* Sect. 6, Vol. 1, edited by C. F. Code, pp. 197–218. American Physiological Society, Washington, D. C.
189. Epstein, A. N. (1971): The lateral hypothalamic syndrome: its implications for the physiological psychology of hunger and thirst. In: *Progress in Physiological Psychology,* edited by E. Stellar and J. M. Sprague, pp. 263–317. Academic Press, New York.
190. Epstein, A. N. (1976): Feeding and drinking in suckling rats. In: *Hunger: Basic Mechanisms and Clinical Implications,* edited by D. Novin, W. Wyrwicka, and G. Bray, pp. 193–213. Raven Press, New York.
191. Epstein, A. N., and Stellar, E. (1955): The control of salt preference in the adrenalectomized rat. *J. Comp. Physiol. Psychol.,* 48:167–172.
192. Epstein, A. N., and Teitelbaum, P. (1962): Regulation of food intake in the absence of taste, smell, and other oropharyngeal sensations. *J. Comp. Physiol. Psychol.,* 55:753–759.
193. Epstein, A. N., and Teitelbaum, P. (1967): Specific loss of the hypoglycemic control of feeding in recovered lateral rats. *Am. J. Physiol.,* 213:1159–1167.
194. Fabry, P. (1955): Studies on the adaptation of metabolism. I. On the glycogen reserves of rats accustomed to interrupted starvation. *Physiol. Bohemoslov.,* 4:33–36.
195. Fabry, P. (1967): Metabolic consequences of the pattern of food intake. In: *Handbook of*

*Physiology,* Sect. 6, Vol. 1, edited by C. F. Code, pp. 31–49. American Physiological Society, Washington, D. C.
196. Fabry, P., Petrasek, R., Braun, T., Bednarek, M., Horakova, E., and Konopasek, E. (1962): Lipogenesis in rats adapted to intermittent starvation or continuous underfeeding. *Experientia,* 18:555–556.
197. Fajan, S. S., and Floyd, J. C., Jr. (1972): Stimulation of islet cell secretion by nutrient and by gastrointestinal hormones released during digestion. In: *Handbook of Physiology,* Sect. 7, Vol. 1, edited by R. O. Greep and E. B. Astwood, pp. 473–494. American Physiological Society, Washington, D. C.
198. Falk, J. L., and Herman, T. S. (1961): Specific appetite for NaCl without postingestional repletion. *J. Comp. Physiol. Psychol.,* 54:405–408.
199. Ferguson, N. B. L., and Keesey, R. E. (1975): Effect of a quinine-adulterated diet upon body weight maintenance in male rats with ventromedial hypothalamic lesions. *J. Comp. Physiol. Psychol.,* 89:478–488.
200. Fernstrom, J. D., and Wurtman, R. J. (1971): Brain serotonin content: Increase following ingestion of carbohydrate diet. *Science,* 174:1023–1025.
201. Fernstrom, J. D., and Wurtman, R. J. (1971): Brain serotonin content: Physiological dependence on plasma tryptophan levels. *Science,* 173:149–152.
202. Fernstrom, J. D., and Wurtman, R. J. (1971): Effect of chronic corn consumption on serotonin content of rat brain. *Nature [New Biol.],* 234:62–64.
203. Fernstrom, J. D., and Wurtman, R. J. (1974): Nutrition and the brain. *Sci. Am.,* 230:84–91.
204. Fibiger, H. C., Phillips, A. G., and Clouston, R. A. (1973): Regulatory deficits after unilateral electrolytic or 6-OHDA lesions of the substantia nigra. *Am. J. Physiol.,* 225:1282–1287.
205. Fibiger, H. C., Zis, A. P., and McGeer, E. G. (1973): Feeding and drinking deficits after 6-hydroxydopamine administration in the rat: Similarities to the lateral hypothalamic syndrome. *Brain Res.,* 55:135–148.
206. Fish, I., and Winick, M. (1969): Effect of malnutrition on regional growth of the developing rat brain. *Exp. Neurol.,* 25:534–540.
207. Fishman, J. (1976): Appetite and sex hormones. In: *Dahlem Workshop on Appetite and Food Intake,* edited by T. Silverstone, pp. 207–218. Dahlem Konferenzen, Berlin.
208. Fleming, D. G. (1969): Food intake studies in parabiotic rats. *Ann. NY Acad. Sci.,* 157:985–1003.
209. Fomon, S. J., Filer, L. J., Thomas, L. N., Anderson, T. A., and Nelson, S. E. (1975): Influence of formula concentration on caloric intake and growth of normal infants. *Acta Paediatr. Scand.,* 64:172–181.
210. Foster, G. M. (1962): *Traditional Cultures and the Impact of Technological Change.* Harper & Row, New York.
211. Frazier, L. E., Wissler, R. W., Stefler, C. H., Woolridge, F. L., and Cannon, P. R. (1947): Studies in amino acid utilization. I. The dietary utilization of mixtures of purified amino acids in protein-depleted adult albino rats. *J. Nutr.,* 33:65–83.
212. Frey, H-H. (1970): p-Chloro-amphetamine—similarities and dissimilarities to amphetamine. In: *Amphetamines and Related Compounds,* edited by E. Costa and S. Garattini, pp. 343–347. Raven Press, New York.
213. Friedman, E., Starr, N., and Gershon, S. (1973): Catecholamine synthesis and the regulation of food intake in the rat. *Life Sci.,* 12:317–326.
214. Friedman, M. I. (1972): Effects of alloxan diabetes on hypothalamic hyperphagia and obesity. *Am. J. Physiol.,* 222:174–178.
215. Friedman, M. I. (1975): Some determinants of milk ingestion in suckling rats. *J. Comp. Physiol. Psychol.,* 89:636–647.
216. Friedman, M. I., and Stricker, E. M. (1976): The physiological psychology of hunger: A physiological perspective. *Psychol. Rev. (in press).*
217. Frohman, L. A., and Bernardis, L. L. (1971): Effect of hypothalamic stimulation on plasma glucose, insulin, and glucagon levels. *Am. J. Physiol.,* 221:1596–1603.
218. Frohman, L. A., Goldman, J. K., Schnatz, J. D., and Bernardis, L. L. (1971): Hypothalamic obesity in the weanling rat: Effect of diet upon the hormonal and metabolic alterations. *Metabolism,* 20:501–506.

219. Fryer, J. H., Moore, N. S., Williams, H. H., and Young, C. M. (1955): A study of the interrelationship of the energy yielding nutrients, blood glucose levels and subjective appetite in man. *J. Lab. Clin. Med.*, 45:684–696.
220. Fujimori, K., and Iwamoto, T. (1974): Mechanisms of hyperglycemic response to chlorpromazine administered into lateral ventricle in rats. II. Secretion of epinephrine from adrenal medulla. *Neuropharmacology*, 13:255–260.
221. Fuller, J. L. (1972): Genetic obesity in animals. *Adv. Psychosom. Med.*, 7:3–24.
222. Fuxe, K. (1965): Evidence for the existence of monoamine-containing neurons in the central nervous system. IV. Distribution of monoamine nerve terminals in the central nervous system. *Acta Physiol. Scand.*, 64:37–85.
223. Galef, B. G. (1976): Mechanism for the transmission of acquired patterns of feeding from adult to weanling rats. In: *Taste and Development: The Genesis of Sweet Preference*, edited by J. M. Weiffenbach. Government Printing Office, Washington, D. C. *(in press).*
224. Galef, B. G., and Clark, M. M. (1971): Parent-offspring interactions determine time and place of first ingestion of solid food by wild rat pups. *Psychonom. Sci.*, 25:15–16.
225. Galef, B. G., and Clark, M. M. (1971): Social factors in the poison avoidance and feeding behavior of wild and domestic rat pups. *J. Comp. Physiol. Psychol.*, 75:358–362.
226. Galef, B. G., and Clark, M. M. (1972): Mother's milk and adult presence: Two factors determining initial dietary selection by weanling rats. *J. Comp. Physiol. Psychol.*, 78:2202–2225.
227. Galef, B. G., and Sherry, D. F. (1973): Mother's milk: A medium for the transmission of cues reflecting the flavor of mother's diet. *J. Comp. Physiol. Psychol.*, 83:374–378.
228. Galicich, J. H., Halberg, F., and French, L. A. (1963): Circadian adrenal cycle in mice kept without food and water for a day and a half. *Nature (Lond.)*, 197:811–812.
229. Garcia, J., and Koelling, R. A. (1967): A comparison of aversion induced by x-rays, toxins, and drugs in the rat. *Radiat. Res.*, 7:439–450.
230. Garcia, J., Ervin, F. R., and Koelling, R. A. (1966): Learning with prolonged delay of reinforcement. *Psychonom. Sci.*, 5:121–122.
231. Garcia, J., Hankins, W. G., and Rusiniak, K. W. (1974): Behavioral regulation of the milieu interne in man and rat. *Science*, 185:824–831.
232. Garcia, J., Kimeldorf, D. J., and Hunt, E. L. (1961): The use of ionizing radiation as a motivating stimulus. *Psychol. Rev.*, 68:383–385.
233. Gentry, R. T., and Wade, G. N. (1976): Androgenic control of food intake and body weight in male rats. *J. Comp. Physiol. Psychol.* 90:18–25.
234. Ghosh, M. N., and Parvathy, S. (1973): The effect of cyproheptadine on water and food intake and on body weight in the fasted adult and weanling rats. *Br. J. Pharmacol.*, 48:328–329.
235. Gibbs, J., Young, R. C., and Smith, G. P. (1973): Cholecystokinin decreases food intake in rats. *J. Comp. Physiol. Psychol.*, 84:488–495.
236. Gilbert, T. F., and James, W. T. (1956): The dependency of cyclical feeding behavior on internal and external cures. *J. Comp. Physiol. Psychol.*, 49:324–344.
237. Gilboe, D. D., and Betz, A. L. (1970): Kinetics of glucose transport in the isolated dog brain. *Am. J. Physiol.*, 219:774–778.
238. Gladfelter, W. E., and Brobeck, J. R. (1962): Decreased spontaneous locomotor activity in the rat induced by hypothalamic lesions. *Am. J. Physiol.*, 203:811–817.
239. Glick, A., and Mayer, J. (1968): Hyperphagia caused by cerebral ventricular infusions of phloridzin. *Nature (Lond.)*, 219:1374.
240. Glickman, N., Mitchell, H. N., Lambert, E. H., and Keeton, R. W. (1948): The total specific dynamic action of high protein and high carbohydrate diets on human subjects. *J. Nutr.*, 36:41–57.
241. Glowinski, J., and Baldessarini, R. J. (1966): Metabolism of norepinephrine in the central nervous system. *Pharmacol. Rev.*, 18:1201–1238.
242. Glucksma, M. L. (1972): Psychiatric observations in obesity. *Adv. Psychosom. Med.*, 7:194–216.
243. Gold, A. M. (1970): Hypothalamic hyperphagia: Males get just as fat as females. *J. Comp. Physiol. Psychol.*, 71:347–356.
244. Gold, A. M. (1973): Hypothalamic obesity following knife cuts that minimize arterial damage. *Physiol. Behav.*, 10:403–406.

245. Gold, R. M. (1973): Hypothalamic obesity: The myth of the ventromedial nucleus. *Science,* 182:488–490.
246. Goldman, H. W., Lehr, D., and Friedman, E. (1971): Antagonistic effects of alpha and beta-adrenergically coded hypothalamic neurons on consummatory behaviour in the rat. *Nature (Lond.),* 231:453–455.
247. Goldman, J. K., Schnatz, J. D., Bernardis, L. L., and Frohman, L. A. (1970): Adipose tissue metabolism of weanling rats after destruction of ventromedial hypothalamic nuclei: Effect of hypophysectomy and growth hormone. *Metabolism,* 19:995–1005.
248. Goldman, J. K., Schnatz, J. D., Bernardis, L. L., and Frohman, L. A. (1972): Effects of ventromedial hypothalamic destruction in rats with pre-existing streptozotocin-induced diabetes. *Metabolism,* 21:132–136.
249. Goldstein, R., Hill, S. Y., and Templer, D. I. (1970): Effect of food deprivation on hypothalamic self-stimulation in stimulus-bound eaters and non-eaters. *Physiol. Behav.,* 5:915–918.
250. Gonzalez, M. F., and Novin, D. (1974): Feeding induced by intracranial and intravenously administered 2-deoxy-D-glucose. *Physiol. Psychol.,* 2:326–330.
251. Grant, L. D., and Jarrard, L. E. (1968): Functional dissociation within hippocampus. *Brain Res.,* 10:392–401.
252. Green, H., Greenberg, S. M., Erickson, R. W., Sawyer, J. L., and Ellison, T. (1962): Effects of dietary phenylalanine and tryptophan upon rat brain amine levels. *J. Pharmacol. Exp. Ther.,* 136:174–178.
253. Greengard, P., and Kababian, J. W. (1974): Role of cyclic AMP in synaptic transmission in the mammalian peripheral nervous system. *Fed. Proc.,* 33:1059–1067.
254. Grossie, J., and Turner, C. W. (1961): Effect of hyperthyroidism on body weight gain and feeding consumption in male and female rats. *Proc. Soc. Exp. Biol. Med.,* 107:520.
255. Grossie, J., and Turner, C. W. (1965): Effect of thyroxine, hydrocortisone, and growth hormone on food intake in rats. *Proc. Soc. Exp. Biol. Med.,* 118:28.
256. Grossman, M. I. (1955): Integration of current views on the regulation of hunger and appetite. *Ann. NY Acad. Sci.,* 63:76–89.
257. Grossman, S. P. (1960): Eating or drinking elicited by direct adrenergic or cholinergic stimulation of hypothalamic mechanisms. *Science,* 132:301–302.
258. Grossman, S. P. (1962): Direct adrenergic and cholinergic blocking agents on hypothalamic mechanisms. *Am. J. Physiol.,* 202:872–882.
259. Grossman, S. P. (1962): Effects of adrenergic and cholinergic blocking drugs on hypothalamic mechanisms. *Am. J. Physiol.,* 202:1230–1236.
260. Grossman, S. P. (1964): Behavioral effects of chemical stimulation of the ventral amygdala. *J. Comp. Physiol. Psychol.,* 57:29–36.
261. Grossman, S. P. (1968): Hypothalamic and limbic influences on food intake. *Fed. Proc.,* 27:1349–1360.
262. Grossman, S. P. (1969): A neuropharmacological analysis of hypothalamic and extrahypothalamic mechanisms concerned with the regulation of food and water intake. *Ann. NY Acad. Sci.,* 157:902–917.
263. Grossman, S. P. (1971): Changes in food and water intake associated with an interruption of the anterior or posterior fiber connections of the hypothalamus. *J. Comp. Physiol. Psychol.,* 75:23–31.
264. Grossman, S. P. (1975): Role of the hypothalamus in the regulation of food and water intake. *Psychol. Rev.,* 82:200–224.
265. Grossman, S. P., and Grossman, L. (1973) Persisting deficits in rats "recovered" from transections of fibers which enter or leave hypothalamus laterally. *J. Comp. Physiol. Psychol.,* 85:515–527.
266. Grunt, J. A. (1964): Effects of adrenalectomy and gonadectomy on growth and development in the rat. *Endocrinology,* 75:446–451.
267. Hahn, P., and Koldovsky, O. (1966): *Utilization of Nutrients During Postnatal Development.* Pergamon Press, Oxford.
268. Hales, C. N., and Kennedy, G. C. (1964): Plasma glucose, nonesterified fatty acids and insulin concentrations in hypothalamic-hyperphagic rats. *Biochem. J.,* 90:620–624.
269. Hall, W. G. (1975): Weaning and growth of artificially reared rats. *Science,* 190:1313–1315.
270. Halpern, B. P. (1967): Some relationships between electrophysiology and behavior in taste.

In: *The Chemical Senses and Nutrition,* edited by M. R. Kare and O. Maller, pp. 213–241. Johns Hopkins Press, Baltimore.

271. Hamilton, C. L. (1963): Interactions of food intake and temperature regulation in the rat. *J. Comp. Physiol. Psychol.,* 56:476–488.

272. Hamilton, C. L. (1964): Rat's preference for high fat diets. *J. Comp. Physiol. Psychol.,* 58:459–460.

273. Hamilton, C. L. (1967): Food and temperature. In: *Handbook of Physiology,* Sect. 6, Vol. 1, edited by C. F. Code, pp. 303–317. American Physiological Society, Washington, D. C.

274. Hamilton, C. L., and Brobeck, J. R. (1962): Temperature response of tube-fed rats. *Am. J. Physiol.,* 203:383–384.

275. Hamilton, C. L., and Brobeck, J. R. (1964): Food intake and temperature regulation in rats with rostral hypothalamic lesions. *Am. J. Physiol.,* 207:291–297.

276. Hamilton, C. L., and Ciaccia, B. J. (1971): Hypothalamus, temperature regulation, and feeding in the rat. *Am. J. Physiol.,* 221:800–807.

277. Han, P. W. (1968): Energy metabolism of tube-fed hypophysectomized rats bearing hypothalamic lesions. *Am. J. Physiol.,* 215:1343–1350.

278. Han, P. W., and Young, T. K. (1964): Obesity in rats without hyperphagia following hypothalamic lesions. *Clin. J. Physiol.,* 19:149–172.

279. Han, P. W., Mu, J. Y., and Lepkovsky, S. (1963): Food intake of parabiotic rats. *Am. J. Physiol.,* 205:1139–1143.

280. Hanson, M. E., and Grossman, M. I. (1948): The failure of intravenous glucose to inhibit food intake in the dog. *Fed. Proc.,* 7:50.

281. Harper, A. E. (1967): Effects of dietary protein content and amino acid pattern on food intake and preference. In: *Handbook of Physiology,* Sect. 6, Vol. 1, edited by C. F. Code, pp. 399–410. American Physiological Society, Washington, D. C.

282. Harper, A. E. (1976): Protein and amino acids in the regulation of food intake. In: *Hunger: Basic Mechanisms and Clinical Implications,* edited by D. Novin, W. Wyrwicka, and G. Bray, pp. 103–113. Raven Press, New York.

283. Harper, A. E., Benevenga, N. J., and Wohlhueter, R. M. (1970): Effects of ingestion of disproportionate amounts of amino acids. *Physiol. Rev.,* 50:428–558.

284. Harrell, L. E., Raubeson, R., and Balagura, S. (1974): Acceleration of functional recovery following lateral hypothalamic damage by means of electrical stimulation in the lesioned areas. *Physiol. Behav.,* 12:897–899.

285. Harris, L. J., Clay, J., Hargreaves, F. J., and Ward, A. (1933): Appetite and choice of diet: The ability of the vitamin-B deficient rat to discriminate between diets containing and lacking the vitamin. *Proc. R. Soc. Lond. [Biol.],* 113:161–190.

286. Harvey, J. A., and McMaster, S. E. (1975): Fenfluramine: Evidence for a neurotoxic action on midbrain and a long-term depletion of serotonin. *Psychopharmacol. Comm.,* 1:217–228.

287. Harvey, J. A., McMaster, S. E., and Yunger, L. M. (1975): p-Chloramphetamine: Selective neurotoxic action in brain. *Science,* 187:841–843.

288. Hausberger, F. X., and Hausberger, B. C. (1960): The etiologic mechanism of some forms of hormonally-induced obesity. *Am. J. Clin. Nutr.,* 8:671–679.

289. Haymaker, W., Anderson, E., and Nauta, W. J. H., editors (1969): *The Hypothalamus.* Charles C Thomas, Springfield, Ill.

290. Heimburg, R. von, and Hollerbeck, G. (1964): Inhibition of gastric secretion in dogs by glucagon given intraportally. *Gastroenterology,* 47:531–535.

291. Herbai, G. (1970): Weight loss in obese-hyperglycemic and normal mice following transauricular hypophysectomy by a modified technique. *Acta Endocrinol. (Kbh.),* 65:712–722.

292. Herberg, L. J., and Blundell, J. E. (1967): Lateral hypothalamus—hoarding behavior elicited by electrical stimulation. *Science,* 155:349–350.

293. Herrero, S. (1969): Radio-frequency-current and direct-current lesions in the ventromedial hypothalamus. *Am. J. Physiol.,* 217:403–410.

294. Hervey, G. R. (1959): The effects of lesions in the hypothalamus in parabiotic rats. *J. Physiol. (Lond.),* 145:336–352.

295. Hervey, G. R. (1969): Regulation of energy balance. *Nature (Lond.),* 222:629–631.

296. Hervey, E., and Hervey, G. R. (1966): The relationship between effects of ovariectomy and progesterone treatment on body weight and composition in the female rat. *J. Physiol. (Lond.),* 187:44–45.

297. Hetherington, A. W. (1943): The production of hypothalamic obesity in rats already displaying chronic hypopituitarism. *Am. J. Physiol.,* 140:89–92.
298. Hetherington, A. W. (1944): Non-production of hypothalamic obesity in the rat by lesions rostral or dorsal to the ventromedial hypothalamic nuclei. *J. Comp. Neurol.,* 80:33–45.
299. Hetherington, A. W., and Ranson, S. W. (1939): Experimental hypothalamo-hypophyseal obesity in the rat. *Proc. Soc. Biol. Med.,* 41:465–466.
300. Hetherington, A. W. and Ranson, S. W. (1940): Hypothalamic lesions and adiposity in the rat. *Anat. Rec.,* 78:149–154.
301. Hetherington, A. W., and Ranson, S. W. (1942): The relation of various hypothalamic lesions to adiposity in the rat. *J. Comp. Neurol.,* 76:475–499.
302. Hetherington, A. W., and Ranson, S. W. (1942): The spontaneous activity and food intake of rats with hypothalamic lesions. *Am. J. Physiol.,* 136:609–617.
303. Himwich, H. E., Bowman, K. M., Davy, C., Fazwkas, J. F., Wortis, J., and Goldfarb, W. (1941): Cerebral blood flow and brain metabolism during insulin hypoglycemia. *Am. J. Physiol.,* 132:640–647.
304. Hirsch, E., and Collier, G. (1974): The ecological determinants of reinforcement in the guinea pig. *Physiol. Behav.,* 12:239–249.
305. Hirsch, J., and Han, R. (1969): Cellularity of rat adipose tissue: Effects of growth, starvation, and obesity. *J. Lipid Res.* 10:77–82.
306. Hirsch, J., and Knittle, J. L. (1970): Cellularity of obese and non-obese human adipose tissue. *Fed. Proc.,* 29:1516–1521.
307. Hochman, C. H. (1964): EEG and behavioral effects of food deprivation in the albino rat. *Electroencephalogr. Clin. Neurophysiol.,* 17:420–427.
308. Hoebel, B. G. (1968): Inhibition and disinhibition of self-stimulation and feeding: Hypothalamic control and postingestional factors. *J. Comp. Physiol. Psychol.,* 66:89–100.
309. Hoebel, B. G. (1969): Feeding and self-stimulation. *Ann. NY Acad. Sci.,* 157:758–777.
310. Hoebel, B. G. (1971): Feeding: Neural control of intake. *Annu. Rev. Physiol.,* 33:533–568.
311. Hoebel, B. G. (1976): Satiety: hypothalamic stimulation, anorectic drugs, and neurochemical substrates. In: *Hunger: Basic Mechanisms and Clinical Implications,* edited by D. Novin, W. Wyrwicka, and G. Bray, pp. 33–50. Raven Press, New York.
312. Hoebel, B. G., and Teitelbaum, P. (1962): Hypothalamic control of feeding and self stimulation. *Science,* 135:375–377.
313. Hoebel, B. G. and Teitelbaum, P. (1966): Weight regulation in normal and hypothalamic hyperphagic rats. *J. Comp. Physiol. Psychol.,* 61:189–193.
314. Hoebel, B. G., and Thompson, R. D. (1969): Aversion to lateral hypothalamic stimulation caused by intragastric feeding or obesity. *J. Comp. Physiol. Psychol.,* 68:536–543.
315. Hokfelt, B., and Bydgeman, R. (1961): Increased adrenaline production following administration of 2-deoxy-D-glucose in the rat. *Proc. Soc. Exp. Biol. Med.,* 106:537–539.
316. Holeckova, E., and Fabry, P. (1959): Hyperphagia and gastric hypertrophy in rats adapted to intermittent starvation. *Br. J. Nutr.,* 13:260–266.
317. Hollifield, G. (1968): Glucocorticoid-induced obesity: A model and a challenge. *Am. J. Clin. Nutr.,* 21:1471–1474.
318. Hollister, A. S., Ervin, G. N., Cooper, B. R., and Breese, G. R. (1975): The roles of monoamine neural systems in the anorexia induced by (+)-amphetamine and related compounds. *Neuropharmacology,* 14:715–723.
319. Hongslo, C. F., Hustvedt, B. E., and Lovo, A. (1974): Insulin sensitivity in rats with ventromedial hypothalamic lesions. *Acta Physiol. Scand.,* 90:757–763.
320. Horton, E. S., Danforth, E., Jr., Sims, E. A. H., and Salans, L. B. (1974): Endocrine and metabolic alterations associated with overfeeding and obesity in man. In: *Obesity Symposium,* edited by W. L. Burland, pp. 229–252. Churchill Livingstone, New York.
321. Horton, E. W. (1969): Hypothesis on physiological roles of prostaglandins. *Physiol. Rev.,* 49:122–161.
322. Houpt, K. A., and Epstein, A. N. (1973): Ontogeny of controls of food intake in the rat: GI fill and glucoprivation. *Am. J. Physiol.,* 225:58–66.
323. Houpt, K. A., and Houpt, T. R. (1975): Effects of gastric loads and food deprivation on subsequent food intake in suckling rats. *J. Comp. Physiol. Psychol.,* 88:764–772.
324. Houpt, T. R., and Hance, H. E. (1971): Stimulation of feed intake in the rabbit and rat by

inhibition of glucose metabolism with 2-deoxy-D-glucose. *J. Comp. Physiol. Psychol.,* 76:395–400.

325. Hunt, C. E., Lindsey, J. R., and Walkley, S. U. (1976): Animal models of diabetes and obesity, including the PBB/Ld mouse. *Fed. Proc.,* 35:1206–1217.
326. Hunter, W. M., Friend, J. A. R., and Strong, J. A. (1966): The diurnal pattern of plasma growth hormone concentration in adults. *J. Endocrinol.,* 34:139–157.
327. Hustvedt, B. E., and Lovo, A. (1972): Correlation between hyperinsulinemias and hyperphagia in rats with ventromedial hypothalamic lesions. *Acta Physiol. Scand.,* 84:29–33.
328. Hustvedt, B. E., and Lovo, A. (1973): Rapid effect of ventromedial hypothalamic lesions on lipogenesis in rats. *Acta Physiol. Scand.,* 87:28A–29A.
329. Inglefinger, F. J. (1944): The late effects of total and subtotal gastrectomy. *N. Engl. J. Med.,* 231:321–327.
330. Jacobs, H. L. (1964): Observations on the ontogeny of saccharine preference in the neonate rat. *Psychonom. Sci.,* 1:105–106.
331. Jacobs, H. L. (1967): Taste and the role of experience in the regulation of food intake. In: *The Chemical Senses and Nutrition,* edited by M. R. Kare and O. Maller, pp. 187–200. Johns Hopkins Press, Baltimore.
332. Jacobs, H. L., and Sharma, K. N. (1969): Taste versus calories: Sensory and metabolic signals in the control of food intake. *Ann. NY Acad. Sci.,* 157:1084–1125.
333. Jalowiec, J. E., Panksepp, J., Shabshelowitz, H., Zolovick, A. J., Stern, W. and Morgane, P. J. (1973): Suppression of feeding in cats following 2-deoxy-d-glucose. *Physiol. Behav.,* 10:805–807.
334. Jankowiak, R., and Stern, J. J. (1974): Food intake and body weight modifications following medial hypothalamic hormone implants in female rats. *Physiol. Behav.,* 12:875–879.
335. Janowitz, H. D. (1958): Hunger and appetite. *Am. J. Med.,* 25:327–332.
336. Janowitz, H. D. (1967): Role of the gastrointestinal tract in regulation of food intake. In: *Handbook of Physiology,* Sect. 6, Vol. 1, edited by C. F. Code, pp. 219–224. American Physiological Society, Washington, D. C.
337. Janowitz, H. D., and Grossman, M. I. (1948): Effect of parenteral administration of glucose and protein hydrolysate on food intake of the rat. *Am. J. Physiol.,* 155:28–32.
338. Janowitz, H. D., and Grossman, M. I. (1948): Relation of blood sugar to spontaneous and insulin-induced hunger sensations. *Am. J. Physiol.,* 155:446–455.
339. Janowitz, H. D., and Grossman, M. I. (1949): Some factors affecting the food intake of normal dogs and dogs with esophagostomy and gastric fistula. *Am. J. Physiol.,* 159:143–148.
340. Janowitz, H. D., and Ivy, A. C., Jr. (1949): Role of blood-sugar levels in spontaneous and insulin-induced hunger in man. *J. Appl. Physiol,* 1:643.
341. Johnson, J. T., and Levine, S. (1973): Influence of water deprivation on adrenocortical rhythms. *Neuroendrocrinology,* 11:268–276.
342. Johnson, M. L., Burke, B. S., and Mayer, J. (1956): Relative importance of inactivity and obesity in the energy balance of obese high school girls. *Am. J. Clin. Nutr.,* 4:37–40.
343. Johnson, P. R., Zucker, L. M., Cruce, J. A. F., and Hirsch, J. (1971): Cellularity of adipose depots in the genetically obese Zucker rat. *J. Lipid Res.,* 12:706–720.
344. Jonsson, G., Malmfors, T., and Sachs, C., editors (1975): *Chemical Tools in Catecholamine Research,* Vol. 1. North Holland Publishing, Amsterdam.
345. Jordan, H. A. (1969): Voluntary intragastric feeding: Oral and gastric contributions to food intake and hunger in man. *J. Comp. Physiol. Psychol.,* 68:498–506.
346. Joseph, S. A., and Kniggle, J. M. (1968): Effects of VMH lesions in adult and newborn guinea pigs. *Neuroendocrinology,* 3:309–331.
347. Kakolewski, J. W., Cox, V. C., and Valenstein, E. S. (1968): Sex differences in body weight change following gonadectomy of rats. *Psychol. Rep.,* 22:547–554.
348. Kakolewski, J. W., Deaux, E., Christensen, J., and Case, B. (1971): Diurnal patterns in water and feed intake and body weight changes in rats with hypothalamic lesions. *Am. J. Physiol.,* 221:711–718.
349. Kanter, G. S. (1957): Hypoglycemic effect of high environmental temperature on dogs. *Am. J. Physiol.,* 188:443–446.
350. Kastin, A. J., Redding, T. W., Hall, R., Besser, G. M., and Schally, A. V. (1975): Lipid

mobilizing hormones of the hypothalamus and pituitary. *Pharmacol. Biochem. Behav.* [*Suppl. 1*], 3:121–126.

351. Kay, D. W. K., and Schapira, K. (1972): Psychiatric observations on anorexia. *Adv. Psychosom. Med.,* 7:277–299.

352. Keesey, R. E., and Boyle, P. C. (1973): Effects of quinine-adulteration upon the body weight of LH-lesioned and intact male rats. *J. Comp. Physiol. Psychol.,* 84:38–46.

353. Keesey, R. E., and Powley, T. L. (1975): Hypothalamic regulation of body weight. *Am. Sci.,* 63:558–565.

354. Kennedy, G. C. (1950): The hypothalamic control of food intake in rats. *Proc. R. Soc. Lond.* [*Biol.*], 137:535–549.

355. Kennedy, G. C. (1953): The role of depot fat in the hypothalamic control of food intake in the rat. *Proc. R. Soc. Lond.* [*Biol.*], 140:549–553.

356. Kennedy, G. C. (1957): The development with age of hypothalamic restraint upon the appetite of the rat. *J. Endocrinol.,* 16:9–17.

357. Kennedy, G. C. (1964): Hypothalamic control of the endocrine and behavioral changes associated with oestrus in the rat. *J. Physiol. (Lond.),* 172:383–392.

358. Kennedy, G. C. (1966): Food intake, energy balance and growth. *Br. Med. Bull.,* 22:216–220.

359. Kennedy, G. C. (1967): Ontogeny of mechanisms controlling food and water intake. In: *Handbook of Physiology,* Sect. 6, Vol. 1, edited by C. F. Code, pp. 337–351. American Physiological Society, Washington, D. C.

360. Kennedy, G. C. (1969): Interactions between feeding behavior and hormones during growth. *Ann. NY Acad. Sci,* 157:1049–1061.

361. Kennedy, G. C., and Mitra, J. (1963): Hypothalamic control of energy balance and the reproductive cycle in the rat. *J. Physiol. (Lond.),* 166:395–407.

362. Kennedy, G. C., and Parker, R. A. (1963): The islets of Langerhans in rats with hypothalamic obesity. *Lancet,* 2:981.

363. Kennedy, G. C., and Parrott, D. M. V. (1958): The effects of increased appetite and of insulin on growth in the hypophysectomized rat. *J. Endocrinal.,* 17:161–166.

364. Kent, M. A., and Peters, R. H. (1973): Effects of ventromedial hypothalamic lesions on hunger-motivated behavior in rats. *J. Comp. Physiol. Psychol.,* 83:92–97.

365. Kim, K. S., Magee, D. F., and Ivy, A. C. (1952): Mechanism of difference in growth rate between male and female rats. *Am. J. Physiol.,* 169:525–530.

366. Kissileff, H. R. (1969): Food-associated drinking in the rat. *J. Comp. Physiol. Psychol.,* 67:284–300.

367. Kissileff, H. R. (1969): Oropharyngeal control of prandial drinking. *J. Comp. Physiol. Psychol.,* 67:309–319.

368. Kissileff, H. R. (1970): Free-feeding in normal and "recovered lateral" rats monitored by a pellet detecting eatometer. *Physiol. Behav.,* 5:163–173.

369. Kissileff, H. R. (1971): Acquisition of prandial drinking in weanling rats and in rats recovering from lateral hypothalamic lesions. *J. Comp. Physiol. Psychol.,* 77:97–109.

370. Kissileff, H. R., and Epstein, A. N. (1962): Loss of salt preference in rats with lateral hypothalamic damage. *Am. Zool.,* 2:533.

371. Kissileff, H. R., and Epstein, A. N. (1969): Exaggerated prandial drinking in the "recovered lateral" rat without saliva. *J. Comp. Physiol. Psychol.,* 67:301–308.

372. Klain, G. J., and Rogers, G. B. (1970): Seasonal changes in adipose tissue lipogenesis in the hibernator. *Int. J. Biochem.,* 1:248–250.

373. Kleiber, M. (1961): *The Fire of Life.* Wiley, New York.

374. Koe, B. K., and Weissman, A. (1966): p-Chlorophenylalanine: Specific depletor of brain serotonin. *J. Pharmacol. Exp. Ther.,* 154:499–516.

375. Kohn, M. (1951): Satiation of hunger from food injected directly into the stomach versus food ingested by mouth. *J. Comp. Physiol. Psychol.,* 44:412–422.

376. Kon, S. K. (1931): The self-selection of food constituents by the rat. *Biochem. J.,* 25:473–481.

377. Kraly, F. S., and Blass, E. M. (1976): Increased feeding in rats in a low ambient temperature. In: *Hunger: Basic Mechanisms and Clinical Implications,* edited by D. Novin, W. Wyrwicka, and G. Bray, pp.77–87. Raven Press, New York.

378. Krasne, F. B. (1962): General disruption resulting from electrical stimulation of the ventro-medial hypothalamus. *Science*, 138:822–823.
379. Krebs, H., and Bindra, D. (1971): Noradrenaline and "chemical coding" of hypothalamic neurones. *Nature [New Biol.]*, 229:178–180.
380. Krebs, H., Bindra, D., and Campbell, J. F. (1969): Effects of amphetamine on neuronal activity in the hypothalamus. *Physiol. Behav.*, 4:685–691.
381. Krecek, J., and Kreckova, J. (1957): The development of the regulation of water metabolism. III. The relation between water and milk intake in infant rats. *Physiol. Bohemoslov.*, 6:26–34.
382. Kruk, Z. L. (1973): Dopamine and 5-hydroxytryptamine inhibit feeding in rats. *Nature [New Biol.]*, 246:52–53.
383. Kujalova, V., and Fabry, P. (1960): Intestinal absorption of glucose, fat, and amino acids in rats adapted to intermittent starvation. *Physiol. Bohemoslov.*, 9:35–41.
384. Kumaresan, P., and Turner, C. W. (1965): Effect of alloxan on feed consumption in rats. *Proc. Soc. Exp. Biol. Med.*, 119:400–402.
385. Kupferman, I. (1974): Feeding behavior in Aplysia: A simple system for the study of motivation. *Behav. Biol.*, 10:1–26.
386. Kurotsu, T., Takeda, M., and Ban, T. (1951): Studies on the gastrointestinal motility and hemorrhage induced by hypothalamic stimulation of rabbits. *Med. J. Osaka Univ.*, 2:97–120.
387. Landau, B. R., and Lubs, H. A. (1958): Animal responses to 2-deoxy-D-glucose administration. *Proc. Soc. Exp. Biol.*, 99:124–127.
388. Larsson, S., and Strom, L. (1957): Some characteristics of gold thioglucose obesity in the mouse. *Acta Physiol. Scand.*, 38: 398–416.
389. Lat, J. (1967): Self-selection of dietary components. In: *Handbook of Physiology*, Sect. 6, Vol. 1, edited by C. F. Code, pp. 367–386. American Physiological Society, Washington, D. C.
390. Lawrence, D. H., and Mason, W. A. (1955): Food intake in the rat as a function of deprivation intervals and feeding rhythms. *J. Comp. Physiol. Psychol.*, 48:267–271.
391. Lawrence, D. H., and Mason, W. A. (1955): Intake and weight adjustments in rats to changes in feeding schedules. *J. Comp. Physiol. Psychol.*, 48:43–46.
392. Leibowitz, S. F. (1970): Hypothalamic β-adrenergic "satiety" system antagonizes an α-adrenergic "hunger" system in the rat. *Nature (Lond.)*, 226:963–964.
393. Leibowitz, S. F. (1970): Reciprocal hunger-regulating circuits involving alpha- and beta-adrenergic receptors located, respectively, in the ventromedial and lateral hypothalamus. *Proc. Natl. Acad. Sci. USA*, 67:1063–1070.
394. Leibowitz, S. F. (1971): Hypothalamic alpha- and beta-adrenergic systems regulate both thirst and hunger in the rat. *Proc. Natl. Acad. Sci. USA*, 68:332–334.
395. Leibowitz, S. F. (1972): Central adrenergic receptors and the regulation of hunger and thirst. In: *Neurotransmitters*, Vol. 50, edited by I. J. Kopin, pp. 327–358. ARNMD, Washington, D. C.
396. Leibowitz, S. F. (1973): Adrenergic receptor mechanisms in eating and drinking. In: *The Neurosciences: Third Study Program*, edited by F. O. Schmitt and F. G. Worden, pp. 713–719. MIT Press, Cambridge, Mass.
397. Leibowitz, S. F. (1975): Amphetamine: Possible site and mode of action for producing anorexia in the rat. *Brain Res.*, 84:160–167.
398. Leibowitz, S. F. (1975): Catecholaminergic mechanisms of the lateral hypothalamus: Their role in the mediation of amphetamine anorexia. *Brain Res.*, 98:529–545.
399. Leibowitz, S. F. (1975): Ingestion in the satiated rat: Role of alpha and beta receptors in mediating effects of hypothalamic adrenergic stimulation. *Physiol. Behav.*, 14:743–754.
400. Leibowitz, S. F. (1975): Pattern of drinking and feeding produced by hypothalamic norepinephrine injection in the satiated rat. *Physiol. Behav.*, 14:731–742.
401. Leibowitz, S. F. (1976): Brain catecholaminergic mechanisms for control of hunger. In: *Hunger: Basic Mechanisms and Clinical Implications*, edited by D. Novin, W. Wyrwicka, and G. Bray, pp. 1–18. Raven Press, New York.
402. Leibowitz, S. F., and Miller, N. E. (1969): Unexpected adrenergic effect of chlorpromazine: Eating elicited by injection into rat hypothalamus. *Science*, 165:609–611.

403. LeMagnen, J. (1956): Hyperphagie provoquee chez le rat blanc par alteration du mecanisme de satiete pheripherique. *C. R. Soc. Biol. (Paris),* 150:32.
404. LeMagnen, J. (1959): Etude d'un phenomene d'appetit provisionnel. *C. R. Acad. Sci. [D] (Paris),* 249:2400–2402.
405. LeMagnen, J. (1960): Effects d'une pluralite de stimuli alimentaires sur le determinisme quantitatif de l'ingestion chez le rat blanc. *Arch. Sci. Physiol.,* 14:411–419.
406. LeMagnen, J. (1967): Habits and food intake. In: *Handbook of Physiology,* Sect. 6, Vol. 1, edited by C. F. Code, pp. 11–30. American Physiological Society, Washington, D. C.
407. LeMagnen, J. (1969): Peripheral and systemic actions of food in the caloric regulation of intake. *Ann. NY Acad. Sci.,* 157:1126–1157.
408. LeMagnen, J. (1972): Regulation of food intake. *Adv. Psychosom. Med.,* 7:73–90.
409. LeMagnen, J., and Devos, M. (1970): Metabolic correlates of the meal onset in the freefood intake of rats. *Physiol. Behav.,* 5:805–814.
410. Le Magnen, J., and Tallon, S. (1966): La periodicite spontanee de la prise d'aliments ad libitum du rat blanc. *J. Physiol. (Paris),* 58:323–349.
411. LeMagnen, J., and Tallon, S. (1968): L'effet du jeune prealable sur les caracteristiques temporelles de la prise d'aliments chez le rat. *J. Physiol. (Paris),* 60:143–154.
412. LeMagnen, J., Devos, M., Gaudilliere, J-P., Louis-Sylvestre, J., and Tallon, S. (1973): Role of a lipostatic mechanism in regulation by feeding of energy balance in rats. *J. Comp. Physiol. Psychol.,* 84:1–23.
413. Lepkovsky, S., Lyman, R., Fleming, D., Nagumo, M., and Dimick, M. M. (1957): Gastrointestinal regulation of water and its effects on food intake and rate of digestion. *Am. J. Physiol.,* 188:327–331.
414. Leshem, M. B., and Blundell, J. E. (1974): Interactive effect of (±)-fenfluramine and (+)-amphetamine on feeding in rats. *J. Pharm. Pharmacol.,* 26:905–906.
415. Leshner, A. I., and Collier, G. (1973): The effects of gonadectomy on the sex differences in dietary self-selection patterns and carcass composition of rats. *Physiol. Behav.,* 11:671–676.
416. Leung, P. M-B., and Rogers, Q. R. (1969): Food intake: Regulation by plasma amino acid pattern. *Life Sci.,* 8:1–9.
417. Leung, P. M-B., and Rogers, Q. R. (1971): Importance of prepyriform cortex in food-intake response of rats to amino acids. *Am. J. Physiol.,* 221:929–935.
418. Levin, R., and Stern, J. M. (1975): Maternal influences on ontogeny of suckling and feeding rhythms in the rat. *J. Comp. Physiol. Psychol.,* 89:711–721.
419. Levine, S. Z., and Kowlessar, O. D. (1962): World nutrition problems. *Annu. Rev. Med.,* 13:41–60.
420. Levison, M. J. Frommer, G. P., and Vance, W. B. (1973): Palatability and caloric density as determinants of food intake in hyperphagic and normal rats. *Physiol. Behav.,* 10:455–462.
421. Levitsky, D. A. (1970): Feeding patterns of rats in response to fasts and changes in environmental conditons. *Physiol. Behav.,* 5:291–300.
422. Liebelt, R. A., and Perry, J. H. (1957): Hypothalamic lesions associated with gold thioglucose-induced obesity. *Proc. Soc. Exp. Biol. Med.,* 95:774–783.
423. Liebelt, R. A., and Perry, J. H. (1967): Action of goldthioglucose on the central nervous system. In: *Handbook of Physiology,* Sect. 6, Vol. 1, edited by C. F. Code, pp. 271–286. American Physiological Society, Washington, D. C.
424. Liebelt, R. A., Schinoe, S., and Nicholson, N. (1965): Regulatory influences of adipose tissue on food intake and body weight. *Ann. NY Acad. Sci.,* 131:559–582.
425. Liebling, D. S., Eisner, J. D., Gibbs, J., and Smith, G. P. (1975): Intestinal satiety in rats. *J. Comp. Physiol. Psychol.,* 89:955–965.
426. Likuski, H. J., Debons, A. F., and Cloutier, R. J. (1967): Inhibition of gold thioglucose induced hypothalamic obesity by glucose analogues. *Am. J. Physiol.,* 212:669–676.
427. Lindvall, O., Bjorklund, A., Nobin, A., and Stenevi, O. (1974): The adrenergic innervation of the rat thalamus as revealed by the glyoxylic acid fluorescence method. *J. Comp. Neurol.,* 154:317–360.
428. Lorber, S., and Shay, H. (1965): The effect of insulin and glucose on gastric motor activity of dogs. *Gastroenterology,* 43:564–574.
429. Lorens, S. A., Sorensen, J. P., and Yunger, L. M. (1971): Behavioral and neurochemical

effects of lesions in the raphe system of the rat. *J. Comp. Physiol. Psychol.,* 77:48–52.

430. Lovett, D., and Booth, D. A. (1970). Four effects of exogenous insulin on food intake. *Q. J. Exp. Psychol.,* 22:406–419.

431. Luckhardt, A. B., and Carlson, A. J. (1915): Contributions to the physiology of the stomach. XVIII. On the chemical control of the gastric hunger mechanism. *Am. J. Physiol.,* 36:37–46.

432. Lynch, H. J. (1971): Diurnal oscillations in pineal melatonin content. *Life Sci.,* 10:791–795.

433. Lytle, L. D., and Campbell, B. A. (1975): Effects of lateral hypothalamic lesions on consummatory behavior in developing rats. *Physiol. Behav.,* 15:323–331.

434. Lytle, L. D., and Keil, F. C. (1974): Brain and peripheral monoamines: possible role in the ontogenesis of normal and drug-induced responses in the immature mammal. In: *Dynamics of Degeneration and Growth in Neurons,* edited by K. Fuxe, L. Olson, and Y. Zotterman, pp. 575–591. Pergamon Press, New York.

435. Lytle, L. D., and Wurtman, R. J. (1976): Neurotransmitter regulatory mechanisms. In: *Dahlem Workshop on Hormone and Antihormone Action at the Target Cell,* edited by J. Clark, Klee, W., Levitski, A., and Wolff, J., pp. 125–145. Dahlem Konferenzen, Berlin.

436. Lytle, L. D., McGuire, R. A., Pettibone, D., Courtright, W., and Schwartz, J. (1975): Developmental effects of 6-hydroxydopamine on temperature regulation in the rat. In: *Chemical Tools in Catecholamine Research,* Vol. 1, edited by G. Jonsson, T. Malmfors, and C. Sachs, pp. 189–196. North Holland Publishing, Amsterdam.

437. Lytle, L. D., Messing, R. B., Fisher, L., and Phebus, L. (1975): Effects of long-term corn consumption on brain serotonin and the response to electric shock. *Science,* 190:692–694.

438. Lytle, L. D., Moorcroft, W. H., and Campbell, B. A. (1971): Ontogeny of amphetamine anorexia and insulin hyperphagia in the rat. *J. Comp. Physiol. Psychol.,* 77:388–393.

439. MacKay, E. M., Calloway, J. W., and Barnes, R. H. (1940): Hyperalimentation in normal animals produced by protamine insulin. *J. Nutr.,* 20:59–66.

440. Makhlouf, G. M. (1974): The neuroendocrine design of the gut. *Gastroentereology,* 67:159–184.

441. Margules, D. L. (1969): Noradrenergic synapses for the suppression of feeding behavior. *Life Sci.,* 8:693–704.

442. Margules, D. L. (1970): Alpha-adrenergic receptors in hypothalamus for the suppression of feeding behavior by satiety. *J. Comp. Physiol. Psychol.,* 73:1–12.

443. Margules, D. L. (1970): Beta-adrenergic receptors in the hypothalamus for learned and unlearned taste aversions. *J. Comp. Physiol. Psychol.,* 73:13–21.

444. Margules, D. L., and Dragovich, J. (1973): Studies on pentolamine-induced overeating and finickiness. *J. Comp. Physiol. Psychol.,* 84:644–651.

445. Margules, D. L., and Olds, J. (1962): Identical "feeding" and "rewarding" systems in the lateral hypothalamus of rats. *Science,* 135:374–375.

446. Margules, D. L., Lewis, M. J., Dragovich, J. A., and Margules, A. S. (1972): Hypothalamic norepinephrine: Circadian rhythms and the control of feeding behavior. *Science,* 178:640–642.

447. Marks, H. E., and Remley, N. R. (1972): The effects of type of lesion and percentage body weight loss on measures of motivated behavior in rats with hypothalamic lesions. *Behav. Biol.,* 7:95–111.

448. Marshall, J. F., and Teitelbaum, P. (1974): Further analysis of sensory inattention following lateral hypothalamic damage in rats. *J. Comp. Physiol. Psychol.,* 86:375–395.

449. Marshall, J. F., Richardson, J. S., and Teitelbaum, P. (1974): Nigrostriatal bundle damage and the lateral hypothalamic syndrome. *J. Comp. Physiol. Psychol.,* 87:808–830.

450. Marshall, J. F., Turner, B. H., and Teitelbaum, P. (1971): Sensory neglect produced by lateral hypothalamic damage. *Science,* 174:523–525.

451. Marshall, N. B., and Mayer, J. (1954): Energy balance in gold thioglucose obesity. *Am. J. Physiol.,* 178:271–279.

452. Marshall, N. B., Barrnett, K. J., and Mayer, J. (1955): Hypothalamic lesions in gold thioglucose injected mice. *Proc. Soc. Exp. Biol. Med.,* 90:240–244.

453. Martin, F. H., and Baile, C. A. (1973): Feeding elicited in sheep by intrahypothalamic injections of PGE$_1$. *Experientia,* 29:306–307.

454. Martin, F. H. Seoane, J. R., and Baile, C. A. (1973): Feeding in satiated sheep elicited by intraventricular injections of CSF from fasted sheep. *Life Sci.,* 13:177–184.

455. Mayer, J. (1953): Glucostatic mechanisms in regulation of food intake. *N. Engl. J. Med.,* 249:13–16.
456. Mayer, J. (1955): Regulation of energy intake and body weight: Glucostatic theory and lipostatic hypothesis. *Ann. NY Acad. Sci.,* 63:15–42.
457. Mayer, J. (1972): General discussion, *Adv. Psychosom. Med.,* 7:322–336.
458. Mayer, J., and Arees, E. A. (1968): Ventromedial glucoreceptors system. *Fed. Proc.,* 27:1345–1348.
459. Mayer, J., and Thomas, D. W. (1967): Regulation of food intake and obesity. *Science,* 156:328–337.
460. McGinty, D., Epstein, A. N., and Teitelbaum P. (1965): The contribution of oropharyngeal sensations to hypothalamic hyperphagia. *Anim. Behav.,* 13:413–418.
461. McKeever, S. (1964): The biology of the golden-mantled ground squirrel Citellus lateralis. *Ecol. Monogr.,* 34:383–401.
462. McLeary, R. A. (1953): Taste and post-ingestion factors in specific hunger behavior. *J. Comp. Physiol. Psychol.,* 46:411–421.
463. Mellinkoff, S. M. (1957): Digestive system. *Annu. Rev. Physiol.,* 19:193–196.
464. Mellinkoff, S. M., Frankland, M., Boyle, D., and Greipel, M. (1956): Relationship between serum amino acid concentration and fluctuations in appetite. *J. Appl. Physiol.,* 8:535–538.
465. Mendelson, J. (1966): Role of hunger in T-maze learning for food by rats. *J. Comp. Physiol. Psychol.,* 62:341–349.
466. Menzel, E. W. (1961): Perception of food size in the chimpanzee. *J. Comp. Physiol. Psychol.,* 54:588–591.
467. Messing, R. B., Phebus, L., Fisher, L., and Lytle, L. D. (1976): Effects of p-chloroamphetamine on locomotor activity and brain 5-hydroxyindoles. *Neuropharmacology,* 15:157–163.
468. Meyer, J. H., and Grossman, M. I. (1972): Release of secretin and cystokinin. In: *Gastrointestinal Hormones,* edited by L. Demling, pp. 43–45. George Thieme Verlag, Stuttgart.
469. Miller, N. E. (1965): Chemical coding of behavior in the brain. *Science,* 148:328–338.
470. Miller, N. E. (1967): Behavioral and physiological technique: rationale and experimental designs for combining their use. In: *Handbook of Physiology,* Sect. 6, Vol. 1, edited by C. F. Code, pp. 51–61. American Physiological Society, Washington, D.C.
471. Miller, N. E., and Kessen, M. L. (1952): Reward effects of food via stomach fistula compared with those of food via mouth. *J. Comp. Physiol. Psychol.,* 45:555–564.
472. Miller, N. E., Bailey, C. J., and Stevenson, J. A. F. (1950): Decreased "hunger" but increased food intake resulting from hypothalamic lesions. *Science,* 112:256–259.
473. Miller, S. N., and Dymsza, H. A. (1963): Artificial feeding of neonatal rats. *Science,* 141:517.
474. Millhouse, O. E. (1969): A Golgi study of the descending medial forebrain bundle. *Brain Res.,* 15:341–363.
475. Millhouse, O. E. (1973): Certain ventromedial hypothalamic afferents. *Brain Res.,* 55:89–105.
476. Millhouse, O. E. (1973): The organization of the ventromedial hypothalamic nucleus. *Brain Res.,* 55:71–87.
477. Miselis, R. R., and Epstein, A. N. (1970): Feeding induced by 2-deoxy-D-glucose injections into the lateral ventricle of the rat. *Physiologist,* 13:262.
478. Molinoff, P. B., and Axelrod, J. (1971): Biochemistry of catecholamines. *Annu. Rev. Pharmacol.,* 40:465–500.
479. Montemurro, D. G., and Stevenson, J. A. F. (1955–1956): The localization of hypothalamic structures in the rat influencing water consumption. *Yale J. Biol. Med.,* 28:396–403.
480. Montgomery, R. G., Singer, G., Purcell, A. T., Narbeth, J., and Bolt, A. G. (1971): The effects of intrahypothalamic injections of desmethylimipramine on food and water intake of the rat. *Psychopharmacologia,* 19:81–86.
481. Mook, D. G., Kenney, N. J., Roberts, S., Nussbaum, A. I., and Rodier, W. I. (1972): Ovarian-adrenal interactions in regulation of body weight by female rats. *J. Comp. Physiol. Psychol.,* 81:198–211.
482. Moorcroft, W. H., Lytle, L. D., and Campbell, B. A. (1971): The ontogeny of hunger-induced arousal in the rat. *J. Comp. Physiol. Psychol.,* 75:59–67.

483. Moore, R. Y. (1970): Brain lesions and amine metabolism. *Int. Rev. Neurobiol.,* 13:67–91.
484. Morgane, P. J. (1961): Alterations in feeding and drinking behavior of rats with lesions in globi pallidi. *Am. J. Physiol.,* 201:420–428.
485. Morgane, P. J. (1961): Differential satiating effects of central self-stimulation and metabolic feedback products on hunger-drive mechanisms. *Am. Psychologist,* 16:414.
486. Morgane, P. J. (1961): Distinct "feeding" and "hunger motivational" systems in the lateral hypothalamus of the rat. *Science,* 133:887–888.
487. Morgane, P. J. (1964): Limbic-hypothalamic midbrain interaction in thirst and thirst motivated behavior. In: *Thirst,* edited by M. J. Wayner, pp. 429–455. Pergamon Press, New York.
488. Morgane, P. J. (1969): The function of the limbic and rhinic forebrain-limbic midbrain systems and reticular formation in the regulation of food and water intake. *Ann. NY Acad. Sci.,* 157:806–848.
489. Morgane, P. J. (1975): Anatomical and neurobiochemical bases of the central nervous control of physiological regulations and behaviour. In: *Neural Integration of Physiological Mechanisms and Behavior,* edited by G. J. Mogenson and F. Calaresu, pp. 24–67. University of Toronto Press, Toronto.
490. Morgane, P. J., and Jacobs, H. L. (1969): Hunger and satiety. *World Rev. Nutr. Diet.,* 10:100–213.
491. Morrison, S. D. (1968): The relationship of energy expenditure and spontaneous activity to the aphagia in rats with lesions in the lateral hypothalamus. *J. Physiol. (Lond.),* 197:325–343.
492. Morrison, S. D., Lin, H. J., Eckel, H. E., Van Itallie, T. B., and Mayer, J. (1958): Gastric contractions in the rat. *Am. J. Physiol.,* 193:4–8.
493. Moskowitz, H. W., Kumaraiah, V., Sharma, K. N., Jacobs, H. L., and Sharma, S. D. (1975): Cross-cultural differences in simple taste preferences. *Science,* 190:1217–1218.
494. Mrosovsky, N. (1974): Hypothalamic hyperphagia without plateau in ground squirrels. *Physiol. Behav.,* 12:259–264.
495. Murphy, J. T., and Renaud, L. P. (1969): Mechanisms of inhibition on the ventromedial nucleus of the hypothalamus. *J. Neurophysiol.,* 32:85–102.
496. Myers, R. D. (1967): Transfusion of cerebrospinal fluid and tissue bound chemical factors between the brains of conscious monkeys: A new neurobiological assay. *Physiol. Behav.,* 2:373–377.
497. Myers, R. D. (1969): Chemical mechanisms in the hypothalamus mediating eating and drinking in the monkey. *Ann. NY Acad. Sci.,* 157:918–932.
498. Myers, R. D. (1975): Brain mechanisms in the control of feeding: A new neurochemical profile theory. *Pharmacol. Biochem. Behav.,* 3:75–83.
499. Myers, R. D. (1975): Impairment of thermoregulation, food and water intakes in the rat after hypothalamic injections of 5,6-dihydroxytryptamine. *Brain Res.,* 94:491–506.
500. Myers, R. D., and Martin, G. E. (1973): 6-OHDA lesions of the hypothalamus: Interaction of aphagia, food palatability, set point for weight regulation, and recovery of feeding. *Pharmacol. Biochem. Behav.,* 1:329–345.
501. Myers, R. D., and Yaksh, T. L. (1968): Feeding and temperature responses in the unrestrained rat after injections of cholinergic and aminergic substances into the cerebral ventricles. *Physiol. Behav.,* 3:917–928.
502. Nachman, M. (1959): The inheritance of saccharin preference. *J. Comp. Physiol. Psychol.,* 52:451–457.
503. Nachman, M. (1962): Taste preferences for sodium salts by adrenalectomized rats. *J. Comp. Physiol. Psychol.,* 55:1124–1129.
504. Nance, D. M., Gorski, R. A., and Panksepp, J. (1976): Neural and hormonal determinants of sex differences in food intake and body weight. In: *Hunger: Basic Mechanisms and Clinical Implications,* edited by D. Novin, W. Wyrwicka, and G. Bray, pp. 257–271. Raven Press, New York.
505. Narang, G. D., Singh, D. V., and Turner, C. W. (1967): Effect of melatonin on thyroid hormone secretion rate and feed consumption of female rats. *Soc. Exp. Biol. and Med.,* 125:184–188.
506. Nauta, W. J. H., and Haymaker, W. (1969): Hypothalamic nuclei and fiber connections. In:

*The Hypothalamus,* edited by W. Haymaker, E. Anderson, and W. J. H. Nauta, pp. 136–209. Charles C Thomas, Springfield, Ill.

507. Neill, D. B., Parker, S. D., and Gold, M. S. (1975): Striatal dopaminergic modulation of lateral hypothalamic self-stimulation. *Pharmacol. Biochem. Behav.,* 3:485–491.

508. Nicolaidis, S., and Meile, M. J. (1972): Cartographie des lesions hypothalamiques supprimant la response alimentaire aux injections intracardiques du 2-deoxy-D-glucose. *J. Physiol. (Paris),* 65:151A.

509. Niijima, A. (1969): Afferent impulse discharges from glucoreceptors in the liver of the guinea pig. Ann. NY Acad. Sci., 157:690–700.

510. Nisbett, R. (1969): Determinants of food intake in human obesity. *Science,* 159:1254–1255.

511. Nisbett, R. (1969): Taste, deprivation, and weight determinants of eating behavior. *J. Person. Soc. Psychol.,* 10:107–116.

512. Nisbett, R. E. (1972): Eating behavior and obesity in men and animals. *Adv. Psychosom. Med.,* 7:173–193.

513. Nisbett, R. E., and Gurwitz, S. (1970): Weight, sex and the eating behavior of human newborns. *J. Comp. Physiol. Psychol.,* 73:245–253.

514. Norgren, R. (1974): Gustatory afferents to ventral forebrain. *Brain Res.,* 81:285–295.

515. Norgren, R., and Leonard, C. M. (1971): Taste pathways in rat brainstem. *Science,* 173:1136–1139.

516. Norgren, R., and Leonard, C. M. (1973): Ascending central gustatory pathways. *J. Comp. Neurol.,* 150:217–237.

517. Novin, D. (1976): Visceral mechanisms in the control of food intake. In: *Hunger: Basic Mechanisms and Clinical Implications,* edited by D. Novin, W. Wyrwicka, and G. Bray, pp. 357–367. Raven Press, New York.

518. Novin, D., Sanderson, J. D., and Vander Weele, D. A. (1974): The effect of isotonic glucose on eating as a function of feeding condition and infusion site. *Physiol. Behav.,* 13:3–7.

519. Novin, D., Vander Weele, D., and Rezek, M. (1973): Hepatic-portal 2-deoxy-D-glucose infusion causes eating: Evidence for peripheral glucoreceptors. *Science,* 181:858–860.

520. Oakley, B., and Pfaffmann, C. (1962): Electrophysiologically monitored lesions in the gustatory thalamic relay of the albino rat. *J. Comp. Physiol. Psychol.,* 55:155–160.

521. Odum, E. P. (1960): Premigratory hyperphagia in birds. *Am. J. Clin. Nutr.,* 8:621–629.

522. Olds, J. (1969): Central nervous system and the reinforcement of behavior. *Am. Psychol.,* 24:114–132.

523. Oltmans, G. A., and Harvey, J. A. (1972): LH syndrome and brain catecholamine levels after lesions of the nigrostriatal bundle. *Physiol. Behav.,* 8:69–78.

524. Oomura, Y., Ono, T., Ooyama, H., and Wayner, M. J. (1969): Glucose and osmosensitive neurons of the rat hypothalamus. *Nature (Lond.),* 222:282–284.

525. Oomura, Y., Ooyama, H., Yamamoto, T., and Naka, F. (1967): Reciprocal relationship of the lateral and ventromedial hypothalamus in the regulation of food intake. *Physiol. Behav.,* 2:97–115.

526. Osborne, T. B., and Mendel, L. B. (1918): The choice between adequate and inadequate diets, as made by rats. *J. Biol. Chem.,* 35:19–27.

527. Palka, Y., Liebelt, R. A., and Critchlow, V. (1971): Obesity and increased growth following partial or complete isolation of ventromedial hypothalamus. *Physiol. Behav.,* 7:187–194.

528. Panksepp, J. (1971): A re-examination of the role of the ventromedial hypothalamus in feeding behavior. *Physiol. Behav.,* 7:385–394.

529. Panksepp, J. (1971): Effects of fats, proteins, and carbohydrates on food intake in rats. *Psychonom. Monogr. (Suppl.),* 4:85–95.

530. Panksepp, J. (1971): Is satiety mediated by the ventromedial hypothalamus? *Physiol. Behav.,* 7:381–384.

531. Panksepp, J. (1972): Hypothalamic radioactivity after intragastric glucose-$^{14}$C in rats. *Am. J. Physiol.,* 223:396–401.

532. Panksepp, J. (1973): Reanalysis of feeding patterns in the rat. *J. Comp. Physiol. Psychol.,* 82:78–94.

533. Panksepp, J. (1973): The ventromedial hypothalamus and metabolic adjustments of feeding behavior. *Behav. Biol.,* 9:65–75.

534. Panksepp, J. (1974): Hypothalamic regulation of energy balance and feeding behavior. *Fed. Proc.*, 33:1150–1165.
535. Panksepp, J. (1975): Central metabolic and humoral factors involved in the neural regulation of feeding. *Pharmacol. Biochem. Behav.*, 3:107–119.
536. Panksepp, J. (1975): Hormonal control of feeding behavior and energy balance. In: *Hormonal Correlates of Behavior, Vol. 2: An Organismic View*, edited by B. E. Eleftheriou and R. L. Sprott, pp. 657–695. Plenum Press, New York.
537. Panksepp, J. (1975): Metabolic hormones and regulation of feeding: A reply to Woods, Decke, and Vasselli. *Psychol. Rev.*, 82:158–164.
538. Panksepp, J. (1976): On the nature of feeding patterns—primarily in rats. In: *Hunger: Basic Mechanisms and Clinical Implications*, edited by D. Novin, W. Wyrwicka, and G. Bray, pp. 369–382. Raven Press, New York.
539. Panksepp, J., and Booth, D. A. (1971): Decreased feeding after injections of amino acids into the hypothalamus. *Nature (Lond.)*, 233:341–342.
540. Panksepp, J., and Nance, D. M. (1972): Insulin, glucose and hypothalamic regulation of feeding. *Physiol. Behav.*, 9:447–451.
541. Panksepp, J., and Nance, D. M. (1974): Effects of para-chlorophenylalanine on food intake in rats. *Physiol. Psychol.*, 2:360–364.
542. Panksepp, J., and Nance, D. M. (1974): The hypothalamic $^{14}$C differential and feeding behavior. *Bull. Psychonom. Soc.*, 3:325–327.
543. Panksepp, J., and Ritter, M. (1975): Mathematical analysis of energy regulatory patterns of normal and diabetic rats. *J. Comp. Physiol. Psychol.*, 89:1019–1028.
544. Panksepp, J., Pollack, A., Krost, K., Meeker, R., and Ritter, M. (1975): Feeding in response to repeated protamine zinc insulin injections. *Physiol. Behav.*, 14:487–493.
545. Panksepp, J., Tonge, D., and Oatley, K. (1972): Insulin and glucostatic control of feeding. *J. Comp. Physiol. Psychol.*, 78:226–232.
546. Park, C. R., Johnson, L. H., Wright, J. H., Jr., and Batsel, K. (1957): Effect of insulin on transport of several hexoses and pentoses into cells of muscle and brain. *Am. J. Physiol.*, 191:13–18.
547. Passmore, R., and Ritchie, F. J. (1957): The specific dynamic action of food and the satiety mechanism. *Br. J. Nutr.*, 11:79–84.
548. Paulson, G., and Gottlieb, G. (1968): Development of reflexes: The reappearance of foetal and neonatal reflexes in aged patients. *Brain*, 91:37–52.
549. Paxinos, G., and Bindra, D. (1972): Hypothalamic knife cuts; Effects on eating, drinking irritability, aggression, and copulation in the male rat. *J. Comp. Physiol. Psychol.*, 79:219–229.
550. Penaloza-Rojas, J. H., and Russek, M. (1963): Anorexia produced by direct current blockade of the vagus nerve. *Nature (Lond.)*, 200:126.
551. Penaloza-Rojas, J. H., Barrera-Mera, B., and Kubli-Garfias, C. (1969): Behavioral and brain electrical changes after vagal stimulation. *Exp. Neurol.*, 23:378–383.
552. Penick, S. B., and Hinkle, L. E. (1961): Depression of food intake induced in healthy subjects by glucagon. *N. Engl. J. Med.*, 264:893–897.
553. Perez-Cruet, J., Tagliamonte, A., Tagliamonte, P., and Gessa, G. L. (1972): Changes in brain serotonin metabolism associated with fasting and satiation in rats. *Life Sci.*, 11:31–39.
554. Perry, J. H., and Liebelt, R. A. (1959): Extra-hypothalamic lesions in goldthioglucose induced obesity in mice. *Anat. Rec.*, 133:322.
555. Perry, J. H., Mori, A., Turner, D., and Martz, D. (1964): Brain lesions, weight change, and food and water intake in alloxanized mice treated with gold-thioglucose. *Anat. Rec.*, 148:321.
556. Pfaff, D. W. (1969): Sex differences in food intake changes following pituitary growth hormone or prolactin injections. In: *Proceedings: 77th Annual Convention, American Psychology Association*, pp. 211–212.
557. Pfaffmann, C. (1936): Differential responses of the new-born cat to gustatory stimuli. *J. Genet. Psychol.*, 49:61–67.
558. Pfaffmann, C. (1952): Taste preference and aversion following lingual denervation. *J. Comp. Physiol. Psychol.*, 45:393.
559. Pfaffmann, C. (1960): The pleasures of sensation. *Psychol. Rev.*, 65:253–268.
560. Pfaffmann, C. (1961): The sensory and motivating properties of the sense of taste. In:

*Nebraska Symposium on Motivation,* edited by M. R. Jones, pp. 71–108. University of Nebraska Press, Lincoln.

561. Phillips, A. G., and Nikaido, A. R. (1975): Disruption of brain stimulation-induced feeding by dopamine receptor blockade. *Nature (Lond.),* 258:750–751.

562. Pilgrim, F. J. (1967): Human food attitudes and consumption. In: *Handbook of Physiology,* Sect. 6, Vol. 1, edited by C. F. Code, pp. 139–146. American Physiological Society, Washington, D.C.

563. Pilgrim, F. J., and Patton, R. A. (1947): Patterns of self-selection of purified dietary components by the rat. *J. Comp. Physiol. Psychol.,* 40:343–348.

564. Plaut, M. S. (1970): Studies of undernutrition in the young rat: Methodological considerations. *Devel. Psychobiol.,* 3:157–167.

565. Pollitt, E. (1975): Failure to thrive: Socioeconomic, dietary intake and mother-child interaction data. *Fed. Proc.,* 34:1593–1597.

566. Pool, R. (1967): Suction lesions and hypothalamic hyperphagia. *Am. J. Physiol.,* 213:31–35.

567. Porter, J. H., Allen, J. D., and Arazie, R. (1974): Reinforcement frequency and body weight as determinants of motivated performance in hypothalamic hyperphagic rats. *Physiol. Behav.,* 13:627–632.

568. Powley, T. L., and Keesey, R. E. (1970): Relationship of body weight to the lateral hypothalamic feeding syndrome. *J. Comp. Physiol. Psychol.,* 70:25–36.

569. Powley, T. L., and Opsahl, C. A. (1974): Ventromedial hypothalamic obesity abolished by subdiaphragmatic vagotomy. *Am. J. Physiol.,* 226:25–33.

570. Powley, T. L., and Opsahl, C. A. (1976): Autonomic components of the hypothalamic feeding syndromes. In: *Hunger: Basic Mechanisms and Clinical Implications,* edited by D. Novin, W. Wyrwicka, and G. Bray, pp. 313–326. Raven Press, New York.

571. Price, J., and Grinker, J. (1973): Effects of degree of obesity, food deprivation, and palatability on eating behavior of humans. *J. Comp. Physiol. Psychol.,* 85:265–271.

572. Pudel, V. E. (1976): Experimental feeding in man. In: *Dahlem Workshop on Appetite and Food Intake,* edited by T. Silverstone, pp. 245–264. Dahlem Konferenzen, Berlin.

573. Putten, L. M. van, van Bekkum, D. W., and Querido, A. (1955): Influences of hypothalamic lesions producing hyperphagia, and of feeding regimens on carcass composition in the rat. *Metabolism,* 4:68–74.

574. Quaade, F., and Juhl, O. (1962): On the glucostatic theory of appetite regulation. II. Arterio-venous glucose and oxygen differences in cerebral blood of normal persons during hunger and satiety. *Am. J. Med. Sci.,* 243:438–445.

575. Quay, W. B. (1968): Individuation and lack of pineal effect in the rat's circadian locomotor rhythm. *Physiol. Behav.,* 3:109–118.

576. Quigley, J. P. (1955): The role of the digestive tract in regulating the ingestion of food. *Ann. NY Acad. Sci.,* 63:6–14.

577. Rabin, B. M. (1972): Ventromedial hypothalamic control of food intake and satiety: A reappraisal. *Brain Res.,* 43:317–342.

578. Rabin, B. M. (1974): Independence of food intake and obesity following ventromedial hypothalamic lesions in the rat. *Physiol. Behav.,* 13:769–772.

579. Rabin, B. M., and Smith, C. J. (1968): Behavioral comparison of the effectiveness of irritative and non-irritative lesions in producing hypothalamic hyperphagia. *Physiol. Behav.,* 3:417–420.

580. Rabinowitz, D., Merimee, T. J., and Burgess, J. A. (1966): Growth hormone-insulin interaction. *Diabetes,* 15:905–910.

581. Rampone, A. J., and Shirasu, M. E. (1956): Temperature changes in the rat in response to feeding. *Science,* 144:317–319.

582. Rayford, P. L., Miller, J. A., and Thompson, J. C. (1976): Secretin, cholecystokinin and newer gastrointestinal hormones. *N. Engl. J. Med.,* 294:1093–1101, 1157–1164.

583. Redding, T. W., Bowers, C. Y., and Schally, A. V. (1966): Effects of hypophysectomy on hypothalamic obesity in CBA mice. *Proc. Soc. Exp. Biol. Med.,* 121:726–729.

584. Redick, J. N., Nussbaum, A. I., and Mook, D. G. (1973): Estradiol induced suppression of feeding in the female rat: Dependence on body weight. *Physiol. Behav.,* 10:543–547.

585. Rehovsky, D. A., and Wampler, R. S. (1972): Failure to obtain sex differences in development of obesity following ventromedial hypothalamic lesions in rats. *J. Comp. Physiol. Psychol.,* 78:102–112.

586. Reinberg, A., and Halberg, F. (1971): Circadian chronopharmacology. *Annu. Rev. Pharmacol.,* 11:455–492.
587. Revusky, S. H. (1967): Hunger level during food consumption: Effects on subsequent preference. *Psychonom. Sci.,* 7:109–110.
588. Reynolds, R. W. (1959): The effect of amphetamine on food intake in normal and hypothalamic hyperphagic rats. *J. Comp. Physiol. Psychol.,* 52:682–684.
589. Reynolds, R. W. (1963): Ventromedial hypothalamic lesions without hyperphagia. *Am. J. Physiol.,* 204:60–62.
590. Reynolds, R. W. (1965): An irritative hypothesis concerning the hypothalamic regulation of food intake. *Psychol. Rev.,* 72:105–116.
591. Reynolds, R. W., and Bryson, G. (1974): Effect of estradiol on the hypothalamic regulation of body weight in the rat. *Res. Chem. Pathol. Pharmacol.,* 7:715–724.
592. Rezek, M., and Kroeger, E. A. (1976): Glucose antimetabolites and hunger (theoretical article). *J. Nutr.,* 106:143–157.
593. Rezek, M., and Novin, D. (1975): The effects of serotonin on feeding in the rabbit. *Psychopharmacologia,* 43:255–258.
594. Richter, C. P. (1922): A behavioristic study of the activity of the rat. *Comp. Psychol. Monogr.,* 1:1–55.
595. Richter, C. P. (1938): Salt taste thresholds of normal and adrenalectomized rats. *Endocrinology,* 24:367–371.
596. Richter, C. P. (1942–43): Total self-regulatory functions in animals and human beings. *Harv. Lect.,* 38:63–103.
597. Richter, C. P. (1956): Salt appetite of mammals: Its dependence on instinct and metabolism. In: *L'Instinct,* edited by M. Autuori, pp. 577–629. Masson, Paris.
598. Richter, C. P. (1967): Sleep and activity: Their relation to the 24-hour clock. *Assoc. Res. Nerv. Ment. Dis.,* 45:8–27.
599. Richter, C. P., and Barelare, B., Jr. (1938): Nutritional requirements of pregnant and lactating rats studied by the self-selection method. *Endocrinology,* 23:15–24.
600. Richter, C. P., and Eckert, J. F. (1938): Mineral metabolism of adrenalectomized rats studied by the appetite method. *Endocrinology,* 22:214–224.
601. Richter, C. P., and Uhlenhuth, G. H. (1954): Comparison of the effects of gonadectomy on spontaneous activity of wild and domesticated Norway rats. *Endocrinology,* 54:323–337.
602. Richter, C. P., Holt, L. E., Jr., and Barelare, B., Jr. (1937): Vitamin B₁ craving in rats. *Science,* 86:354–355.
603. Richter, C. P., Holt, L. E., Jr., and Barelare, B., Jr. (1938): Nutritional requirements for normal growth and reproduction in rats studied by the self-selection method. *Am. J. Physiol.,* 122:734–744.
604. Richter, C. P., Holt, L. E., Jr., Barelare, B., Jr., and Hawkes, C. D. (1938): Changes in fat, carbohydrate, and protein appetite in vitamin B deficiency. *Am. J. Physiol.,* 124:596–602.
605. Ritter, R. C., and Epstein, A. N. (1975): Control of meal size by central noradrenergic action. *Proc. Natl. Acad. Sci. USA,* 72:3740–3743.
606. Ritter, S., Wise, C. D., and Stein, L. (1975): Neurochemical regulation of feeding in the rat: Facilitation by α-noradrenergic, but not dopaminergic, receptor stimulants. *J. Comp. Physiol. Psychol.,* 88:778–784.
607. Roberts, S., Kenney, N. J., and Mook, D. G. (1972): Over-eating induced by progesterone in the ovariectomized, adrenalectomized rat. *Horm. Behav.,* 3:267–276.
608. Roberts, W. W., and Carey, R. J. (1965): Rewarding effect of performance of gnawing aroused by hypothalamic stimulation in the rat. *J. Comp. Physiol. Psychol.,* 59:317–324.
609. Roberts, W. W., Steinberg, M. L., and Means, L. W. (1967): Hypothalamic mechanisms for sexual, aggressive, and other motivational behaviors in the opossum, Didelphis virginiana, *J. Comp. Physiol. Psychol.* 64:1–15.
610. Robson, J. R. K. (1976): Commentary: Changing food habits in developing countries. *Ecol. Food Nutr.,* 4:251–256.
611. Rodgers, W. H. (1967): Specificity of specific hungers. *J. Comp. Physiol. Psychol.,* 64:49–58.
612. Rodgers, W. H., Epstein, A. N., and Teitelbaum, P. (1965): Lateral hypothalamic aphagia: Motor failure or motivational deficit? *Am. J. Physiol.,* 268:334–342.

613. Rodin, J. (1975): Causes and consequences of time perception differences in overweight and normal weight people. *J. Person. Soc. Psychol.,* 31:898–904.
614. Rodin, J. (1976): The relationship between external responsiveness and the development and maintenance of obesity. In: *Hunger: Basic Mechanisms and Clinical Implications,* edited by D. Novin, W. Wyrwicka, and G. Bray, pp. 409–419. Raven Press, New York.
615. Rodin, J. (1976): The role of perception of internal and external signals on the regulation of feeding in overweight and non-obese individuals. In: *Dahlem Workshop on Appetite and Food Intake,* edited by T. Silverstone, pp. 265–284. Dahlem Konferenzen, Berlin.
616. Rogers, Q. R., and Leung, P. M-B. (1973): The influence of amino acids on the neuroregulation of food intake. *Fed. Proc.,* 32:1709–1726.
617. Rolls, E. T. (1976): Neurophysiology of feeding. In: *Dahlem Workshop on Appetite and Food Intake,* edited by T. Silverstone, pp. 21–42. Dahlem Konferenzen, Berlin.
618. Rosenquist, A. R., and Hoebel, B. G. (1968): Wheel running elicited by electrical stimulation of the brain. *Physiol. Behav.,* 3:563–566.
619. Ross, L. (1974): Effects of manipulating the salience of food upon consumption by obese and normal eaters. In: *Obese Humans and Rats,* edited by S. Schacter and J. Rodin, pp. 89–95. Erlbaum/Halsted, Washington, D.C.
620. Roth, J., Glick, S. M., Yalow, R. S., and Berson, S. A. (1963): Secretion of growth hormone: Physiologic and experimental modification. *Metabolism,* 12:577–579.
621. Roth, S. R., Schwartz, M., and Teitelbaum, P. (1973): Failure of recovered lateral hypothalamic rats to learn specific food aversions. *J. Comp. Physiol. Psychol.,* 83:184–197.
622. Rowe, J. C., Maxwell, G. M., Castillo, C. A., Freeman, D. J., and Crumpton, C. W. (1959): A study in man of cerebral blood flow and cerebral glucose lactate and pyruvate metabolism before and after eating. *J. Clin. Invest.,* 38:2154–2158.
623. Rowland, N. E., and Antelman, S. M. (1976): Stress-induced hyperphagia and obesity in rats: A possible model for understanding human obesity. *Science,* 191:310–312.
624. Rozin, P. (1967): Specific hunger for thiamine: Recovery from deficiency and thiamine preference. *J. Comp. Physiol. Psychol.,* 59:98–101.
625. Rozin, P. (1967): Thiamine specific hunger. In: *Handbook of Physiology,* Sect. 6, Vol. 1, edited by C. F. Code, pp. 411–431. American Physiological Society, Washington, D.C.
626. Rozin, P. (1968): Specific aversions and neophobia as a consequence of vitamin deficiency and/or poisoning in half-wild and domestic rats. *J. Comp. Physiol. Psychol.,* 66:82–88.
627. Rozin, P., and Kalat, J. W. (1971): Specific hungers and poison avoidance as adaptive specializations of learning. *Psychol. Rev.,* 78:459–486.
628. Rozin, P., and Rodgers, W. H. (1967): Novel diet preferences in vitamin deficient rats and rats recovered from vitamin deficiencies. *J. Comp. Physiol. Psychol.,* 63:421–428.
629. Ruiter, L. de (1967): Feeding behavior of vertebrates in the natural environment. In: *Handbook of Physiology,* Section 6, Vol. 1, edited by C. F. Code, pp. 97–116. American Physiological Society, Washington, D.C.
630. Rusak, B., and Zucker, I. (1974): Fluid intake of rats in constant light and during feeding restricted to the light or dark portion of the illumination cycle. *Physiol. Behav.,* 13:91–100.
631. Russek, M. (1970): Demonstration of an hepatic glucosensitive mechanism on food intake. *Physiol. Behav.,* 5:1207–1209.
632. Russek, M. (1976): A conceptual equation of intake control. In: *Hunger: Basic Mechanisms and Clinical Implications,* edited by D. Novin, W. Wyrwicka, and G. Bray, pp. 327–347. Raven Press, New York.
633. Russek, M., and Morgane, J. P. (1963): Anorexic effect of intraperitoneal glucose in the hypothalamic hyperphagic cat. *Nature (Lond.),* 199:1004–1005.
634. Russek, M., and Stevenson, J. A. F. (1972): Correlation between the effects of several substances on food intake and on the hepatic concentration of reducing sugars. *Physiol. Behav.,* 8:245–249.
635. Russek, M., and Tina, S. (1962): Conditioning of adrenalin anorexia. *Nature (Lond.),* 193:1296–1297.
636. Russek, M., Mogenson, G. J., and Stevenson, J. A. F. (1967): Calorigenic, hyperglycemic, and anorexigenic effects of adrenaline and noradrenaline. *Physiol. Behav.,* 2:429–436.
637. Rutman, R. J., Lewis, F. S., and Bloomer, W. D. (1966): Bipiperidyl mustard, a new obesifying agent in the mouse. *Science,* 153:1000–1002.

638. Salans, L. B., Cushman, S. W., Horton, E. S., Danforth, E., Jr., and Sims, E. A. H. (1974): Hormones and the adipocyte: Factors influencing the metabolic effects of insulin and adrenaline. In: *Obesity Symposium,* edited by W. L. Burland, pp. 204–216. Churchill Livingstone, New York.
639. Saller, C. F., and Stricker, E. M. (1976): Hyperphagia and increased growth after intraventricular injection of 5,7-dihydroxytryptamine. *Science,* 192:385–387.
640. Salter, J. M. (1960): Metabolic effects of glucagon in the Wistar rat. *Am. J. Clin. Nutr.,* 8:535–539.
641. Samanin, R., Ghezzi, D., Valzelli, L., and Garattini, S. (1972): The effects of selective lesioning of brain serotonin or catecholamine containing neurones on the anorectic activity of fenfluramine and amphetamine. *Eur. J. Pharmacol.,* 19:318–322.
642. Sanders-Bush, E., and Sulser, F. (1970): p-Chloramphetamine: In vivo investigations on the mechanism of action of the selective depletion of cerebral serotonin. *J. Pharmacol. Exp. Ther.,* 175:419–426.
643. Sanghvi, I. S., Singer, G., Friedman, E., and Gershon, S. (1975): Anorexigenic effects of d-amphetamine and l-dopa in the rat. *Pharmacol. Biochem. Behav.,* 3:81–86.
644. Schacter, S. (1968): Obesity and eating. *Science,* 161:751–756.
645. Schacter, S. (1971): Some extraordinary facts about obese humans and rats. *Am. Psychologist,* 26:129–144.
646. Schacter, S., and Gross, L. (1968): Manipulated time and eating behavior. *J. Person. Soc. Psychol.,* 10:98–106.
647. Scharrer, E. C., Baile, A., and Mayer, J. (1970): Effect of amino acids and protein on food intake of hyperphagic and recovered aphagic rats. *Am. J. Physiol.,* 218:400–404.
648. Schildkraut, J. J., and Kety, S. S. (1967): Biogenic amines and emotion. *Science,* 156:21–30.
649. Schmitt, M. (1973): Influences of hepatic portal receptors on hypothalamic feeding and satiety centers. *Am. J. Physiol.,* 225:1089–1095.
650. Schulman, J. L., Carleton, J. L., Whitney, G., and Whitehorn, J. C. (1957): Effect of glucagon on food intake and body weight in man. *J. Appl. Physiol.,* 11:419–421.
651. Schuman, S. H., and Williams, G. W. (1974): Biochemical profiles during a Michigan heat wave: Suggestion of nutritional disturbance. *Ecol. Food Nutr.,* 3:117–123.
652. Schwartz, M., and Teitelbaum, P. (1974): Dissociation between learning and remembering in rats with lesions in the lateral hypothalamus. *J. Comp. Physiol. Psychol.,* 87:384–398.
653. Sclafani, A., and Grossman, S. P. (1969): Hyperphagia produced by knife cuts between the medial and lateral hypothalamus in the rat. *Physiol. Behav.,* 4:533–537.
654. Sclafani, A., and Maul, G. (1974): Does the ventromedial hypothalamus inhibit the lateral hypothalamus? *Physiol. Behav.,* 12:157–162.
655. Sclafani, A., Berner, C. N., and Maul, G. (1973): Feeding and drinking pathways between medial and lateral hypothalamus in the rat. *J. Comp. Physiol. Psychol.,* 85:29–51.
656. Sclafani, A., Berner, C. N., and Maul, G. (1975): Multiple knife cuts between the medial and lateral hypothalamus in the rat: A reevaluation of hypothalamic feeding circuitry. *J. Comp. Physiol. Psychol.,* 88:210–217.
657. Scott, E. M. (1946): Self selection of diet. I. Selection of purified components. *J. Nutr.,* 31:397–406.
658. Scott, E. M., and Quint, E. (1946): Self selection of diet. III. Appetites for B vitamins. *J. Nutr.,* 32:285–291.
659. Scott, E. M., and Verney, E. L. (1947): Self-selection of diet. 6. The nature of appetites for B vitamins. *J. Nutr.,* 34:471–480.
660. Scott, E. M., and Verney, E. L. (1947): Self selection of diet. IX. The appetite for thiamine. *J. Nutr.,* 37:81–92.
661. Scott, N. W., Scott, C. C., and Luckhardt, A. B. (1938): Observations on the blood sugar level before, during, and after hunger periods in animals. *Am. J. Physiol.,* 123:243–247.
662. Seaver, R. L., and Binder, H. J. (1972): Anorexia nervosa and other anorectic states in man. *Adv. Psychosom. Med.,* 7:257–276.
663. Seoane, J. R., and Baile, C. A. (1973): Ionic changes in cerebrospinal fluid and feeding, drinking and temperature of sheep. *Physiol. Behav.,* 10:915–923.
664. Shah, N. M. (1968): A double-blind study on appetite stimulation and weight gain with

cyproheptadine as adjunct to specific therapy in pulmonary tuberculosis. *Curr. Med. Pract.*, 12:961–964.

665. Shapiro, S. (1968): Adrenal catecholamine response of the infant rat to insulin-provoked hypoglycemia. *Endocrinology*, 82:1065–1067.
666. Share, I., Martyniuk, E., and Grossman, M. I. (1952): Effect of prolonged intragastric feeding on oral food intake in dogs. *Am. J. Physiol.*, 169:229–235.
667. Sharma, K. N. (1967): Receptor mechanisms in the alimentary tract: their excitation and functions. In: *Handbook of Physiology*, Sect. 6, Vol. 1, edited by C. F. Code, pp. 225–237. American Physiological Society, Washington, D.C.
668. Shoulson, I., and Chase, T. N. (1975): Fenfluramine in man: Hypophagia associated with diminished serotonin turnover. *Clin. Pharmacol. Ther.*, 17:616–621.
669. Simpson, C. W., and Dicara, L. V. (1973): Estradiol inhibition of catecholamine elicted eating in the female rat. *Pharmacol. Biochem. Behav.*, 1:413–419.
670. Sims, E. A. H. (1974): Studies in human hyperphagia. In: *Treatment and Management of Obesity*, edited by G. A. Bray and J. E. Bethune, pp. 28–43. Harper & Row, Hagerstown, Md.
671. Singh, D. (1973): Effects of preoperative training on food-motivated behavior of hypothalamic hyperphagic rats. *J. Comp. Physiol. Psychol.*, 84:47–52.
672. Simoons, F. J. (1974): Fish as forbidden food: The case of India. *Ecol. Food Nutr.*, 3:185–201.
673. Simoons, F. J. (1974): Rejection of fish as human food in Africa: A problem in history and ecology. *Ecol. Food Nutr.*, 3:89–105.
674. Slangen, J. L., and Miller, N.E. (1969): Pharmacological tests for the function of hypothalamic norepinephrine in eating behavior. *Physiol. Behav.*, 4:543–552.
675. Smart, J. L., and Dobbing, J. (1971): Vulnerability of developing brain. II. Effects of early nutritional deprivation on reflex ontogeny and development of behaviour in the rat. *Brain Res.*, 28:85–95.
676. Smith, C. J. V. (1972): Hypothalamic glucoreceptors—the influence of gold thioglucose implants in the ventromedial and lateral hypothalamic areas of normal and diabetic rats. *Physiol. Behav.*, 9:391–396.
677. Smith, D. A. (1972): Incentive as a factor in the behaviors of rats given lateral hypothalamic stimulation. *Physiol. Behav.*, 8:1077–1086.
678. Smith, G. P., and Epstein, A. N. (1969): Increased feeding in response to decreased glucose utilization in rat and monkey. *Am. J. Physiol.*, 217:1083–1084.
679. Smith, G. P., and Gibbs, J. (1975): Cholecystokinin: A putative satiety signal. *Pharmacol. Biochem. Behav.*, 3:135–138.
680. Smith, G. P., and Gibbs, J. (1976): Cholecystokinin and satiety: theoretic and therapeutic implications. In: *Hunger: Basic Mechanisms and Clinical Implications*, edited by D. Novin, W. Wyrwicka, and G. Bray, pp. 349–355. Raven Press, New York.
681. Smith, G. P., and Root, A. W. (1969): Effect of feeding on hormonal responses to 2-deoxy-D-glucose in conscious monkeys. *Endocrinology*, 85:963–968.
682. Smith, G. P., Gibbs, J., and Young, R. C. (1974): Cholecystokinin and intestinal satiety in the rat. *Fed. Proc.*, 33:1146–1149.
683. Smith, G. P., Gibbs, J., Strohmayer, A. J., and Stokes, P. (1972): Threshold doses of 2-deoxy-D-glucose for hypoglycemia and feeding in rats and monkeys. *Am. J. Physiol.*, 222:77–81.
684. Smith, M. (1966): Effects of intravenous injections on eating. *J. Comp. Physiol. Psychol.*, 61:11–14.
685. Smith, M., and Duffy, M. (1957): Some physiological factors that regulate eating behavior. *J. Comp. Physiol. Psychol.*, 48:387–391.
686. Smith, M., Pool, R., and Weinberg, H. (1962): The role of bulk in the control of eating. *J. Comp. Physiol. Psychol.*, 55:115–120.
687. Smith, M., Salisbury, R., and Weinberg, H. (1961): The reaction of hypothalamic-hyperphagic rats to stomach preloads. *J. Comp. Physiol. Psychol.*, 54:660–664.
688. Smith, O. A. (1956): Stimulation of lateral and medial hypothalamus and food intake in the rat. *Anat. Rec.*, 124:363–364.
689. Smith, P. E. (1927): The disabilities caused by hypophysectomy and their repair: The

tuberal (hypothalamic) syndrome in the rat. *JAMA,* 88:158–161.

690. Snowdon, C. T. (1969): Motivation, regulation, and the control of meal parameters with oral and intragastric feeding. *J. Comp. Physiol.,* 69:91–100.
691. Snyder, S. (1974): Drugs, neurotransmitters, and schizophrenia. *Science,* 184:1243–1253.
692. Soulairac, A. (1967): Control of carbohydrate intake. In: *Handbook of Physiology,* Sect. 6, Vol. 1, edited by C. F. Code, pp. 387–398. American Physiological Society, Washington, D.C.
693. Soulairac, A., and Soulairac, M. L. (1960): Action de la reserpine, de la serotonine et de l'iproniazide sur le comportement alimentaire du rat. *C. R. Soc. Biol.,* 154:510–513.
694. Spector, N. H., Brobeck, J. R., and Hamilton, C. L. (1968): Feeding and core temperature in albino rats: Changes induced by preoptic heating and cooling. *Science,* 161:286–288.
695. Spector, S., Gordon, R., Sjoerdsma, A., and Udenfriend, S. (1967): End-product inhibition of tyrosine hydroxylase as a possible mechanism for regulation of norepinephrine synthesis. *Mol. Pharmacol.,* 3:549–555.
696. Spiegel, T. A. (1973): Caloric regulation of food intake in man. *J. Comp. Physiol. Psychol.,* 84:24–37.
697. Stark, P. and Totty, C. W. (1967): Effects of amphetamine on eating elicited by hypothalamic stimulation. *J. Pharmacol. Exp. Ther.,* 158:272–278.
698. Stefanik, P. A., Heald, F. P., Jr., and Mayer, J. (1959): Calorie intake in relation to energy output of obese and non-obese adolescent boys. *Am. J. Clin. Nutr.,* 7:55–62.
699. Steffens, A. B. (1969): Blood glucose and FFA levels in relation to the meal pattern in the normal rat and the ventromedial hypothalamic lesioned rat. *Physiol. Behav.,* 4:215–225.
700. Steffens, A. B. (1969): The influence of insulin injections and infusions on eating and blood glucose level in the rat. *Physiol. Behav.,* 4:823–828.
701. Steffens, A. B. (1970): Plasma insulin content in relation to blood glucose level and meal pattern in the normal and hypothalamic hyperphagic rat. *Physiol. Behav.,* 5:147–151.
702. Stellar, E. (1954): The physiology of motivation. *Psychol. Rev.,* 61:5–22.
703. Stellar, E. (1967): Hunger in man: Comparative and physiological studies. *Am. Psychologist,* 22:118–130.
704. Stellar, E., Hyman, R., and Samet, S. (1954): Gastric factors controlling water and salt solution drinking. *J. Comp. Physiol. Psychol.,* 47:220–226.
705. Stephan, F. K., Valenstein, E. S., and Zucker, I. (1971): Copulation and eating during electrical stimulation of the rat hypothalamus. *Physiol. Behav.,* 7:587–593.
706. Stern, J. J., and Greenwood, M. R. C. (1974): A review of development of adipose cellularity in man and animals. *Fed. Proc.,* 33:1952–1955.
707. Stern, J. J. and Zwick, G. (1973): Effects of intraventricular norepinephrine and estradiol benzoate on weight regulatory behavior in female rats. *Behav. Biol.,* 9:605–612.
708. Stern, J. J., Porterfield, A. L., and Krupa, R. J. (1974): Endocrine interactions in regulation of body weight by female rats. *J. Comp. Physiol. Psychol.,* 86:926–929.
709. Stevenson, J. A. F. (1969): Neural control of food and water intake. In: *The Hypothalamus,* edited by W. Haymaker, E. Anderson, and W. J. H. Nauta, pp. 524–621. Charles C Thomas, Springfield, Ill.
710. Stevenson, J. A. F., and Franklin, C. (1970): Effects of ACTH and corticosteroids in the regulation of food and water intake. *Prog. Brain Res.,* 32:512–515.
711. Stevenson, J. A. F., and Montemurro, D. G. (1963): Loss of weight and metabolic rate of rats with lesions in the medial and lateral hypothalamus. *Nature (Lond.),* 198:92.
712. Storlien, L. H., and Albert, D. J. (1972): The effect of VMH lesions, lateral cuts and anterior cuts on food intake, activity level, food motivation, and reactivity to taste. *Physiol. Behav.,* 9:191–197.
713. Stowe, F. R., and Miller, A. T. (1957): The effect of amphetamine on food intake in rats with hypothalamic hyperphagia. *Experientia,* 13:114–115.
714. Stricker, E. M., and Wolf, G. (1967): The effects of hypovolemia on drinking in rats with lateral hypothalamic damage. *Proc. Soc. Exp. Biol. Med.,* 124:816–820.
715. Stricker, E. M., and Zigmond, M. J. (1974): Effects on homeostasis of intraventricular injections of 6-hydroxydopamine in rats. *J. Comp. Physiol. Psychol.,* 86:973–994.
716. Stricker, E. M., and Zigmond, M. J. (1976): Brain catecholamines and the lateral hypothalamic syndrome. In: *Hunger: Basic Mechanisms and Clinical Implications,* edited by D. Novin, W. Wyrwicka, and G. Bray, pp. 19–32. Raven Press, New York.

717. Stricker, E. M., and Zigmond, M. J. (1976): Recovery of function following brain damage: implications for motivated ingestive behaviors. In: *Dahlem Workshop on Appetite and Food Intake,* edited by T. Silverstone. Dahlem Konferenzen, Berlin *(in press).*
718. Stricker, E. M., Friedman, M. I., and Zigmond, M. J. (1975): Glucoregulatory feeding by rats after intraventricular 6-hydroxydopamine or lateral hypothalamic lesions. *Science,* 189:895–897.
719. Strominger, J. L., and Brobeck, J. R. (1953): A mechanism of regulation of food intake. *Yale J. Biol. Med.,* 25:383–390.
720. Strominger, J. L., Brobeck, J. R., and Cort, R. L. (1953): Regulation of food intake in normal rats and in rats with hypothalamic hyperphagia. *Yale J. Biol. Med.,* 26:55–74.
721. Stunkard, A. J. (1968): Environment and obesity: Recent advances in our understanding of regulation of food intake in man. *Fed. Proc.,* 27:1367–1373.
722. Stunkard, A. J. (1974): New treatments for obesity: behavior modification. In: *Treatment and Management of Obesity,* edited by G. A. Bray and J. E. Bethune, pp. 103–116. Harper & Row, Hagerstown, Md.
723. Stunkard, A. J., and Fox, S. (1971): The relationship of gastric motility and hunger. *Psychosom. Med.,* 33:123–134.
724. Stunkard, A. J., Clovis, W. L., and Free, S. M. (1962): Skin temperature after eating, evidence bearing upon a thermostatic control of food intake. *Am. J. Med. Sci.,* 244:126–130.
725. Sturdevant, R. A. L., and Goetz, H. (1976): Cholecystokinin both stimulates and inhibits human food intake. *Nature (Lond.),* 267:713–715.
726. Sudsaneh, S., and Mayer, J. (1959): Relation of metabolic events to gastric contractions in the rat. *Am. J. Physiol.,* 197:269–273.
727. Sullivan, A. C., and Triscari, J. (1976): Possible interrelationships between metabolic flux and appetite. In: *Hunger: Basic Mechanisms and Clinical Implications,* edited by D. Novin, W. Wyrwicka, and G. Bray, pp. 115–125. Raven Press, New York.
728. Swanson, L. W., and Hartman, B. K. (1975): The central adrenergic system: An immuno-fluorescence study of the location of cell bodies and their efferent connections in the rat utilizing dopamine-$\beta$-hydroxylase as a marker. *J. Comp. Neurol.,* 163:467–505.
729. Szabo, O., and Szabo, J. (1972): Evidence for an insulin-sensitive receptor in the central nervous system. *Am. J. Physiol.,* 223:1349–1353.
730. Tannenbaum, G. A., Paxinos, G. and Bindra, D. (1974): Metabolic and endocrine aspects of the ventromedial hypothalamic syndrome in the rat. *J. Comp. Physiol. Psychol.,* 86:404–413.
731. Tartellin, M. F., and Gorski, R. A. (1971): Variations in food and water intake in the normal and acyclic female rat. *Physiol. Behav.,* 7:847–852.
732. Tartellin, M. F., Shryne, J. E., and Gorski, R. A. (1975): Patterns of body weight change in rats following neonatal hormone manipulation. *Acta. Endocrinol (Kbh.),* 79:177–191.
733. Teitelbaum P. (1955): Sensory control of hypothalamic hyperphagia. *J. Comp. Physiol. Psychol.,* 48:156–163.
734. Teitelbaum, P. (1957): Random and food directed activity in hyperphagic and normal rats. *J. Comp. Physiol. Psychol.,* 50:486–490.
735. Teitelbaum, P. (1961): Disturbances in feeding and drinking behavior after hypothalamic lesions. In: *Nebraska Symposium on Motivation,* edited by M. R. Jones, pp. 39–65. University of Nebraska Press, Lincoln.
736. Teitelbaum, P. (1967): Motivation and control of food intake. In: *Handbook of Physiology,* Sect. 6, Vol. 1, edited by C. F. Code, pp. 319–335. American Physiological Society, Washington, D.C.
737. Teitelbaum, P. (1969): Stages of recovery and development of lateral hypothalamic control of food and water intake. *Ann. NY Acad. Sci.,* 157:849–860.
738. Teitelbaum, P. (1971): The encephalization of hunger. In: *Progress in Physiological Psychology,* edited by E. Stellar and J. M. Sprague, pp. 319–350. Academic Press, New York.
739. Teitelbaum, P., and Campbell, B. A. (1958): Ingestion patterns in hyperphagic and normal rats. *J. Comp. Physiol. Psychol.,* 51:135–141.
740. Teitelbaum, P., and Cytawa, J. (1965): Spreading depression and recovery from lateral hypothalamic damage. *Science,* 147:61–63.
741. Teitelbaum, P., and Epstein, A. N. (1962): The lateral hypothalamic syndrome: Recovery

of feeding and drinking after lateral hypothalamic lesions. *Psychol. Rev.,* 69:74–90.

742. Teitelbaum, P., Cheng, M-F., and Rozin, P. (1969): Development of feeding parallels its recovery after hypothalamic damage. *J. Comp. Physiol. Psychol.,* 67:430–441.

743. Tenen, S. S., and Miller, N. E. (1964): Strength of electrical stimulation of lateral hypothalamus, food deprivation and tolerance for quinine in food. *J. Comp. Physiol. Psychol.,* 58:55–62.

744. Tepperman, H. M., and Tepperman, J. (1964): Adaptive hyperlipogenesis. *Fed. Proc.,* 23:73–75.

745. Tepperman, J., and Tepperman, H. M. (1964): Effects of antecedent food intake on hepatic lipogenesis. *Am. J. Physiol.,* 193:55–64.

746. Tepperman, J., and Tepperman, H. M. (1965): Adaptive hyperlipogenesis—late 1964 model. *Ann. NY Acad. Sci.,* 131:404–411.

747. Ter Haar, M. B. (1972): Circadian and estrual rhythms in food intake in the rat. *Horm. Behav.,* 3:213–220.

748. Thoenen, H. (1974): Trans-synaptic enzyme induction. *Life Sci.,* 14:223–235.

749. Thomas, D. W., and Mayer, J. (1968): Meal taking and regulation of food intake by normal and hypothalamic hyperphagic rats. *J. Comp. Physiol. Psychol.,* 66:642–653.

750. Titlebaum, L. F., Falk, J. L., and Mayer, J. (1960): Altered acceptance and rejection of NaCl in rats with diabetes insipidus. *Am. J. Physiol.,* 199:72–74.

751. Tongue, D. A., and Oatley, K. (1973): Feeding and arteriovenous differences of blood glucose in the rat after injection with 2-deoxy-D-glucose and after food deprivation. *Physiol. Behav.,* 10:497–505.

752. Tsang, Y. C. (1938): Hunger motivation in gastrectomized rats. *J. Comp. Psychol.,* 26:1–17.

753. Ungerstedt, U. (1971): Adipsia and aphagia after 6-hydroxydopamine induced degeneration of the nigro-striatal dopamine system. *Acta Physiol. Scand.,* 367:95–121.

754. Ungerstedt, U. (1971): Stereotaxic mapping of the monoamine pathways in the rat brain. *Acta Physiol. Scand.,* 367:1–48.

755. Valenstein, E. S., and Cox, V. C. (1970): Influence of hunger, thirst, and previous experience in the test chamber on stimulation-bound eating and drinking. *J. Comp. Physiol. Psychol.,* 70:189–199.

756. Valenstein, E. S., Cox, V. C., and Kakolewski, J. W. (1969): Sex differences in hyperphagia and body weight following hypothalamic damage. *Ann. NY Acad. Sci.,* 157:1030–1048.

757. Valenstein, E. S., Cox, V. C., and Kakolewski, J. W. (1970): Reexamination of the role of the hypothalamus in motivation. *Psychol. Rev.,* 77:16–31.

758. Valenstein, E. S., Kakolewski, J. W., and Cox, V. C. (1967): Sex differences in taste preference for glucose and saccharin solutions. *Science,* 156:942–943.

759. Vance, W. B. (1965): Observations on the role of salivary secretions in the regulation of food and fluid intake in the white rat. *Psychol. Monogr.,* 79:1–15.

760. Vander Weele, D. A., and Sanderson, J. D. (1976): Peripheral glucosensitive satiety in the rabbit and the rat. In: *Hunger: Basic Mechanisms and Clinical Implications,* edited by D. Novin, W. Wyrwicka, and G. Bray, pp. 383–393. Raven Press, New York.

761. Vander Weele, D. A., Novin, D., Rezek, M., and Sanderson, J. D. (1974): Duodenal satiety mechanism. *Physiol. Behav.,* 12:467–473.

762. Van Itallie, T. B., Beaudoin, R., and Mayer, J. (1952): Arterovenous glucose differences, metabolic hypoglycemia and food intake in man. *J. Clin. Nutr.,* 1:208–217.

763. Van Veen, A. G., Hong, L. G., and Nio, O. K. (1971): Some nutritional and economic considerations of Javanese dietary patterns. *Ecol. Food Nutr.,* 1:39–43.

764. Vilberg, T. R., and Beatty, W. W. (1975): Behavioral changes following VMH lesions in rats with controlled insulin levels. *Pharmacol. Biochem. Behav.,* 3:377–384.

765. Wade, G. N. (1972): Gonadal hormones and behavioral regulation of body weight. *Physiol. Behav.,* 8:523–534.

766. Wade, G. N. (1974): Interaction between estradiol-17β and growth hormone in control of food intake in weanling rats. *J. Comp. Physiol. Psychol.,* 86:359–362.

767. Wade, G. N. (1975): Some effects of ovarian hormones on food intake and body weight in female rats. *J. Comp. Physiol. Psychol.,* 88:183–193.

768. Wade, G. N., and Zucker, I. (1969): Hormonal and developmental influences on rat saccharin preferences. *J. Comp. Physiol. Psychol.*, 69:291–300.
769. Wade, G. N., and Zucker, I. (1969): Taste preferences of female rats: Modification by neonatal hormones, food deprivation, and prior experience. *Physiol. Behav.*, 4:935–943.
770. Wade, G. N., and Zucker, I. (1970): Development of hormonal control over food intake and body weight in female rats. *J. Comp. Physiol. Psychol.*, 70:213–220.
771. Wade, G. N., and Zucker, I. (1970): Hormonal modulation of responsiveness to an aversive taste stimulus in rats. *Physiol. Behav.*, 5:269–273.
772. Wade, G. N., and Zucker, I. (1970): Modulation of food intake and locomotor activity in female rats by diencephalic hormone implants. *J. Comp. Physiol. Psychol.*, 72:328–336.
773. Wagner, J. W., and De Groot, J. (1963): Changes in feeding behavior after intracerebral injections in the rat. *Am. J. Physiol.*, 204:483–487.
774. Walker, D. W., and Remley, N. R. (1970): The relationships among percentage body weight loss, circulating free fatty acids and consummatory behavior in rats. *Physiol. Behav.*, 5:301–309.
775. Walsh, J. H., and Grossman, M. I. (1973): Gastrin. *N. Engl. J. Med.*, 292:1324–1334.
776. Wampler, R. S. (1971): Regulatory deficits in rats following unilateral lesions of the lateral hypothalamus. *J. Comp. Physiol. Psychol.*, 75:190–199.
777. Wampler, R. S. (1973): Increased motivation in rats with ventromedial hypothalamic lesions. *J. Comp. Physiol. Psychol.*, 84:275–285.
778. Wampler, R. S., and Gier, H. T. (1974): Continuing gonadal function in rats with ventromedial hypothalamic area lesions. *J. Comp. Physiol. Psychol.*, 87:831–841.
779. Wangensteen, O. H., and Carlson, H. A. (1931): Hunger sensations in a patient after total gastrectomy. *Proc. Soc. Exp. Biol. Med.*, 28:545–547.
780. Waxler, S. H., and Brecher, G. (1950): Obesity and food requirement in albino mice following administration of gold thioglucose. *Am. J. Physiol.*, 162:428–439.
781. Wayner, M. J., Cott, A., Millner, T., and Tartaglione, R. (1971): Loss of 2-deoxy-D-glucose induced eating in recovered lateral rats. *Physiol. Behav.*, 7:881–884.
782. Weil-Malherbe, H., Axelrod, J., and Tomchick, R. (1959): Blood-brain barrier for adrenaline. *Science*, 129:1226–1227.
783. Weiner, I. H., and Stellar, E. (1951): Salt preference of the rat determined by a single-stimulus method. *J. Comp. Physiol. Psychol.*, 44:394–401.
784. Weiss, B. (1961): Effects of brief exposure to cold on performance and food intake. *Science*, 127:467–468.
785. Whichelow, M. J. (1974): Peripheral metabolism of carbohydrate in obesity and diabetes. In: *Obesity Symposium*, edited by W. L. Burland, pp. 217–228. Churchill Livingstone, New York.
786. Whishaw, I. Q., and Veale, W. L. (1974): Comparison of the effect of prostaglandin $E_1$ and norepinephrine injected into the brain on ingestive behavior in the rat. *Pharmacol. Biochem. Behav.*, 2:421–425.
787. Wilkinson, H. A., and Peele, T. L. (1962): Modification of intracranial self-stimulation by hunger or satiety. *Am. J. Physiol.*, 203:537–540.
788. Williams, R. R. (1961): *Toward the Conquest of Beri-Beri*. Harvard University Press, Cambridge, Mass.
789. Wilson, E. O. (1975): *Sociobiology: The New Synthesis*. Belknap Press, Cambridge, Mass.
790. Winick, M., and Noble, A. (1966): Cellular response in rats during malnutrition at various ages. *J. Nutr.*, 89:300–306.
791. Winick, M., and Rosso, P. (1969): The effect of severe early malnutrition on cellular growth of human brain. *Pediatr. Res.*, 3:181–189.
792. Winslow, C. E. A., and Herrington, L. P. (1949): *Temperature and Human Life*. Princeton University Press, Princeton.
793. Wise, R. A. (1974): Lateral hypothalamic electrical stimulation: Does it make animals "hungry"? *Brain Res.*, 67:187–209.
794. Wolf, G., and Steinbaum, E. A. (1965): Sodium appetite elicited by subcutaneous formalin: Mechanism of action. *J. Comp. Physiol. Psychol.*, 59:335–339.
795. Wolgin, D. L., Cytawa, J., and Teitelbaum, P. (1976): The role of activation in the regulation of food intake. In: *Hunger: Basic Mechanisms and Clinical Implications*, edited

by D. Novin, W. Wyrwicka, and G. Bray, pp. 179–189. Raven Press, New York.

796. Woods, S. C., and Shogren, R. E., Jr. (1972): Glycemic responses following conditioning with different doses of insulin in rats. *J. Comp. Physiol. Psychol.*, 81:220–228.

797. Woods, S. C., Decke, E., and Vasselli, J. R. (1974): Metabolic hormones and regulation of body weight. *Psychol. Rev.*, 81:26–43.

798. Woodward, E. (1970): Clinical experience with fenfluramine in the United States. In: *Amphetamines and Related Compounds,* edited by E. Costa and S. Garattini, pp. 685–691. Raven Press, New York.

799. Wooley, O. (1971): Long-term food regulation in the obese and non-obese. *Psychosom. Med.*, 33:436–444.

800. Wooley, O., and Wooley, S. (1976): The experimental psychology of obesity. In: *Obesity: Pathogenesis and Management,* edited by T. Silverstone and J. Fincham. Technical and Medical Publishing Co., Lancaster, England *(in press).*

801. Wooley, S. C. (1971): Long-term food regulation in the obese and nonobese. *Psychosom. Med.*, 33:436–444.

802. Wurtman, R. J. (1963): *Catecholamines.* Little, Brown, Boston.

803. Wurtman, R. J. (1974): Effects of physiologic variations of brain monoamines. In: *Frontiers of Neurology and Neuroscience Research,* edited by P. Seeman and G. M. Brown, pp. 16–25. University of Toronto Press, Toronto.

804. Wurtman, R. J., and Fernstrom, J. D. (1972): L-Tryptophan, L-tyrosine, and the control of brain monoamine biosynthesis. In: *Perspectives in Neuropharmacology,* edited by S. H. Snyder, pp. 143–193. Oxford University Press, New York.

805. Wurtman, R. J., and Fernstrom, J. D. (1974): Effects of the diet on brain neurotransmitters. *Nutr. Rev.*, 32:193–200.

806. Wurtman, R. J., Axelrod, J., and Kelly, D. E. (1968): *The Pineal.* Academic Press, New York.

807. Wyrwicka, W. (1967): Conditioned behavioral analysis of feeding mechanisms. In: *Handbook of Physiology,* Sect. 6, Vol. 1, edited by C. F. Code, pp. 63–78. American Physiological Society, Washington, D.C.

808. Wyrwicka, W. (1969): Sensory regulation of food intake. *Physiol. Behav.*, 4:853–858.

809. Wyrwicka, W., and Dobrzecka, C. (1960): Relationship between feeding and satiation centers of the hypothalamus. *Science,* 132:805–806.

810. Wyrwicka, W., Dobrzecka, C., and Tarnecki, R. (1960): The effect of electrical stimulation of the hypothalamus on the conditioned reflexes, type II. *Acta Biol. Exp.*, 20:121–136.

811. Yaksh, T. L., and Myers, R. D. (1972): Hypothalamic "coding" in the unanesthetized monkey of noradrenergic sites mediating feeding and thermoregulation. *Physiol. Behav.*, 8:251–257.

812. Yalow, R. S., Glick, S. M., Roth, J., and Berson, S. A. (1965): Plasma insulin and growth hormone levels in obesity and diabetes. *Ann. NY Acad. Sci.*, 131:357–373.

813. Yin, T. H., Hamilton, C. L., and Brobeck, J. R. (1970): Food intake of rats given hypertonic solutions by gavage and water intravenously. *Proc. Soc. Exp. Biol. Med.*, 133:83–85.

814. York, D. A., and Bray, G. A. (1972): Dependence of hypothalamic obesity on insulin, the pituitary and the adrenal gland. *Endocrinology,* 90:885–894.

815. Young, P. T. (1955): The role of hedonic processes in motivation. In: *Nebraska Symposium on Motivation,* edited by M. R. Jones, pp. 193–238. University of Nebraska Press, Lincoln.

816. Young, P. T. (1966): Hedonic organization and regulation of behavior. *Psychol. Rev.*, 73:59–86.

817. Young, P. T. (1967): Palatability: The hedonic response to foodstuffs. In: *Handbook of Physiology,* Sect. 6, Vol. 1, edited by C. F. Code, pp. 353–366. American Physiological Society, Washington, D.C.

818. Young, P. T., and Falk, J. L. (1956): The relative acceptability of sodium chloride solutions as a function of concentration and water need. *J. Comp. Physiol. Psychol.*, 49:569–575.

819. Young, R. C., Gibbs, J., Antin, J., Holt, J., and Smith, G. P. (1974): Absence of satiety during sham feeding in the rat. *J. Comp. Physiol. Psychol.*, 87:795–800.

820. Young, T. K., and Liu, A. C. (1965): Hyperphagia, insulin, and obesity. *Chin. J. Physiol.*, 19:247–253.

821. Young, V. R., and Scrimshaw, N. S. (1971): The physiology of starvation. *Sci. Am.,* 225:14–21.
822. Zigmond, M. J., and Stricker, E. M. (1972): Deficits in feeding behavior after intraventricular injection of 6-hydroxydopamine in rats. *Science,* 177:1211–1214.
823. Zigmond, M. J., and Stricker, E. M. (1973): Recovery of feeding and drinking by rats after intraventricular 6-hydroxydopamine or lateral hypothalamic lesions. *Science,* 182:717–720.
824. Zigmond, M. J., and Stricker, E. M. (1974): Ingestive behavior following damage to central dopamine neurons: implications for homeostasis and recovery of function. In: *Neuropsychopharmacology of Monoamines and Their Regulatory Enzymes,* edited by E. Usdin, pp. 385–402. Raven Press, New York.
825. Zis, A. P., and Fibiger, H. C. (1975): Neuroleptic-induced deficits in food and water regulation: Similarities to the lateral hypothalamic syndrome. *Psychopharmacologia,* 43:63–68.
826. Zucker, I. (1969): Hormonal determinants of sex differences in saccharine preference, food intake, and body weight. *Physiol. Behav.,* 4:595–602.
827. Zucker, I. (1971): Light-dark rhythms in rat eating and drinking behavior. *Physiol. Behav.,* 6:115–126.

*Nutrition and the Brain*, Vol. 2,
edited by R. J. Wurtman and
J. J. Wurtman. Raven Press,
New York © 1977.

# Effect of Undernutrition on Brain Morphology

## William J. Shoemaker and Floyd E. Bloom

*Arthur Vining Davis Center for Behavioral Neurobiology, The Salk Institute,
San Diego, California 92112*

## I. INTRODUCTION

The brain, like all other tissues, needs building blocks of amino acids, vitamins, minerals, energy substrates, and fatty acids to construct and maintain its $10^{10}$ neurons and $10^{11}$ other cells. A reasonable hypothesis then would be that a deficit in one or more of these essential nutrients could affect the initial development and subsequent maintenance of a tissue as structurally complex as the brain. Such a hypothesis is not easy to test. This chapter reviews the results of studies that attempted to answer the question of nutritional effects on brain morphology; we propose that only quantitative morphological methods can answer this question.

Without *a priori* knowledge of this field, a convenient way to organize the important variables is as follows:

1. Nutritional
   a. Nutritional insult, i.e., the qualitative and quantitative departure from optimum nutrition
   b. Time in the life span of the individual when this insult is applied
   c. Duration of the nutritional insult
2. Anatomical
   a. Region of the brain affected
   b. Nature and extent of the lesion, e.g., necrotic, hemorrhagic, hyperplastic, deformation
   c. Cellular and noncellular elements involved
   d. Whether the lesion is reversible or irreversible with rehabilitation
   e. Possible functional deficits expected

Although this outline appears reasonable and straightforward, there are many reasons why this ideal cannot be met. Some of these reasons are:

1. In all of the studies to be discussed, the nutritional deprivation was imposed early in life, either prenatally or during the early postnatal period. This is the period of development and rapid growth of the brain so that almost all of our discussion concerns nutritional effects on brain development with only brief reference to nutritional effects on function or structure in a brain already normally developed. The question of whether undernutrition or nonlethal starvation alters the structure of an adult brain will remain moot until more research has been done on this important aspect.

2. Because the dietary manipulation is imposed very early in development, the restriction almost always is one of total nutrient intake rather than a specific item of the diet. Total nutrient deprivation is usually done by feeding the mother diets differing in amount or protein content during gestation and/or lactation, or restricting the time that each offspring in the litter has access to the nipple. The small number of reports dealing with essential dietary fat deficiency to the mother on the composition of the offspring's brain (17,18,80, 97) are not considered here nor are any studies on vitamin or mineral deficiency.

3. The neuropathology resulting from nutritional insult is quite unconventional in that there is no focal lesion. There is no site of trauma, hemorrhage, or malformation as is usual in developmental neuropathology. Rather, undernutrition as a generalized detriment to brain development leads to a "distortion and deficit" pathology of the brain (33). The damage is spread evenly, perhaps imperceptibly, throughout the entire tissue, altering it subtly; this produces distortions in ways that belie prediction of functional consequences but which definitely are not normal.

4. The current status of knowledge in brain structure-function relationships is such that no one morphological element can yet be indicated as primarily essential for a certain function. Therefore studies of brain structure after undernutrition include analyses of almost all structural parameters using a wide variety of methods.

We have not restricted our discussions of brain morphology to the rat but have included studies on many different species, including man. Similarly, we do not discriminate against different methods of experimental undernutrition, although some methods are believed to offer certain advantages over others (85). Although other reviews of this general topic include studies on the peripheral nervous system (111), the effects of nutritional rehabilitation (6), and the relationship to behavior (69), we chose to limit our discussion by not including these aspects. We begin by briefly describing the major structural elements of the central nervous system (CNS) susceptible to alteration by undernutrition. Much evidence for the latter presumption must still be speculative as the susceptibility of each structural element has not been studied in detail. Following this, we offer a review of the various methods useful in the study of morphological alterations after nutritional insult, the data base available from the major studies, and a critical commentary on the interpretation of their findings. We include some unpublished work of our own and others which used quantitative methods that hold promise for new insights into this important question. Finally, we conclude with some comments concerning appropriate expectations of the future of this field.

## II. STRUCTURAL ELEMENTS OF THE CNS AND THEIR POTENTIAL FOR ALTERATION BY UNDERNUTRITION

### A. Neurons

Neurons are nerve cells; they have the ability to conduct bioelectrical impulses over long distances without any loss of signal strength. Although neurons possess the structural elements of most other cells in the body (nucleus, nucleoli, endoplasmic reticulum, Golgi apparatus, etc.), they have special properties that allow them to function as components within a rapid communications network. One of these properties is the ability to form and maintain intimate structural connections with other specific cells over distances which can be very long. These connections depend on long processes known to be extensions of the cell cytoplasm surrounded by the cell membrane, somewhat like an enormous pseudopod. Neuronal processes are basically of two types: Each neuron possesses one *axon,* which may subsequently give off multiple collateral branches; axons conduct the electrical impulses away from the cell. It is the *dendrites,* of which each neuron may have several, that carry impulses toward the cell body. Another important property of differentiated neurons is that they do not again undergo cell division. Indeed, a cell which has 90% of its cytoplasm tied up in lengthy extended processes would be hard pressed to divide. One relevant implication of this restrictive property is that once a neuron is fatally damaged, that particular neuron and its multiple connections are lost for the life of the animal. In addition, after early development, germinal stem cell populations for neurons become inactive, making repopulation after neuronal loss impossible.

When viewing the brain microscopically, only the neuronal cell body, or perikaryon, can ordinarily be identified unambiguously at the light microscopic level. This is because the processes emerging from the cell body (Fig. 1) can be traced only a short distance before they are lost in a great tangle of

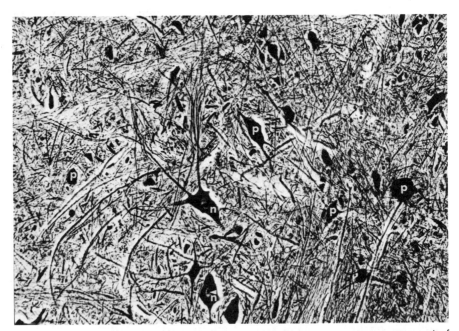

**FIG. 1.** Stained section from monkey spinal cord illustrating a common arrangement of neuron cell bodies and their processes. Much of the space between cell bodies is occupied by the neuropil, (the fibrous network of the axonal and dendritic processes from these neurons) and a large number of incoming, branched axon terminals. The perikaryons of several neurons are indicated (p), and in certain neurons the nucleus (n) and the nucleolus within it are visible. Bodian silver stain, ×150. [Reprinted with permission of Dr. David Bodian (Johns Hopkins University) and of Rockefeller University Press.]

processes from many other cells (the neuropil). Some of the features of neuronal perikarya that can be studied are the position of the cell nucleus in the cell body, the prominence and number of nucleoli within the nucleus, the shape and condition of the cell membrane, and of course the position of cell bodies relative to other anatomical features in the brain. Although most of these indices could possibly be altered by undernutrition, there is little evidence that they are. What is perhaps more relevant is that early undernutrition can restrict the formation, existence, and eventual final position of certain neurons. In the cerebellum, which continues neurogenesis after birth in both rats and man, undernutrition applied during the period of neurogenesis results in a deficit in the width of the short-lived external granular layer. This deficit is reflected in, *inter alia,* a reduction in cerebellar granule cells. Granule cells bud from the external granule layer and migrate to a position deep to the Purkinje cells. Undernutrition during these events, the first 3 weeks of life in the rat, has been shown to retard or permanently prevent some cells from migrating (Fig. 2).

The electron microscope is required to view changes in the fine details of axons and dendrites. Dendrites and axons (Fig. 3) could develop changes in shape, appearance of the membrane, and condition and number of mitochondria; in addition, axons could have their numerous synaptic vesicles altered. Although such alterations do occur in certain disease states, they have not been described in undernourished animals.

However, between the ordinary surface detail of perikaryal size, number, and location visualized by conventional microscopy and the unfathomable depths of ultrastructural detail visualized in the electron microscope lies a sea of intermediate detail in important neuronal structure, chemistry, and circuitry. These intermediate features require that the anatomy of an individual neuron be revealed selectively, but more or less in entirety, so that its structural configuration can be traced over considerable distances. It is necessary to be able to trace neuronal processes within or between regions of the brain without their being obscured by the cytological details of the innumerable neurons and glia whose boundaries are traversed. To accomplish this objective, neurons must be "stained" by methods which can select individual cells on the basis of a general cytoplasmic chemical or structural component. Some stains (e.g., the metallic impregnation stains of Golgi or Bodian) operate selectively on chemical principles not yet understood. Others (e.g., the cytochemical methods of fluorescence histochemistry or enzyme immunocytochemistry) select various specific chemical components relevant to neurotransmitter synthesis or storage.

Recent work (53,81) using the Golgi stain showed that Purkinje cells of undernourished rat cerebellum possess abnormal dendritic processes, altered in both number and length (Fig. 4). It is not known if the cytoplasmic constituents of these shortened dendrites are also abnormal.

The synapse is the functional point of anatomical contact between directly communicating neurons. Most such functional interneuronal communication

**CONTROL**          **EXPERIMENTAL**

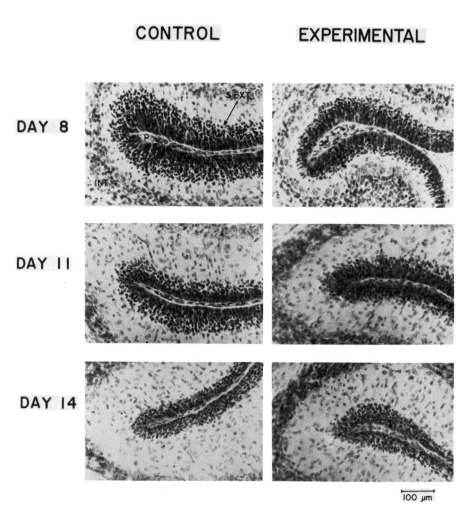

DAY 8

DAY II

DAY 14

100 μm

**FIG. 2.** Photomicrographs of the external granular layer (EXT) of the subfolium of the rat cerebellar uvula from control and experimental (undernourished from birth) rats. Cell-stained sections from three different stages of postnatal cerebellar development are shown for both groups. The internal granular cell layer (INT) and Purkinje cells (P) are also indicated. At day 8 the external granular layer is smaller in the undernourished brains (0.19 ± 0.01 vs. 0.23 ± 0.02 mm² by areal measurements). However, at day 11 the regions are the same size (0.21 ± 0.04 vs. 0.20 ± 0.04 mm²), and at day 14 the undernourished rat exhibits a larger external layer [0.11 ± 0.01 (experimental) vs. 0.02 ± 0.01 (control)]. The bar indicates the magnification. (Courtesy of S. Griffin, ref. 54.)

in mammalian brains depends on the conversion of propagated electrical potentials into the physically triggered release of a specific chemical transmitter. Naturally, a great deal of attention has focused on the ultrastructure of the synapse with respect to size, shape, transmitter content, and transmitter storage vesicle, as well as on the overall location and occurrence of synapses. In

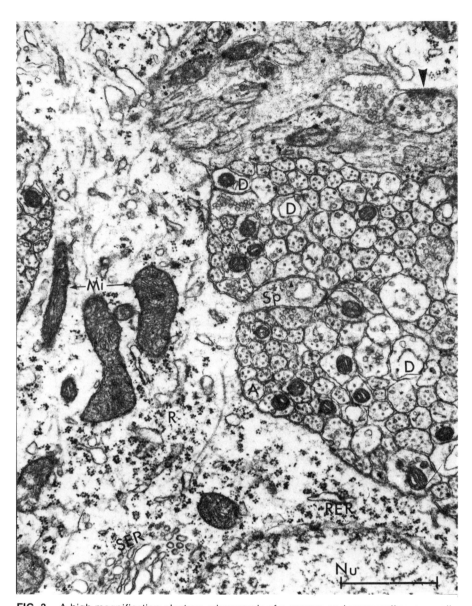

**FIG. 3.** A high-magnification electron micrograph of a neuron and surrounding neuropil. The apical portion of the neuron can be seen across the bottom of the field with a portion of its nucleus visible (Nu). The cytoplasm of this neuron is filled with normal cellular organelles such as ribosomes (R), ribosomes attached to endoplasmic reticulum (RER), and smooth endoplasmic reticulum (SER) of the Golgi network; also visible are several mitochondria (Mi). The apical dendrite of the neuron continues upward along the left edge of the micrograph and passes out of view; from its right surface a small dendritic spine (Sp) can be seen on which are one or (possibly) two specialized contacts from small terminal axons (small arrowhead). Three or four other probable dendrites are cut in cross section (D), each exhibiting a saccule of slightly dilated smooth endoplasmic reticulum. The most numerous elements of the neuropil are fine unmyelinated axons (A). The large dendrite at the upper right has a very pronounced specialized contact (presumably synaptic) made by a vesicle-filled terminal (large arrowhead). The bar equals 1 $\mu$m.

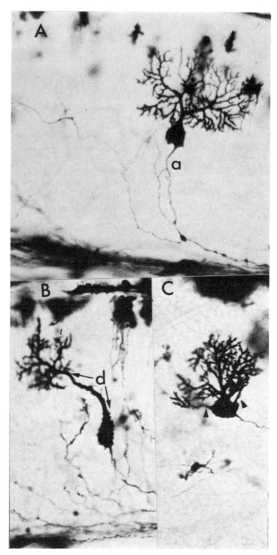

**FIG. 4.** Golgi-Cox stained Purkinje cells from rats sacrificed at 11 days postnatal. **A:** A typical cell from well-nourished controls. It features an oval-shaped perikaryon having a single thin axonal process (a), a large main dendrite that branches within 0.5 mm of the perikaryon, and profuse dendritic branching. **B:** A Purkinje cell from an undernourished rat's brain. Note the elongated dendritic process (d), the lack of dendritic bifurcation, and the small amount of terminal dendritic branching. **C:** Another cell from an undernourished rat demonstrating extrasomal dendrites (arrowheads), a situation seen much more frequently in the under-nourished rats than in controls. (This figure was generously provided by Griffin and Wood-ward, ref. 53.)

particular, nutritionists have focused on synapses; on the one hand, this is because under certain conditions synapses show plasticity—i.e., a change in their pattern of structural or functional connectivity (39); and on the other hand, a deficit in synaptic connections provides a simple causal explanation for the relationship between undernutrition and intellectual impairment. This increased attention to synapses may be unwarranted: The plastic changes in synapses described to date occur only under specific experimental conditions but not yet under conditions of altered nutrition. Similarly, a functional deficit of the brain can be caused by changes in neurons, dendrites, or glial cells, or even by changes not mirrored morphologically.

Nevertheless, several investigators, ourselves included, have studied one or more aspects of synapses after early undernutrition. At this point it appears that both the frequency of synapses, as well as some of their staining properties, can be modified by nutrition. Of all the neuronal structural elements amenable to study by current methods, synapses are perhaps still the most promising for the nutritionist.

### B. Nonneural Cells

The nonneural cells of the brain, including those constituting the lining of the blood vessels, are classified into several types (Fig. 5) but are considered here as a group. These cells surround and support the neurons—hence their name, glia, which means "glue." They do not ordinarily generate electrical impulses. Paradoxically, although the glial cells of the brain outnumber the neurons by manyfold, much less is known about them. Glial cells, unlike neurons, have a defined lifespan and are slowly replaced throughout the life of the animal (5,29). The nonneural cells of the brain also develop later than the neurons (Fig. 6) so that the majority of nonneural cells are formed after birth for many species (32). It is very likely that almost all of the brain cell deficit seen after undernutrition during the first 10 postnatal days in the rat is a deficit of glial cells. Interestingly, although glial cells replace themselves throughout life, the large deficit in glial cells due to early undernutrition is not restored if the return to adequate feeding is later than 2–3 weeks of age (129). Many of these same findings have been shown to be true for undernourished children (128). However, it should be pointed out that even if the cellular deficit caused by early undernutrition were shown to be restricted chiefly to nonneural cells, behavioral and intellectual impairment could still be affected.

Some of the evidence that glial cells play a role in the overall function of the nervous system arises from studies of myelinated axons. In the peripheral nervous system, axons normally encased by the myelin sheath function abnormally if that sheath is insufficient. Myelin is composed of cholesterol, phospholipid, and glycolipid, and is produced by nonneural cells in a pattern that appears to insulate the long axonal processes of neurons (Fig. 5). In the

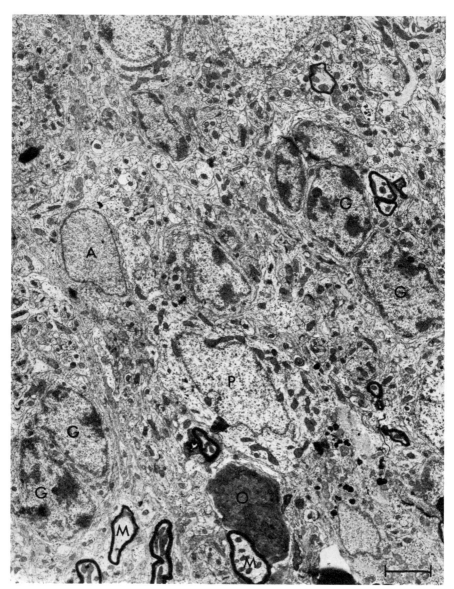

**FIG. 5.** This low-power electron micrograph from normal rat cerebellum contains cross-sections through two types of glia cells, an astrocyte (A) and an oligodendrocyte (O). It also indicates the intimate association between glial cells and neurons. P, a Purkinje cell; G, small granule cells. The plasma membrane of the oligodendrocyte can be seen to envelop a myelinated axon (M) at bottom center. The bar equals 5 $\mu$m.

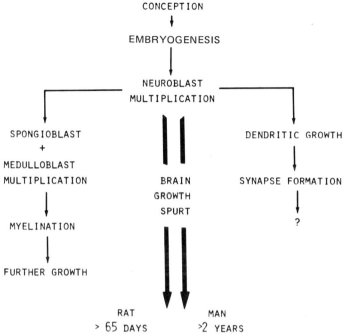

CONCEPTION

EMBRYOGENESIS

NEUROBLAST
MULTIPLICATION

SPONGIOBLAST
+
MEDULLOBLAST
MULTIPLICATION

BRAIN
GROWTH
SPURT

DENDRITIC GROWTH

SYNAPSE FORMATION

MYELINATION

?

FURTHER GROWTH

RAT
> 65 DAYS

MAN
>2 YEARS

**FIG. 6.** A diagrammatic representation of the primary events in neurogenesis. The time axis, from top to bottom, runs from conception to the final stages of brain development. This is a generalized scheme, applicable to any species. Brain growth is indicated as being complete at just over 65 days of age for the rat and 2 years for humans. Pre- and postnatal development are represented as a continuum; the point of birth in this representation varies according to the species. The events in glial cell formation are shown on the left, those of neuronal formation on the right. Both neurons and glia derive from neuroblasts; the diagram attempts to show that the formation of neurons is complete at a time when glial cell precursors (spongioblasts and medulloblasts) are still being formed. The heavy arrows represent the time of the "brain growth spurt" or rapid increase in brain mass. Adapted from a similar diagram of J. Dobbing.

brain the myelin, which makes up almost one-half of the dry weight of the brain, is produced by a certain glial cell type, the oligodendrocyte. Presumably these glia are deficient in number after undernutrition because a substantial deficit in myelin has been seen after early life undernutrition. It is possible, but has not been demonstrated, that the myelinated brain axons (not all axons in the brain are normally myelinated) decrease their conductance speed when the myelination is deficient; this could account for a functional deficit.

Another possible role of glial cells in brain function involves cellular nutrition. Wigglesworth (124) and Treherne (119) assembled both morphological and biochemical evidence that glial cells in insect nervous systems store nutrient material that is passed on to the neurons when needed. Under conditions of food restriction, carbohydrates stored in glial cells are released and then taken up by neurons. The histological arrangement of neurons and glial cells in mammalian nervous systems also suggest such functions for glial cells. In mammals neurons are rarely in direct contact with the blood capillaries but rather are separated from the blood vessels by glial cells. This "interposed" arrangement between the neurons and their blood supply has frequently suggested a nutritive or metabolic regulator function for the glia. Unfortunately, there is no evidence to fortify this attractive hypothesis.

## C. Summary

The overwhelming structural feature of the brain is its complexity. We know from functional studies that each region of the brain is organized to process very specific information. Neuroscientists are just beginning to bring order out of the millions of cells and the billions of connections these cells make with each other. Although specific diseases (e.g., parkinsonism) are associated with degenerative changes in specific brain regions, undernutrition causes no obvious morphological pathology. It appears that the initial formation of neurons is susceptible to undernutrition if the period of experimentally imposed undernutrition coincides with their period of neuronogenesis. Since almost all neurons develop very early in embryogenesis, only particular regions of the cerebellum, hippocampus, and olfactory system could be affected by postnatal undernutrition. A deficit in cerebellar granule cells after early undernutrition has been seen by several investigators. Another aspect of neurons that appears to be susceptible to undernutrition is the outgrowth of neuronal processes. Golgi-stained preparations show quite stunted dendritic processes on cerebellar Purkinje cells.

What has not yet been seen are abnormalities in the fine structure of neurons with normal or abnormal processes. However, the electron microscope has been useful in studies of synapses in undernourished animals. These structures, because of their structural unity and functional importance, are a reasonable target for further studies on anatomical alterations due to undernutrition.

## III. METHODS FOR STUDYING NUTRITIONAL EFFECTS ON CNS STRUCTURES

### A. Gross Measurements

"Gross measurements" here is used to indicate structural studies of the brain not utilizing the microscope. The earliest studies of undernutrition and brain development used brain size and weight as the measured variables. These studies were done at the turn of the century when microscopic methods for examining brain tissue were crude (57–59,65).

Gross measurements are necessary in most human studies because postmortem deterioration of the tissue ensues rapidly. Nevertheless, considerable information can be obtained from measurements of size and weight of the brain and its various components. Furthermore, certain brain measurements can be made in the intact subject, providing the added benefit of doing prospective studies on the same individual. Cranial transillumination has been used to view the brain and its ventricles (93); echoencephalography has been used to determine dimensions of the ventricular system (41,42), and head circumference is often taken as an index of brain size (19).

## B. Microscopic Methods

### 1. Conventional Light Microscopy

Cell stains of brain tissue (cresyl violet, hematoxylin and eosin, thionine) stain the nucleus and perinuclear cytoplasm of most of the larger cells, but few of the axonal or dendritic processes stain regularly. Furthermore, only fortuitous sections permit visualization of long processes in the same section as the cell body. To visualize myelin selectively requires that special stains be used either as counterstains or on adjacent sections. Thus a comprehensive view of brain tissue at the light microscopic level is quite difficult to obtain routinely. What can be seen with such preparations is the relative positions of the major cell groups (termed nuclei) and, under favorable circumstances, the quantification of areas occupied by certain cell types. Standard histological preparations provide the necessary orientation for other morphological procedures (e.g., Golgi studies, fluorescence microscopy, and histochemistry) and are an adjunct to autoradiographic methods.

Golgi-stained material offers the researcher the opportunity to view single neurons with all their processes stained. This stain penetrates to very few cells in the tissue but makes visible the details of axonal and dendritic ramifications not seen with usual histological techniques. When the investigator can identify specific neurons from animal to animal (e.g., cerebellar Purkinje cells), the Golgi-impregnated material allows him to compare fine details of axonal or dendritic morphology between normal and experimental animals (Fig. 4, for example).

### a. Cytochemical microscopy.

Histochemical techniques combine the detection of a cellular constituent, usually an enzyme, with a stain so that the location of the stain on the tissue section indicates the enzyme location. In addition, the practitioners of histochemistry believe that the intensity of the staining reaction provides quantitative information on the amount of the enzyme or whatever constituent is studied. Such semiquantitative studies have been applied to malnourished animals for comparison with controls (74,75,82). The chief criticism of these studies is that stain intensity may be influenced by extraneous factors such as the intracellular distribution of the enzyme, competing reactions, and the light-refracting properties of other cellular constituents.

*b. Immunocytochemical microscopy.*

Immunocytochemistry provides still another tool to the morphologist by using the immunological specificity of the antigen-antibody reaction to help visualize specific compounds in tissue·sections. This relatively new technique requires purification of the substance to be localized so that specific antibodies can be produced against it. The antigen-antibody reaction is then carried out on the tissue section and visualized by the use of secondary antibodies. These secondary antibodies are usually tagged with a substance that can be visualized easily (peroxidase) or one that fluoresces. One advantage of immunocytochemistry over the conventional staining approach is that the stainable substances are those that the experimenter selected as playing a significant role in neuronal transmission. It is not surprising, therefore, that the substances studied with this elegant technique are tyrosine hydroxylase, tryptophan hydroxylase, dopamine-$\beta$-hydroxylase, enzymes of the GABA system, and cyclic AMP. However, for present purposes, quantification of these reaction products for use in experimental studies remains problematic, and to our knowledge this set of techniques has not been applied to brains of undernourished animals either qualitatively or quantitatively.

*c. Autoradiography.*

Another method that relies on the light microscope to localize specific reactions in tissue sections is autoradiography. In this case high-energy radiation particles emitted from labeled tissue sources are marked by their passage through special photographic emulsions spread in a thin layer over the section. These penetrations result in latent images within silver halide particles in the emulsion. When photographically developed, the visible grains are located directly over that region of the cell which contained the isotope emitting the particle. Two kinds of experiments take advantage of this precise localization: uptake of specific substances (drugs, hormones, etc.) labeled by a radioisotope so that the cells that accumulate the substance can be seen; alternatively, autoradiography can be used when giving the animal a radiolabeled substance that will be incorporated into cellular constituents (nuclear DNA, cytoplasmic polypeptides, or glycoproteins) differentially to reveal the state of certain cells. Great advantage has been taken of this latter approach with labeled thymidine, a precursor for DNA synthesis. Immediately preceding cell division, cells double the amount of DNA in the nucleus. If labeled thymidine is present, it is incorporated into the DNA of the two daughter cells resulting from the mitotic cycle. By timing the injection of the labeled thymidine so that it is present in the tissue for a very short time, only those cells undergoing mitosis within that time span pick up the label. Furthermore, those cells that incorporate labeled thymidine and continue to divide dilute the label to insignificant levels. Therefore those cells that divide when the label is present, but not thereafter, develop silver grains in the overlayed emulsion. It is by this method that investigators are able to determine the "birthdays" of neurons, i.e., the date of final cell division after which they begin to differentiate but do not again divide. A few investigators have applied autoradiographic analysis to undernourished rat brains (72,81).

### 2. Electron Microscopy

The electron microscope is capable of much higher resolution than is attainable with the light microscope; paradoxically, despite this gain in resolution, experimental studies are far more difficult to interpret than those done with light microscopy. With the high magnification and greater resolution of the electron microscope come major difficulties stemming primarily from sampling because of the very small area of tissue observed and from uncertainty over the identification of the structures seen. Although the electron microscope can provide the investigator with great detail in the material under examination, the deficits in undernourished brain tissue have been too subtle to be identified readily.

Nevertheless, studies on undernourished brains utilizing the electron microscope have often reported differences, as compared to control brains, that are primarily differences of frequency. An increased frequency of certain intracellular bodies, for instance, could be ascribed to undernourishment (134). Often these studies assume the good will of their audience in accepting the observers' conclusions since strict quantitative comparisons of large samples are rarely attempted. This practice, while common among descriptive morphologists, may be less acceptable to quantitatively oriented nutritionists.

Statistically sound sampling procedures and counting paradigms—whether it be cells, synapses, neuropil area, etc.—done in a blind fashion must be instituted to assure both the investigator and the scientific community that the results are valid. [See articles by Cragg (27) and Sima (108) for examples of quantitative electron microscopy.] The type of quantitative morphology proposed here is both tedious and time-consuming to do. There is available equipment to aid in quantitative image processing which could well hasten the quantifying of morphological material. These computer-like devices can be used either on-line (such as a vidicon-tube attached to the microscope) or work from negative or positive photographic images. At present these devices are rather expensive, but as their use spreads and their value becomes realized it is hoped that they can be a common adjunctive procedure for all electron microscopists.

### C. Indirect Methods

Under "indirect methods" we include those studies measuring CNS constituents that can infer morphological entities. For example, in cases where brain lipid and cholesterol are measured by chemical extraction after undernutrition, the results infer alterations in extent of brain myelination. Similarly, when brain DNA and RNA are measured, the results infer modification of cell number and size, not genetic alterations. The following components illustrate the results of biochemical measures after undernutrition which relate to morphological alterations.

### 1. DNA, RNA, and Protein: Ratios and Inferences

The very extensive use of DNA measurements to assess the number of brain cells after undernutrition was initiated by Winick and Noble (126,127) and has been widely imitated. The use of DNA levels to indicate the number of cells in a tissue assumes the following: (a) The amount of DNA in each diploid cell is constant for all cells. (b) There are very few polyploid cells in the brain. (c) The assay employed measures DNA reliably and is not influenced by other compounds present.

Winick's use of 6.2 pg DNA per cell nucleus, obtained from the work of Enesco and Leblond (40), seems to fit with averages from a number of tissues (31). Regarding polyploidy in brain cells, Heller and Elliot (60) found very little in nuclei from several different brain regions. The assay used by Winick and Noble in their studies was Burton's diphenylamine reaction (22). Although Munro (77) cautioned against using diphenylamine and recommends reacting deoxypentane with indole, this modification may not substantially alter the findings.

Measurements of RNA and protein, often used in combination with DNA assays, have not been examined carefully for their assumptions and weaknesses. Measurement of RNA levels in brain tissue so far has not allowed distinction among the various classes of RNA (e.g., ribosomal, messenger, transfer) and has lumped them together. Perhaps the greatest problem in dealing with biochemical extractions of DNA, RNA, and protein from well- or undernourished brains is that the data do not distinguish between neurons and glial cells. Total DNA deficits may indicate a lower number of cells but do not indicate which cells are lacking. Similarly, low RNA/protein ratios, in a general way, may indicate decreased metabolic activity. Even if measured from a specific brain region, the RNA/protein ratio of neurons alone may be quite different from the ratio for the entire tissue but may be obscured by the much larger proportion contributed by the nonneuronal cells.

### 2. Myelin Constituents

The criticisms levelled at DNA assays, etc. can be overcome when extracting compounds closely associated with specific structural elements. That is the case with myelin representing a major share of the oligodendrocytes in the brain. In a thorough study of myelination using histological, autoradiographic, histochemical, and biochemical means, Schonback et al. (94) convincingly demonstrated the relationship between these specialized glial cells and myelin formation. Furthermore, their work indicates that cholesterol levels are a reasonable indicator of the accumulation of myelin in the developing brain. The unusual lipids found in myelin are even more precise indicators.

### 3. Transmitter Levels and Enzymes

Neurotransmitters and the enzymes involved in their metabolism are important chemical indicators of structure for two reasons. First, determining the transmitter levels can give information about the functional differentiation of neurochemically specific populations of neurons or axonal terminals in a given anatomical region. Used in combination with other techniques (e.g., electron microscopy), the measurement of several different transmitter substances in a given region can help determine whether a specific subset of neurons has been altered by the treatment or a nonspecific generalized defect has occurred.

Secondly, it is obvious from Table 2 (see below) that a great deal of work has already been done combining undernutrition and measurements of one or more transmitters or related enzymes. With the increased sophistication and miniaturization of the methods, it is clear that measurements of neurotransmitters will play a major role in future research efforts on this question.

We do not dwell on the methodology of transmitter or enzyme quantitation. The methods used are generally based on well-founded chemical procedures. They offer two distinct advantages over histochemical or other methods: (a) a high degree of specificity derived from molecular structural studies, and (b) quantitative results. The last point, quantitative results, is very attractive to researchers in this area because of the subtle nature of the deficits after undernutrition. It is now possible to analyze a region of brain approximately 1 $mm^3$ in size, and weighing only a few milligrams, for several transmitters. The results could indicate deficits as small as 20–30% below control values in certain transmitters, a situation not likely to be detected by any of the more conventional morphological methods. If the transmitter results are then combined with what is known about the types of neurons and terminals in the given region, a reasonable picture of the distortion due to nutritional deficiencies begins to emerge.

### 4. Summary

The complexity of the brain is such that no one method can provide sufficient information to describe adequately the changes that occur during and after nutritional deficiencies. Keeping in mind that nutritional lesions in the brain are the "distortion and deficit" type, the need for quantitative data becomes more obvious. This need is now being met by morphometric studies using either light or electron microscopy. New computer-aided devices will also help in this respect. Another tack is that taken by combining a morphological measure with biochemical measures. This combination of tools provides chemical specificity and quantitation to the cellular or subcellular observations.

## IV. WHAT HAS BEEN DEMONSTRATED

### A. Morphological Results

#### 1. Early Workers

A study of the literature relating morphological alterations to early undernutrition (Table 1) reveals that critical studies were performed very early. The first paper to appear in the American scientific literature was published in 1904 by Hatai of the University of Chicago (57). There followed several papers by Hatai (58,59) and Jackson and Stewart (65). Some of the early observations have a very familiar ring, as for example this quotation from a paper by Stewart: "It is interesting to note that the marked growth of the brain in rats stunted by underfeeding occurs only at a period when the normal increase in size is still due partly to cell multiplication, especially in the cerebellum. This is a phase of the inanition problem worthy of further investigation" (114).

Stewart anticipated Winick and Noble by almost 50 years. Even more remarkable is a 1918 paper by Sugita (117). One of the interesting aspects of Sugita's paper is that he compared three methods of obtaining undernourished rats. He carried out an extensive histological examination of the brains of animals undernourished by either separation from the mother, placing 17–18 pups on one mother, or reducing the amount of food to the lactating mother. Regardless of method, Sugita found that the undernourished pups had smaller cerebral cortical volumes and increased cortical thickening. He concluded that the reduced size of the brain was due to a reduction in neuron size, as well as myelination, but that the total number of neurons is the same as in the well-nourished controls.

Not only has no one since done a morphological study on brain comparing different methods for undernourishing rats, but with only a few exceptions the results obtained in 1918 have not been improved on. Thus the following evidence that early undernutrition affects brain morphology has been available since the end of World War I (compiled from these references: 57–59, 65,114,115,117).

1. Undernutrition early in the life of the animal results in decreased brain size, especially cortical tissue.

2. The decrease in brain size is not nearly as great as the decrease in other organs and whole body size.

3. Brain neurons are "born," in most cases, before the birth of the animal, and therefore:

4. Postnatal undernutrition should not affect the number of neurons but should reduce their size.

5. Another cause of the reduction in brain size is a deficit in myelination.

6. Those brain regions that undergo neurogenesis postnatally (e.g., the cerebellum) are more likely to develop deficits in neuron number and be more affected by the undernutrition.

We might add that these early workers did not know whether these morphological deficits had a detrimental effect on the animal's functioning. This very important question seems not to have been answered. Our state of ignorance, as well as our state of knowledge, has not changed greatly over the years.

## 2. Renaissance: The Work of Winick

For unknown reasons, research in this area was inactive for many years. Much of the credit for the increase in research activity on these fundamentally important questions over the last decade must be given to Winick. In a series of papers over several years (125–127,129) Winick helped to focus interest on the nutrition-brain-development problem. Using biochemical techniques familiar to nutritionists, Winick defined the phases of brain growth in terms of hyperplasia and hypertrophy, determined which phases were critical for both brain stunting and rehabilitation, and demonstrated that these essential features are true in undernourished children as well as in rats (128,130).

The impetus given by Winick's work to the entire field has resulted in increased interest not only from nutritionists, but also from histologists, electron microscopists, and biochemists. Tables 1 and 2 list nearly all of the contributions made by these various disciplines to the study of nutritional effects on brain structure.

## 3. Quantitative Microscopic Studies

To overcome the criticisms mentioned above, histologists frequently employ quantitative procedures with their microscopy. These methods may be as simple as counting manually the number of neurons and glial cells in histological sections (36,66,107) or using the eyepiece reticule for measuring individual cells (36,117).

The use of areal measurements on photomicrographs probably shortens the time required to quantitate histological preparations. However, the region chosen must be one with discriminable cell populations as in the cerebellum (9,10,54) (Fig. 2, for example).

Electron microscopists, perhaps because of sampling problems, frequently require quantitative morphology. Cragg (27) used a counting procedure to

TABLE 1. Compilation of reports from the literature on alterations of brain morphology after or during nutritional deprivation

| Findings | Species | Method of undernutrition[a] | Reference |
|---|---|---|---|
| *Gross measurements[b]* | | | |
| In weanling rats undernutrition reduced brain size, but not by as much as other organs. | Rat | 1 | Hatai (57) |
| Size and weight of brain lower when undernutrition began early in life. | Rat | 2 | Jackson and Stewart (65) |
| Brain weight of malnourished Ugandan children at autopsy was significantly lower than both nonmalnourished Ugandan and a reference group of children. | Human | c | Brown (19) |
| Decreased brain size and increased CSF space was seen by transillumination in severe marasmic children. | Human | c | Rozovski et al. (93) |
| Children with marasmus had reduced head circumference, delayed brain size increase as measured by transillumination, and normal ventricular index as determined by echoencephalography. | Human | c | Engsner et al. (41) |
| Children with kwashiorkor had reduced head circumference, abnormal transillumination findings, and an increased ventricular index. | Human | c | Engsner et al. (42) |
| *Standard histology and histochemistry* | | | |
| Using three different methods of undernourishing newborn rats, the author demonstrated smaller cerebral cortex volumes and greater cortical thickness in the undernourished rats. The growth of neuron size was retarded, as was myelination, but the total number of neurons was the same as controls. | Rat | 2,3,6 | Sugita (117) |
| No nerve degeneration, but cell density was greater and the dendritic development reduced. | Rat | 2 | Eayrs and Horn (37) |
| Reduction of the dietary protein (6%) during gestation resulted in an apparant loss of large multipolar neurons in brain and spinal cord at term; several enzymes, tested histochemically, showed no difference in the neurons of the undernourished. | Rat | 4 | Shrader and Zeman (106) |
| Reduced cell counts in cerebral cortex; predominantly nonneural cells. | Rat | 4/3 | Siassi and Siassi (107) |
| Retarded outgrowth of apical dendritic tree of cerebellar Purkinje cells. | Rat | 6 | Sima and Persson (109) |

| Findings | Species | No. | Reference |
|---|---|---|---|
| No evidence of degenerative changes in nerve cells or fibers; but cells contained less cytoplasm, myelin sheaths were thinner, and dendritic development was reduced. | Rat | 5 | Stewart et al. (116) |
| Reduced cell number in germinal external granular layer and internal granular layer of cerebellum. | Rat | 6 | Barnes and Altman (9) |
| Reduced numbers of stellate, basket, granule, and Purkinje cells in undernourished cerebellum. | Rat | 6 | Barnes and Altman (10) |
| Using DNA contents and areal measurements of histological preparations, undernourished rats were shown to have a slowing of cell production in the external granular layer of the cerebellum. | Rat | 3 | Griffin et al. (54) |
| Using quantitative microscopic means, undernourished rats had fewer neurons in both cerebral and cerebellar cortex; specifically noted was a 21% loss in Purkinje cells and 31% deficit in granule cells. | Rat | 3 | Dobbing et al. (36) |
| Young monkeys given 2% protein diets for 15 weeks had a drastically altered distribution of thiamine pyrophosphatase, inosine diphosphatase, acid phosphatase, and ATPase in motor neurons of the spinal cord. | Squirrel monkey | 1 | Manocha and Olkowski (74) |
| After 15 weeks of low-protein diets, monkey cerebellum showed alterations in a number of cytochemically demonstrable enzymes. Purkinje, stellate, and basket cells were more sensitive to the undernutrition. Most oxidative enzymes were decreased, but liposomal enzymes were increased. | Squirrel monkey | 1 | Manocha and Olkowski (75) |
| Microscopic examination of undernourished pig spinal cord revealed swollen myelin sheaths but no degeneration. There was an absolute increase in the number of neuroglial cells. Motor neurons showed loss of chromatin and occasionally an eccentric nucleus. There were minimal changes in higher levels of the nervous system (brain). | Pig | 1 | Platt et al. (83) |
| Loss of Nissl substances from the motor cells of the anterior horns of the spinal cord. Less severe changes were seen in thalamus, caudate, and cerebral cortex, but these regions also showed increased satellitosis, ghost cells, and loss of cells. | Dog | 3 | Platt and Stewart (84) |
| Counting neurons and glial cells in the lateral vestibular nucleus after 1 month of undernutrition from birth showed the neuron size to be unchanged, but there were increases in density of small and medium-sized neurons and glial cells. | Rat | 5[d] | Johnson and Yoesle (66) |

TABLE 1. (*continued*)

| Findings | Species | Method of undernutrition[a] | Reference |
|---|---|---|---|
| *Golgi-stained preparations* | | | |
| Golgi-Cox stained preparations of cerebellum from undernourished rats showed significantly more dendritic aberrations involving branching and shape. This demonstrates that undernutrition can affect the nonmitotic growth of neurons. | Rat | 3 | Griffin and Woodward (53) |
| Undernutrition from birth to day 35 resulted in reduced Purkinje cell packing density in cerebellar vermis. Golgi stain revealed a 20% loss of dendritic field area of Purkinje cells. | Mouse | 3 | Pysh and Perkins (87) |
| The large cortical pyramidal cells of layer V in frontal and occipital cortex had reduced number of spines, less basilar dendritic density, and reduced dendritic thickness in undernourished rats. Neuronal process deficits documented by quantification. | Rat | 2 | Salas et al. (136) |
| Layer V cortical pyramidal neurons were studied at 35 days of age after pre- and post-weaning nutritional deprivation. The undernourished rats displayed a decrease in the number and span of dendritic basilar processes. | Rat | 3/1 | Cordero et al. (137) |
| *Autoradiographic methods* | | | |
| Autoradiographic analysis reveals a late maturing external granular layer, implying depressed cell formation and loss of germinal cells. | Rat | 6 | Lewis et al. (72) |
| Autoradiography with $^{14}$C-thymidine revealed, in the cerebral cortex, that the mitotic rate is much slower in undernourished rats; but, as if in compensation, the rate of cell loss is also slower. | Rat | 6 | Patel et al. (81) |
| *Electron microscopy* | | | |
| Qualitative differences in the free and membrane-bound ribosomes of the endoplasmic reticulum and in synaptic membranes of cortex and hippocampus. | Rhesus monkey | 1 | Ordy (79) |
| The density of neuronal cell bodies in visual and frontal cortex was higher by 22–33% owing to retarded neuropil development. Axon terminals and other neuronal structures were not abnormal by EM measurement but the number of axon terminals associated with one neuron was reduced (by ca. 40%). | Rat | 2/3 | Cragg (27) |
| Undernourished rat cerebellar molecular layer contained fewer glial cell processes as determined by morphometric analysis. | Rat | 2 | Clos et al. (25) |

| Description | Species | | Reference |
|---|---|---|---|
| Using quantitative measurements at the ultrastructural level, undernourished somatosensory cortex had a higher density of neurons, a diminished size and density of presynaptic endings. | Rat | 5 | Gambetti et al. (51) |
| Found lamellar whorls and aggregation of synaptic vesicles in presynaptic elements of undernourished rats (believed to be a sign of degeneration). | Rat | 1 | Yu et al. (134) |
| The deposition of myelin as determined by counting myelin lamellae in EM sections was impaired in optic nerve and ventral and dorsal lumbar roots. The axonal radial growth is disproportionately more affected in optic nerves than spinal roots. | Rat | 6 | Sima (108) |
| Phosphotungstic acid stain in the molecular layers of the cerebellum and dentate gyrus of hippocampus in undernourished rats revealed deficits (of 9% and 24%, respectively) in the number of synapses per unit area. | Rat | 5 | Shoemaker and Bloom (101) |
| Similar profiles of synapses were noted with the phosphotungstic acid stain; no qualitative difference was observed between well- and undernourished brains, and no quantitation was attempted. | Rat | 5 | Burns et al. (21) |

*Indirect measurements: DNA, RNA, and protein*

| Description | Species | | Reference |
|---|---|---|---|
| Reduced brain DNA, RNA, and protein when the rats were undernourished from birth to weaning, implying a reduced cell number but normal cell size. | Rat | 3 | Winick and Noble (127) |
| Lower DNA in cerebellum of undernourished rats. | Rat | 3 | Chase et al. (23) |
| Decreases in glial proliferation and migration in cerebrum; also decrease in neuronal fiber proliferation. | Rat | 3[e] | Bass et al. (11) |
| Reduced cell proliferation and number in cerebellum, but not cell size. | Rat | 2 | Gourdon et al. (52) |
| Reductions in brain DNA, RNA, lipid, protein, cholesterol, phospholipid, and cerebroside when undernourished. | Rat | 2 | Cully and Lineberger (28) |
| Reduced cerebral and cerebellar DNA and cholesterol. | Mouse | 2 | Howard and Granoff (62) |
| Reduced brain DNA, RNA, cholesterol, and phospholipid phosphorus. | Rat | 3 | Guthrie and Brown (55) |
| Reduced DNA content of whole brain at birth after undernutrition of the mother before and during pregnancy: presumed to be a deficit in neurons. | Rat | 4 | Zamenhof et al. (135) |
| DNA content of cerebellum, cerebrum, hippocampus, and brainstem were lower than control, and marked in cerebrum and cerebellum. | Rat | 3 | Fish and Winick (46) |
| DNA levels in normal and undernourished children showed deficits in cells in all brain regions; but compared to the rat, greater deficits in cerebrum and brainstem. | Human | d | Winick et al. (130) |

TABLE 1. (continued)

| Findings | Species | Method of undernutrition[a] | Reference |
|---|---|---|---|
| *Indirect measurements: myelin constituents* | | | |
| The concentration of myelin in the optic tract was reduced by 20% as measured spectrophotometrically. | Rat | 1 | Buchanan and Roberts (20) |
| Myelin constituents measured showed no change when rats were undernourished after weaning. | Rat | 1 | Dobbing and Widdowson (35) |
| Myelin reduction was inferred from neurochemical findings on whole brain homogenates. | Rat | 3 | Benton et al. (13) |
| In cerebral cortex and white matter, myelination was greatly retarded—thought to be due to decrease in glial cell precursors. Both histological and biochemical methods were used. | Rat | 3[e] | Bass et al. (12) |
| Reduced cerebroside and plasmalogen levels in white matter from four malnourished children. | Human | [c] | Fishman et al. (47) |
| Reduced synthesis of whole brain myelin protein, especially proteolipid protein, shown by isotope incorporation. | Rat | 2/3 | Wiggins et al. (123) |
| Neurochemical composition of brain myelin constituents unaffected when undernourished after the ninth postnatal week. | Pig | 1 | Fishman et al. (48) |
| Reduced cerebral and cerebellar DNA and cholesterol. | Mouse | 2 | Howard and Granoff (62) |
| Reduced brain DNA, RNA, cholesterol, and phospholipid phosphorus. | Rat | 3 | Guthrie and Brown (55) |
| *Measurements on single isolated neuronal cell bodies* | | | |
| Lowered dry mass and RNA content in spinal motor neurons. | Rat | 2 | Haltia (56) |

[a]The different methods used to produce undernourished animals are coded as follows: (1) Animals were undernourished by dietary means only after they were weaned from the mother. (2) Animals were separated from the lactating mother for various lengths of time; the well-nourished controls were kept with the mother constantly. (3) Animals (usually rodents) were placed in litters of 16 or more young per mother (a normal litter size for rats is 10–11 young); the well-nourished control litters usually numbered 8 or less. (4) Prenatal "undernutrition" was achieved by reducing the protein content or total diet of the mother during gestation. (5) Litter size was kept constant in both control and undernourished groups (usually 8 for rodents); the undernutrition was produced by feeding some of the lactating mothers a lower-percent-protein diet that reduced milk production. (6) Similar to (5) except that the lactating mothers are fed a restricted amount of normal diet. Studies using a combination method or more than one method are indicated as "x"/"y" and "x," "y," respectively.

[b]The data were arranged according to methodology, e.g., gross measurements.

[c]Human studies are not experimental but are gathered from clinical presentations or at autopsy. In many cases the severity and duration of undernutrition cannot be determined precisely. Refer to the individual papers for details.

[d]In this study, inexplicably, no figure is given for the number of rat pups nursing on each mother.

[e]In these studies the undernutrition was produced by nursing in litters of 12.

TABLE 2. *Compilation of studies that use assays of neurotransmitters, neurotransmitter-related enzymes, or similar biochemical measurements*

| Findings[a] | Species | Method of undernutrition[b] | Reference |
|---|---|---|---|
| **Acetylcholine** | | | |
| Brain acetylcholinesterase activity, NE concentration and content, and 5-HT concentration and content were lower than in controls during the first few weeks of life in undernourished rats. | Rat | 3 | Sereni et al. (98) |
| Acetylcholinesterase activity was elevated in undernourished, rehabilitated rats at 16 weeks of age. | Rat | 6 | Adlard and Dobbing (1) |
| Acetylcholinesterase activity per brain was lower at weaning in undernourished rats. | Rat | 6 | Adlard and Dobbing (2) |
| Total brain cholinesterase activity was lower at 3 and 7 weeks in the undernourished brains but specific activity (per gram of brain or per milligram of N) was increased at 7 weeks. | Rat | 5 | Im et al. (63) |
| Weanling pigs, malnourished for 11 weeks (3% protein), had less total cholinesterase activity in the brain but higher specific activity in the cerebrum. | Pig | 1 | Im et al. (64) |
| No difference in acetylcholinesterase and choline acetyltransferase activity from synaptosomal fractions of cerebral cortex in normal and undernourished rats. | Rat | 5 | Gambetti et al. (50) |
| Undernourished rats' brains had decreased choline acetyltransferase and dopamine-$\beta$-hydroxylase but increased tyrosine hydroxylase levels. | Rat | 5 | Shoemaker et al. (105) |
| Previously undernourished rats had lower levels of synaptosomal protein but not of acetylcholinesterase activity after rehabilitating at 12 weeks of age. | Rat | 6 | Adlard et al. (3) |
| Previously undernourished rats had higher specific activity of acetylcholinesterase but not of choline acetyltransferase 4 weeks after rehabilitation. Also see Sobotka et al. (110) below. | Rat | 5 | Eckhert et al. (38) |
| **Serotonin** | | | |
| Previously undernourished rats had higher turnover rates of 5-HT in pons-medulla, hippocampus, and striatum but not in hypothalamus, midbrain, or cerebrum after rehabilitation at 20 weeks of age. | Rat | 6 | Tricklebank and Adlard (120) |

171

TABLE 2. (continued)

| Findings | Species | Method of undernutrition[b] | Reference |
|---|---|---|---|
| 5-Hydroxytryptophan decarboxylase activity and 5-HT levels were lower at 21 days in the undernourished rats. | Rat | 3 | Hernandez (61) |
| Rats undernourished from conception through 140 days of age had higher concentrations (μg/g wet weight) of NE and 5-HT in several brain areas, but total brain NE content was lower. | Rat | 4/5 | Stern et al. (112) |
| Feeding rats for 6 weeks on a tryptophan-deficient diet (corn) results in reduced 5-HT levels in whole brain, which could be restored by a single injection of tryptophan (50 mg/kg). | Rat | 1 | Fernstrom and Hirsch (45) |
| *Norepinephrine* | | | |
| Undernourished rat brains contained 25% less NE than controls, but tyrosine hydroxylase levels were increased. | Rat | 5 | Shoemaker and Wurtman (103) |
| NE and DA levels were lower in the malnourished compared to the control, crowded, or infected groups. | Mouse | 5 | Lee and Dubos (71) |
| Undernourished rats regained whole brain levels of NE after rehabilitation, by 90 days of age. | Rat | 5 | Wiener (122) |
| Undernourished rats had higher 5-HT and NE concentrations and contents at birth when the low protein diet was begun prior to mothers' matings. By 21 days (weaning) several brain regions showed increased concentrations of amines, but the whole brain content of 5-HT and NE was 10–15% lower compared to controls on laboratory chow. | Rat | 4/5 | Stern et al. (113) |
| Undernourished pups had lower brain cholesterol, cerebellar DNA, cerebellar acetylcholinesterase activity, telencephalic NE and DA content; brainstem 5-HT concentration, however, was significantly increased. | Rat | 5 | Sobotka et al. (110) |

Also see Sereni et al. (98), Stern et al. (112), and Shoemaker et al. (105), above.

172

| | | | |
|---|---|---|---|
| *Dopamine* | | | |
| Both NE and DA were decreased in undernourished rat brain; DA was low in basal ganglia (where it is a transmitter); uptake of labeled NE unchanged. Also see Sobotka et al. (110), above. | Rat | 5 | Shoemaker and Wurtman (104) |
| *GABA* | | | |
| Glutamate dehydrogenase and glutamate decarboxylase, enzymes involved with GABA metabolism, had lower activity per gram of brain at 4 weeks of age in neonatal undernourished rats. Most of this deficit was due to failure to increase during the second week after birth. | Rat | 3 | Rajalakshmi et al. (88) |
| *Histamine* | | | |
| Feeding weanling guinea pigs and rats 3% and 0.5% protein diets, respectively, for 3 weeks resulted in two- to fourfold increases in brain histamine levels. Brain histidine, the precursor amino acid, was similarly elevated. | Guinea pig and rat | 1 | Enwonwu and Worthington (43) |
| Weanling rats, fed 0.5% lactalbumin diets for several weeks, accumulated two to four times as much brain histamine as controls on normal protein diets. Refeeding with adequate protein reversed this increase to normal levels in ca. 1 week. | Rat | 1 | Enwonwu and Worthington (44) |
| *Miscellaneous constituents* | | | |
| NE-binding but not DA-binding protein was reduced: could be protein of storage granules or part of the postsynaptic receptor. | Mouse | 5 | Lee (70) |
| Reduced Na$^+$-K$^+$-ATPase activity in isolated synaptosomes in cerebral and cerebellar cortices of undernourished rats. | Rat | 5 | Kissane and Hawrylewicz (68) |
| Miniature pigs, weaned at either 5, 21, or 35 days of age, and fed either low (5%) or adequate (20%) protein diets, showed differing patterns of brain amino acids: these vary according to time of weaning, level of protein in the diet, and brain region analyzed. | Miniature pig | 1 | Badger and Tumbleson (8) |

Abbreviations: NE, norepinephrine. 5-HT, serotonin. DA, dopamine.
[a]Most of these works infer brain structural alterations from the chemical results. They are arranged according to the neurotransmitter system involved.
[b]See footnote [a] in Table 1 for explanation.

determine the density of neuronal cell bodies and the number of axon terminals associated with one neuron. Both are greatly altered in undernourished
brains. Sima (108) quantified the number of myelin lamellae in electron
microscopic sections to show that myelination was more reduced in brain than
peripheral nerves. Gambetti et al. (51) also found increased cell density in
brain after undernutrition; their methods also allowed them to observe a
decrease in the size and density of presynaptic endings.

We used a slightly different approach by employing a stain (ethanolic
phosphotungstic acid) that selectively reveals synaptic complexes (4,16) (Fig.
7). This procedure allows us to sample wide areas for synaptic quantification
easily. Undernourishing rats as previously described by Shoemaker and
Wurtman (103), we found a deficit in the number of synapses in the cerebellar
molecular layer and the molecular layer of the hippocampal dentate gyrus
(Table 3). In addition, by making area measurements on the tissue blocks with
the light microscope, we were able to determine the decrease in overall tissue
area in the undernourished brains. The area figure is transposed into a volume
figure by assuming the third dimension was reduced by the average reduction
of the other two dimensions. By combining the synapse deficit percentage
with the volume reduction, one can estimate the hypothetical total deficit in
synapses in that tissue (the numbers in brackets in Table 3). Finally, in a
further attempt at numerical rigor, the authors applied the standard $t$-test to
the results. This was possible by using each photograph for either the control
or the undernourished brain as a sample of that type brain. There is variability
from one sample region to another on the grid and an $n$ of 20–30 was obtained
for each group.

## 4. Summary of Morphological Experiments

Taken as an entity, the compiled microscopic evaluations of undernourished brains can be summarized using data from several species and many

TABLE 3. *Quantification of PTA-stainable synaptic complexes in the molecular*
*layers of the cerebellum and hippocampal dentate*

| Measurement | | Dentate gyrus | Cerebellum |
|---|---|---|---|
| Total no. of synapses counted | | 1,700 | 1,600 |
| Synapses per 100 $\mu^2$ | | | |
| ($\pm$ SEM) | Control | 23.4 $\pm$ 0.8 | 28.2 $\pm$ 2.3 |
| | Undernourished | 17.8 $\pm$ 1.4[a] | 26.1 $\pm$ 1.7 |
| % Difference | | −24 | −9 |
| % Difference in width of tissue | | −14 | −23 |
| Hypothetical deficit in total no. of | | | |
| synapses (%) | | [52] | [59] |

From Shoemaker and Bloom (101).
[a]Significantly different from well-nourished controls ($p < 0.05$ by $t$-test).

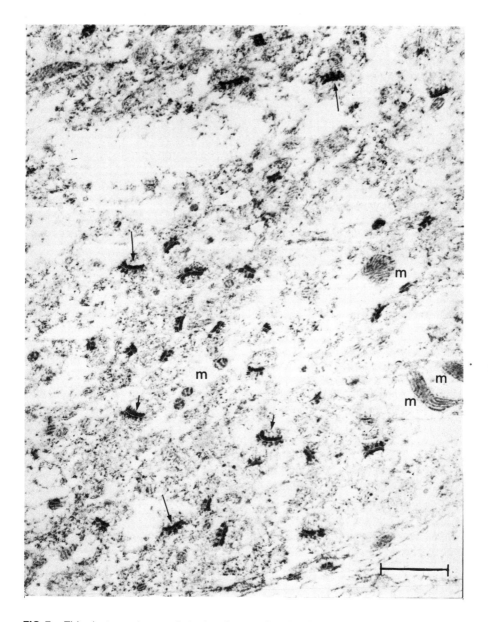

**FIG. 7.** This electron micrograph depicts the cytochemical detection of specialized synaptic contacts by block staining with ethanolic phosphotungstic acid. A slightly overreacted field was selected in order to visualize more fully the background elements. The most numerous and heavily stained elements seen are the synaptic junctional complexes (some indicated by arrows), but some electron-dense stain also has been deposited in mitochondria (m). Note that despite the relatively heavy stained background, the synaptic junctions are easily discernible for tabulation. The bar equals 1 μm. (See Bloom, ref. 14, for detailed discussion.)

different methods of undernutrition. The formative steps of neuron formation in mammals (i.e., cell formation, migration, differentiation, and death) occur prenatally, with certain exceptions. Only two reports, one using DNA as a measure of neurons (135), the other using nonquantitative histology (106), claim to modify the number of neurons by prenatal undernutrition. All other reports use chiefly postnatal undernutrition paradigms; the predominant finding is that the number of neurons is not decreased. The exceptions referred to above are the cerebellum, the hippocampus, and the olfactory bulb. These regions undergo a certain amount of neurogenesis postnatally in a number of species. Consequently a great deal of work has been done on cerebellar development under conditions of nutritional deprivation. It was found very early that the cerebellum was more drastically affected than other regions of the brain (36,46,117). Later detailed studies showed that there are deficits in granule cells (9,36), Purkinje cells (10,36), and stellate and basket cells (10); decreases in germinal cell activity and number (9,10,54,72); decreased glial cell processes (25); and abnormal and stunted Purkinje cell dendrites (53,87) (Fig. 4).

Another brain region that has been utilized for studies of neuronal development during undernutrition is layer V of the frontal and occipital cortex. The large cortical pyramidal cells of layer V have been visualized with the Golgi stain and subjected to morphometric analysis by two different groups (136, 137). Both groups found deficits in number of basilar dendritic processes; other deficits seen were decreased numbers of dendritic spines and decreased dendritic thickness. The neurons of cortical layer V are late-maturing; hence, the authors attribute the retarded growth of the processes to the nutritional deficiency instituted after birth. We would agree with this interpretation but wish to know if the axonal processes are equally as affected as the dendrites. Similarly, it would be important to determine whether incoming fibers form fewer synapses on the reduced number of dendrites of these pyramidal cells or whether they make the normal number of synaptic connections on a smaller dendritic volume.

Although these studies of rat cerebral cortex with the Golgi stain show unequivocal differences from controls in the growth and pattern of dendrites, similar differences in dendritic branching of cortical layer V are seen between rats reared for 30 days after weaning in complex or isolated environments (138,139). This latter finding indicates that environmental differences more subtle than nutrition can affect delicate neural patterns such as fine dendritic morphology. Nutritionists will need to be more aware of other aspects of the animals' environment that can mimic the changes seen with undernutrition, and design their experiments to eliminate or control for nonnutritional differences between groups.

The use of the Golgi stain technique in nutritional research is quite recent. It has been concluded in studies of undernutrition that neuronal number is generally not decreased while the density of neurons is generally increased

(27,37,51,66,107,117). Recently more detailed reports on the nature of the ultrastructural distortion have appeared. Gambetti et al. (51), using quantitative methods in the somatosensory cortex, determined that the density of presynaptic endings was diminished. As mentioned above, we (101) detected deficits in the number of synaptic contacts in hippocampal dentate and the cerebellar molecular layer, regions that develop their synapses postnatally. This information, coupled with the Golgi-stained material discussed above (53,87,136,137), make a case for deficits in the postmitotic growth of neuronal processes, both dendritic and axonal.

## B. Interpretation of Neurotransmitter Alterations

Based on the observation that undernutrition inhibits the growth of processes, as discussed above, one might expect that measurements of neurotransmitters would be a useful method of identifying specific neuronal terminal deficits. No doubt this is what motivated the many studies described in Table 2. Before reviewing the findings, however, some caution must be inserted on interpreting neurotransmitter levels and their enzymes as markers for neurons and neuronal processes.

First, there is the problem of expressing the amount of a chemical substance (transmitter or enzyme) in the appropriate anatomical base unit; i.e., is the most appropriate expression of data in units of grams (or moles) per brain, grams per gram of brain, grams per milligram of protein, etc.? Although this issue has been discussed in the literature before (103,104,113) and while no imposed edict is intended here, it is quite important that the problem be understood as being nontrivial. The full meaning of any such expression is obviously a function of both numerator and denominator, so that one can obtain lower values for the concentration of a substance either by having an absolute lower amount of the substance or by having more of the normalizing substance. Thus an absolute whole brain content of 300 ng norepinephrine is noted as half the concentration of norepinephrine in a brain weighing 1 g as compared to a brain weighing 0.5 g if transmitter content is expressed per gram of brain.

When one of us (W.J.S.) initially became involved in measuring transmitters in undernourished brains, both the transmitter amount and the weight of the brain were found to be altered from control values: They were both decreased. For several reasons, however, this paired decrease seemed to be more a coincidence than a coupled-interlocking phenomenon. Firstly, although the cause for the decrease in norepinephrine was unknown, it seemed reasonable that the decrease in brain weight was due, to a considerable extent, to lack of myelin (see "myelin" section of Table 1) and deficits in glial cells. These changes bear no direct relationship to catecholamines. Secondly, some of the chemical components specific to the catecholamine neurons (i.e., the enzyme tyrosine hydroxylase) increased in absolute amount rather than decreasing as the norepinephrine content did. This divergent result speaks against the notion that the undernourished brain is a normally constituted but smaller version of the control brain.

Finally, if the two indices in question (i.e., norepinephrine amount and brain weight) were tightly coupled, they should covary in some regular fashion under different experimental conditions. However, this was clearly not the case: Although undernourished rats had less norepinephrine on the average, the most undernourished rats, which had the smallest brains, did not always have the lowest amount of norepinephrine.

In these animals the norepinephrine level, if expressed as concentration per gram of brain, would actually be higher than control values. While literally true, expressing the data as increases in concentration would also be extremely misleading. However, it is possible to test the strength of the relationship between transmitter amount and brain size in a series of normal animals of the same age and sex. A correlation coefficient ($r$) was calculated between several chemical constituents measured in a given whole brain or brain region and the weight of the tissue from which it was measured. Those correlations are seen in Table 4. From analogous tissue we measured the same components in undernourished rats of the same age as the normals. The only

TABLE 4. *Correlation coefficient between a chemical constituent measured in a tissue and the weight of that tissue*

| Constituent measured | Tissue from normal animals[a] | Tissue from undernourished animals[a] |
|---|---|---|
| Rat whole brain norepinephrine (assayed 1969) | .101 | .340 |
| Rat whole brain norepinephrine (assayed 1971) | .099 | −.433 |
| Rat whole brain dopamine | −.568 | .403 |
| Rat corpus striatum dopamine | .670 | −.012 |
| Rat whole brain tyrosine | .630 | .141 |
| Rat whole brain protein | .976 | |

Modified from Shoemaker (100).

The correlation coefficient ($r$) is a useful measure of the relatedness between two variables from a sample set. Values for $r$ range from +1 to −1. A value of zero would indicate no correlation between variables, +1 would be a perfect positive correlation, −1 would indicate an inverse correlation. Since perfect correlations are rarely achieved, an indication of the strength of correlation can be obtained by determining $r^2$. This value estimates the portion of one variable "explained" by the other variable. For instance, a correlation $r = .70$ would mean that approximately 50% of the variability in one measure can be "explained" by variability in the other measure; a correlation of $r = .80$ can "explain" 64% of variability, etc.

[a]Ten to 20 tissues used in each correlation.

substance that correlated well with brain weight is brain protein ($r = .976$). The total amount of brain tyrosine, an amino acid found in all brain cells, correlates weakly with the weight of the brain ($r = .630$). (See footnote to Table 4 for an explanation of the strength of $r$.) There is some suggestion that if the tissue is more homogeneous, as in the tissue of the corpus striatum, that correlations with a substance found there in high amounts (dopamine) are better ($r = .670$), but this is still a not very compelling correlation. Also, note the poor relative correlation of these same two variables in the undernourished rats ($r = -.012$). The correlation coefficient of the other substances with brain weight indicates no relationship between them; i.e., large brains do not contain more norepinephrine, and small brains do not contain less. If the reported transmitter levels in some of the studies listed in Table 2 are recalculated, as we have done, the reader can compare both per-gram and per-brain levels and make an individual decision as to which index is the more meaningful.

There are still more reasons for caution in interpreting neurotransmitter and enzyme changes after undernutrition, arising from the complex metabolism of these substances. This subject is discussed in detail elsewhere in this volume (see chapter by Nowak and Munro, *this volume*) but is relevant here when using these substances as morphological markers. Most known neurotransmitters are small molecules, enzymatically converted from available precursors, chiefly amino acids. The enzymatic steps involved are under multiple control by precursors, cofactors, cosubstrates, intermediate compounds, and endproducts. Unless one knows the precise role played by all of the controlling factors, it is difficult to predict the new steady-state level of any of the components when one of them is altered.

Here is but one example from our own experience: When early undernutrition was found to result in lowered brain norepinephrine levels, we also measured the amount of tyrosine hydroxylase (103). Tyrosine hydroxylase is the rate-limiting enzymatic step in norepinephrine formation (121), and we fully expected the level of the enzyme also to be decreased. After repeated measurements it was clear that our expectations were wrong; although norepinephrine levels were decreased, tyrosine hydroxylase activity was increased (103). This "paradoxical" situation now has a rational metabolic explanation (96); but if we had measured only the enzyme as a marker for that system, we would have had to assume that undernutrition causes increases in the adrenergic neurons, measured either per brain or per gram of brain.

This dynamic aspect of neurotransmitters and their enzymes requires the nutritional investigator to alter his experimental approach when using these substances as morphological markers. Unlike most morphological entities, the levels of these biochemical substances vary according to the time of day (89), nature of the previous meal (26,95,133), endocrine status (73), and state of arousal (90). We advise that when these substances are used as markers for neurons or terminals that, in addition to environmental constancy, a microscopic observation of the tissue also be included in the study so that the quantitative chemical change can be reasonably interpreted. Of course this does not apply to purely metabolic studies of neurotransmitters after undernutrition.

### C. Summary of Neurotransmitter Findings

The published findings on brain neurotransmitter alterations due to undernutrition include alterations in the putative neurotransmitters: norepinephrine (71,98,103,104,110,112,113), dopamine (71,104,110), and serotonin (61,98, 110,112,113,120). On reviewing the data for each of these transmitters, one is confronted by a variety of methods used to produce the undernutrition, differences in the age of the animal at sacrifice, the brain regions assayed, and the methods of assay, not to mention the way the data are finally expressed. No attempt is made here to resolve the conflicting results, if indeed such a process were possible. However, certain observations appear to be more consistent than others and these deserve comment.

### 1. Norepinephrine

Most of the studies dealing with transmitter levels report deficits in the catecholamines norepinephrine and dopamine when measured up to the time of weaning and expressed as content per brain. Determination of the levels of two of the enzymes involved in that pathway, tyrosine hydroxylase (103,105) and dopamine-$\beta$-hydroxylase (105), shows increases in the former and decreases in the latter. This points out the difficulties, discussed previously, of relying on enzyme levels alone to indicate structural alterations. One study reported the turnover rate of norepinephrine in undernourished rat brains at weaning (104), but this measure is difficult to translate into structural terms. Still another report measured the catecholamine-binding protein in undernourished mice (70). Here norepinephrine-binding protein was found to be reduced compared to that in well-nourished mice, but dopamine-binding protein was unaffected. These amine-binding proteins are of interest for morphological reconstruction of the undernourished brain in that they could represent the binding proteins of the amine-storage granules or possibly the postsynaptic receptor for the amine. This recent report has not yet been followed up, but it is difficult to see how the various alternatives could be distinguished by other than morphological means.

### 2. Acetylcholine

Changes in the acetylcholine system are difficult to interpret because the transmitter itself decays rapidly within seconds of decapitation; no study of undernutrition on acetylcholine itself has used assay methods—e.g., the microwave fixation method (24)—that avoid this problem. Furthermore, two well-known enzymes are involved in acetylcholine metabolism, choline acetyltransferase (the synthetic enzyme) and acetylcholinesterase (a degradative enzyme); the latter, however, is not useful as a marker because its location does not appear to coincide with acetylcholine neurons and processes (67,92). Of the few studies in Table 2 that measured choline acetyltransferase, one measured the activity of the enzyme in the synaptosomal fraction of cerebral cortex (50), and another was carried out 4 weeks after rehabilitation (38). Both studies found no difference in this enzyme in undernourished compared to control animals. Only the measurement at weaning on whole brain levels (105) revealed significant deficits in choline acetyltransferase activity.

### 3. γ-Aminobutyric Acid

Of the other substances suspected of being neurotransmitters, only γ-aminobutyric acid (GABA) has received attention. Rajalakshmi et al. (88) measured the levels of glutamate dehydrogenase and glutamate decarboxylase at weaning in rats. The activities of both of these enzymes were lowered in the undernourished brains. These authors showed that the deficit in the enzymes was not evenly accumulated over 4 weeks but was due almost entirely to the lack of a large increase during the second postnatal week.

As we have seen previously, it is difficult to ascribe much meaning to enzyme changes, and no work has been published as yet on GABA levels themselves in undernourished animals. Careful regional studies, however, might attribute the enzyme changes to a specific neuronal population that develops dramatically during the second postnatal week. GABA appears to be worthy of further study in that some work already indicates vulnerability to undernutrition and GABA neurons are approximately 10,000-fold more numerous in mammalian brain than any of the catecholamine neurons. Too little work has been done on dopamine neurons to advance a judgment about that system, and the results of studies on serotonin are almost equally divided between decreased and increased levels after undernutrition.

There are other substances believed to function as neurotransmitters; some would be difficult to work with because they are amino acids (glycine, glutamate, aspartate) (15) or are stored in cells other than neurons (histamine) (43,44,76). Recently several small brain peptides were discovered to possess neurotransmitter-like activity (15). There have been no studies of these peptides under conditions of nutritional deprivation. Although perinatal undernutrition is believed to be primarily a deficit of dietary amino acids, one cannot assume that amino acid-derived constituents are universally decreased. While most of the known neurotransmitters are derived from amino acid precursors, so too are the enzymes involved in their metabolism, some of which have been shown to increase under conditions of nutrient deprivation.

## V. QUANTIFICATION OF MORPHOLOGICAL ALTERATIONS IN UNDERNOURISHED BRAINS

The question arises whether the neurotransmitter findings, when combined with the view of the undernourished brain given us by morphologists, contribute to our understanding of the deficits. In other words, do we have quantitative corroboration for the decreased postmitotic growth of certain neurons by undernutrition? The most likely candidate, perhaps because it has been studied most often, is the noradrenergic neuronal system. These brainstem neurons, which are actually quite few in number, send processes to all other parts of the brain, some traversing many millimeters (7). The consistency of the reports of lowered levels of brain norepinephrine in undernourished animals points to this neuronal system as one whose total growth of processes has been impaired. Unfortunately this prime candidate has a skeleton or two in its closet.

After Shoemaker and Wurtman observed the deficit in brain norepinephrine levels, they tried to determine whether there was a decrease in the number of noradrenergic terminals or in the amount of transmitter in a normal complement of terminals by doing an uptake study (104). In catecholamine pharmacologists' hands, the uptake by the tissues of $^3$H-norepinephrine introduced into the cerebrospinal fluid is a good indicator of the number of synaptic terminals that release norepinephrine as a transmitter. However, after repeated attempts, no difference could be found in uptake capability between well- and undernourished brains when expressed per brain. Although we excluded discussions of rehabilitation effects in this chapter, studies of norepinephrine levels in brains of previously-undernourished rats, given several months of an adequate diet, provide another piece of evidence. In two separate studies of norepinephrine levels in undernourished-rehabilitated rats (105,122), the catecholamine level returned to control values by 90 days of age. These two facts (i.e., that undernourished rats have a deficit of transmitter but a normal amount of terminal uptake ability, and that when rehabilitated their transmitter levels return to normal) deal a severe blow to the belief that noradrenergic neuronal processes are permanently stunted by undernutrition.

Recently another piece of evidence was added. Fluorescence microscopy of the locus coeruleus and its fiber system in undernourished and control rats (Shoemaker and Bloom, *unpublished observations*) revealed no difference between the size and shape of the nucleus, or in the number or characteristics of its processes.

If undernutrition affected primarily the growth of processes, those neurons so affected should have lower amounts of the transmitter substances that are transported and stored in these processes. It is this kind of reasoning that led researchers to assay most of the known neurotransmitters (or their enzymes) during and after undernutrition. Most of the studies report deficits per brain of these important substances. However, interpreting the enzyme changes is risky, and the best transmitter candidate for demonstrating deficits, norepinephrine, must overcome much evidence against a true morphological deficit. The way out of this quagmire of information and interpretation may be quite simple. If the brain region chosen for study is delimited to include known populations of neurons and fiber bundles, the assay of several transmitters (or their enzymes) could be revealing. Gaetani et al. (49) studied catecholamine and acetylcholine markers in the mouse sympathetic ganglion. Although the structures they chose are not part of the brain, these workers were able to make reasonable assumptions about the growth and development of the ganglia in undernourished mice because much is known about ganglia neurons and their connections. The only study we are aware of in which several transmitters are measured in a region of relatively well-known structural relationships is our own work on the dentate gyrus of the hippocampus. This work is still in progress but when completed will include measures of norepinephrine, dopamine, GABA, and choline acetyltransferase on a very defined region of the brain. It is hoped this combined study will complement the electron microscopic findings in this same region (Table 3). Combining descriptive morphology and neurotransmitter level measurements in one study offers a chance for increasing our insight into the complex arrangement of cells and processes. One of the other points emerging here is that the sites of possible distortion by undernutrition most likely will require use of the electron microscope. The importance and vulnerability of synapses has already been demonstrated. Furthermore, the completely unexplored area of neuron-glia relationships altered by undernutrition holds promise if means can be found to quantitate the fine-structure analysis necessary for such an investigation.

## VI. CONCLUSIONS: NEW METHODS FOR THE FUTURE AND A FINAL QUESTION

Why has progress in this field been so slow? This is a fair question in view of the insight of the earliest workers in this field. It certainly deserves an answer, but if we were to answer it in detail it would appear either as whining or as a justification of our ignorance—neither burden of which we wish to place on the reader. Rather, we want only to stipulate awareness of the extreme complexity of the brain and the broad void of knowledge concerning the relationships which living cells express in the brain by their formation of specific synapses under normal conditions.

### A. Two New Approaches

We conclude with a description of two new approaches for morphological quantification. Neither of these methods of study has been applied as yet to undernourished brain material. There is no guarantee that they will be able to capture what has eluded many, although both include the ingredients we believe essential to success in this area: One method is analysis at the electron microscopic level, and the other is a means of quantifying the images produced by the electron microscope.

The first is a program we have been involved in for several years. Basically it involves automated morphometric analysis of synapses visualized by the electron microscope. The material under study is stained with ethanolic-phosphotungstic acid (E-PTA) to stain synapses selectively. The photographic negatives of the tissue sections obtained by electron microscopy are then digitized onto magnetic tape for computer image processing. Because E-PTA stains synaptic complexes almost exclusively, the resultant picture of the tissue is nearly a black and white image. This situation is ideal for processing the digitized image as there is little possibility of mistaking extraneous images for synapses. Ultimately a program will be written to enable the computer to identify the synapses in a field, count them, measure several characteristics (e.g., width, arch of curvature, length, number of dense projections), and perform appropriate statistical analysis on all of these. Although conceptually simple, the task is not an easy one and is still incomplete. To give an idea of some of the steps involved, Fig. 8 shows the four stages in the sequence from

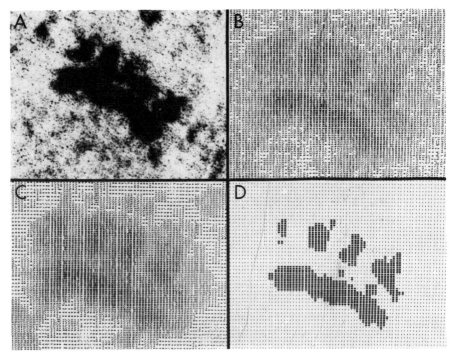

**FIG. 8.** The four stages from a high-magnification photographic image of an ethanolic phosphotungstic acid-stained synapse (**A**), to the initial digitization of a synapse onto computer tape (**B**), to that same image after a geometric smoothing operation (**C**), and finally to that image both smoothed and thresholded for gray levels (**D**). This resultant image would then be the object of further computer-aided morphometric analyses.

photographic image of an E-PTA-stained synapse (a), a similar synapse after digitization onto a computer tape (b), the same image after a smoothing operation (c), and the resultant image after both smoothing and thresholding of gray levels (d). This series of photographs was obtained with the help of our collaborators at the Division of Computer Research and Technology of N.I.H., Judith Prewitt and Ann Barber. The program was developed by Prewitt et al. (86) and utilizes the PDP-10 computer. The final digitized image would be the subject of further morphometric analysis.

The marriage between the electron microscope and computer-aided image processing is relatively new, but some medical centers are already providing computer facilities to their members by time-sharing. Thus this powerful tool will be increasingly available to microscopists to use in studies such as the one we described.

Another existing approach is that taken by Dr. Joe Wood at the University of Texas. In a series of papers (131,132), Wood and his collaborators described their use of the analytical electron microscope (AEM) for the detection of neurotransmitters at the level of the synaptic vesicle. The AEM is primarily a scanning electron microscope with a high-energy probe to determine elemental analysis of small areas of the section. Wood demonstrated that the dichromate stain for biogenic amines can be utilized to determine the precise location of the amine in a high-power electron micrograph. Furthermore, the spectrum given off by the microscope's interaction with the tissue section can be quantified to register the amount of substance under the probe. This elegant and expensive technique has not yet been applied to the problems we are discussing here, but AEM promises to answer the question of whether deficits in transmitter levels are due to less transmitter per terminal or fewer normally loaded terminals.

## B. An Important Consideration

A final question arises which cannot be ignored. The question is posed most eloquently by the British neuropathologist Dobbing in a recent article (34); simply stated, it asks if all this study of brain distortion by undernutrition is really necessary. While not condemning such studies outright, Dobbing raises several valid points. These are: (a) Many of the anatomical deficits documented in undernourished animals probably have very little functional significance. He states: "It is scarcely conceivable that a permanent 15% deficit in glial cells, or a few laminas missing from a myelin sheath of perhaps 200 laminations, can make much difference to brain function. Glial cell number and myelin lipids have been measured because they were easy to measure and for no other reason" (34). Furthermore, he feels minor deficits in the number of neurons may be unimportant in the face of an enormous functional reserve. (b) Dobbing expresses a strong disbelief in the usefulness of quantitative histology. This seems chiefly to be because of the great complexity of the brain. (c) What contribution do animal experiments make, Dobbing asks, when the only medically proper and humane course to take with undernourished children is to feed them as soon as possible? (d) Having decried morphological means as a way of deducing the function consequences of undernutrition, Dobbing turns to behavioral studies. Although stating that the evidence for learning deficits due to undernutrition is equivocal, he offers several other possible behavioral differences between well- and undernourished animals, much of it work from his own laboratory.

These are indeed provocative ideas, and all those working in this area should consider them seriously. While we agree with much that they contain, we feel that Dobbing's influence may mislead some into considering the behavioral abnormality as the sole indicator of nutritional insult to the animal. Although certainly unintended by Dobbing, this misconception can lead to two possible fallacies. One is that abnormal behavior "infers" altered brain structure, and the other is that the absence of behavioral consequences "infers" normal brain development. We also are aware of the complexities of the brain and the difficulties in untangling the many possible consequences of altered nutrient supply, but it is important to determine if the altered function is actually due to a "distorted" brain. Abnormal behavior can be the consequence of early experiences by the young (30,78), the altered endocrine status of the undernourished (91,99,102,118), a biochemical alteration of the brain without morphological consequences, or a primary structural alteration of the cells of the brain.

What can occasionally be overlooked is that altered brain structure can have consequences other than behavioral ones. The brain plays a major role in controlling the endocrine system of the body via the hypothalamus-pituitary system and other pathways. These possible effects of undernutrition could have grave implications for the well-being and reproductive capacity of the individual.

The long-range psychological and endocrine consequences of undernutrition on neurobiological processes have not yet been documented. It would be unwise for fundamental scientists to neglect any of these problems, no matter how difficult their solution may be.

## ACKNOWLEDGMENTS

The authors acknowledge the generosity of Drs. Sue Griffin and Don Woodward of the University of Texas Medical Center, Dallas, for providing Figs. 2 and 4; and Dr. David Bodian, Johns Hopkins Medical School, and Rockefeller University Press for permission to use Fig. 1. Thanks are also extended to Judith Prewitt and Ann Barber of N.I.H. for their assistance in obtaining parts of Fig. 8. A debt of gratitude is owed the following individuals who, as collaborators and discussants, contributed to the contents of this chapter: Drs. Joseph T. Coyle, Jr., James Nathanson, Margret Schlumpf, Sandra Wiener, and Elena Battenberg. A special note of thanks goes to Mr.

Hamilton Poole for help in preparing the figures, and to Dee Estep and Pat Millhouse for many hours of expert typing.

*Note Added in Proof*

Several newly published articles merit comment. (1) C. D. West and T. L. Kemper (*Brain Res., 107:*221–237, 1976) examined Golgi-impregnated neurons in the occipital cortex of 30-day-old undernourished rats; their results indicate a decrease in synaptic spine density, thereby suggesting a decreased synaptic termination on the reduced dendritic lengths. (2) J. W. T. Dickerson and S.-K. Pao (*Biol. Neonate, 25:*114–124, 1975), anticipating one of our suggestions, measured several neurotransmitters in specific brain regions. However, they report neurotransmitter levels on a per gram basis, and this, as we have discussed above, can obscure deficits in the absolute amount of these substances because the loss of glial cells and myelin decreases the total tissue weight. Had the results been expressed as neurotransmitter content per brain region, there would have been reported large deficits in GABA, glutamate, NE, and 5-HT in the 21-day-old undernourished rat forebrain, cerebellum, and brainstem. (3) S. E. Dyson and D. G. Jones (*Brain Res., 114:*365–378, 1976; *Exp. Neurol., 51:*529–535, 1976), using PTA stain to visualize synaptic junctions in the occipital cortex, report significant deficits in synaptic density in 20-day-old undernourished rats, similar to our data in Table 4. In addition, these authors performed morphometric analysis of the synaptic profiles, demonstrating that both pre- and postsynaptic densities were diminished in the undernourished rats.

## REFERENCES

1. Adlard, B. P. F., and Dobbing, J. (1971): Elevated cholinesterase activity in adult rat brain after undernutrition in early life. *Brain Res.*, 30:198–199.
2. Adlard, B. P. F., and Dobbing, J. (1971): Vulnerability of developing brain. III. Development of four enzymes in the brains of normal and undernourished rats. *Brain Res.*, 28:97–107.
3. Adlard, B. P. F., Dobbing, J., and Smart, J. L. (1974): Adult brain nerve-ending content and acetylcholinesterase activity in rats growth retarded for different periods in early life. *Biochem. Soc. Trans.*, 2:124–127.
4. Aghajanian, G., and Bloom, F. E. (1967): The formation of synaptic junctions in developing rat brain: A quantitative electron microscopic study. *Brain Res.*, 6:716.
5. Allen, E. (1912): The cessation of mitosis in the central nervous system of the albino rat. *J. Comp. Neurol.*, 22:547.
6. Altman, J., Das, G. D., and Sudarshan, K. (1970): The influence of nutrition on neural and behavioral development. I. Critical review of some data on the growth of the body and the brain following dietary deprivation during gestation and lactation. *Dev. Psychobiol.*, 3:281–301.
7. Anden, N-E., Dahlstrom, A., Fuxe, K., Larsson, K., Olson, L., and Ungerstedt, U. (1966): Ascending monoamine neurons to the telencephalon and diencephalon. *Acta Physiol. Scand.*, 67:313–326.
8. Badger, T. M., and Tumbleson, M. E. (1974): Protein-calorie malnutrition in young miniature swine: Brain free amino acids. *J. Nutr.*, 104:1329–1338.
9. Barnes, D., and Altman, J. (1973): Effects of different schedules of early undernutrition on the preweaning growth of the rat cerebellum. *Exp. Neurol.*, 38:406–419.
10. Barnes, D., and Altman, J. (1973): Effect of two levels of gestational-lactational undernutrition on the postweaning growth of the rat cerebellum. *Exp. Neurol.*, 38:420–428.
11. Bass, N. H., Netsky, M. G., and Young, E. (1970): Effect of neonatal malnutrition on developing cerebrum. I. Microchemical and histologic study of cellular differentiation in the rat. *Arch. Neurol.*, 23:289–302.
12. Bass, N. H., Netsky, M. G., and Young, E. (1970): Effect of neonatal malnutrition on developing cerebrum. III. Micro-chemical and histologic study of myelin formation in the rat. *Arch. Neurol.*, 23:303–313.
13. Benton, J. W., Moser, H. W., Dodge, P. R., and Carr, S. (1966): Modification of the schedule of myelination in the rat by early nutritional deprivation. *Pediatrics*, 38:801–807.
14. Bloom, F. E. (1972): The formation of synaptic junctions in developing brain. In: *Structure and Function of Synapses*, edited by G. D. Pappas and D. P. Purpura, pp. 101–120. Raven Press, New York.
15. Bloom, F. E. (1973): Amino acids and polypeptides in neuronal function. *Neurosci. Res. Prog. Bull.*, 10:No. 2.

16. Bloom, F. E., and Aghajanian, G. K. (1968): Fine structural cytochemical analysis of the staining of synaptic junctions with phosphotungstic acid. *J. Ultrastruct. Res., 22*:361–375.

17. Borgman, R. F., Bursey, R. G., and Caffrey, B. C. (1975): Influence of dietary fat upon rats during gestation and lactation. *Am. J. Vet. Res., 36*:795–798.

18. Borgman, R. F., Bursey, R. G., and Caffrey, B. C. (1975): Influence of maternal dietary fat upon rat pups. *Am. J. Vet. Res., 36*:799–805.

19. Brown, R. E. (1966): Organ weight in malnutrition with special reference to brain weight. *Dev. Med. Child. Neurol., 8*:512–522.

20. Buchanan, A. R., and Roberts, J. E. (1948): Relative lack of myelin in optic tracts as result of underfeeding in the young albino rat. *Proc. Soc. Exp. Biol. Med., 69*:101–104.

21. Burns, E. M., Richards, J. G., and Kuhn, H. (1975): An ultrastructural investigation of the effects of perinatal malnutrition on E-PTA stained synaptic junctions. *Experientia, 32*:1451–1453.

22. Burton, K. (1956): A study of the conditions and mechanisms of the diphenylamine reaction for the colorimetric estimation of deoxyribonucleic acid. *Biochem. J., 62*:315.

23. Chase, H. P., Lindsley, W. F. B., and O'Brien, D. (1968): Undernutrition and cerebellar development. *Nature (Lond.), 221*:554–555.

24. Cheney, D. L., Racagni, G., Zsilla, G., and Costa, E. (1976): Differences in the action of various drugs on striatal acetylcholine and choline content in rats killed by decapitation or microwave radiation. *J. Pharm. Pharmacol., 28*:75–77.

25. Clos, J., Rebiere, A., and Legrand, J. (1973): Differential effects of hypothyroidism and undernutrition on the development of glia in the rat cerebellum. *Brain Res., 63*:445–449.

26. Cohen, E. L., and Wurtman, R. J. (1976): Brain acetylcholine: Control by dietary choline. *Science, 191*:561–562.

27. Cragg, B. G. (1972): The development of cortical synapses during starvation in the rat. *Brain, 95*:143–150.

28. Culley, W. J., and Lineberger, R. O. (1968): Effect of undernutrition on the size and composition of the rat brain. *J. Nutr., 96*:375–381.

29. Dalton, M. M., Hommes, O. R., and Leblond, C. P. (1968): Correlation of glial proliferation with age in the mouse brain. *J. Comp. Neurol., 134*:397.

30. Daly, M. (1973): Early stimulation of rodents: A critical review of present interpretations. *Br. J. Psychol., 64*:435–460.

31. Davidson, J. N., and Leslie, I. (1950): Nucleic acids in relation to tissue growth: A review. *Cancer Res., 10*:587.

32. Dobbing, J. (1968): Effects of experimental undernutrition on development of the nervous system. In: *Malnutrition, Learning, and Behavior,* edited by N. S. Scrimshaw and J. Gordon. M.I.T. Press, Cambridge.

33. Dobbing, J., and Smart, J. L. (1973): Early undernutrition, brain development, and behavior. In: *Ethology and Development,* edited by S. A. Barnett, pp. 16–36. Lippincott, Philadelphia.

34. Dobbing, J., and Smart, J. L. (1974): Vulnerability of developing brain and behavior. *Br. Med. Bull., 30*:164–168.

35. Dobbing, J., and Widdowson, E. (1965): The effect of undernutrition and subsequent rehabilitation on myelination of rat brain as measured by its composition. *Brain, 88*:357–366.

36. Dobbing, J., Hopewell, J. W., and Lynch, A. (1971): Vulnerability of developing brain. VII. Permanent deficit of neurons in cerebral and cerebellar cortex following early mild undernutrition. *Exp. Neurol., 32*:439–447.

37. Eayrs, J. T., and Horn, G. (1955): Development of cerebral cortex in hypothyroid and starved rats. *Anat., Rec., 121*:53.

38. Eckhert, C. D., Levitsky, D. A., and Barnes, R. H. (1975): Postnatal stimulation: The effects on cholinergic enzyme activity in undernourished rats. *Proc. Soc. Exp. Biol. Med., 149*:860–863.

39. Eidelberg, E., and Stein, D. G. (1974): Functional recovery after lesions of the nervous system. *Neurosci. Res. Prog. Bull., 12*:No. 2.

40. Enesco, M., and Leblond, C. P. (1962): Increase in cell number as a factor in the growth of the organs of the young male rat. *J. Embryol. Exp. Morphol., 10*:530.

41. Engsner, G., Belete, S., Sjogren, I., and Vahlquist, B. (1974): Brain growth in children with marasmus. *Ups. J. Med. Sci., 79*:116–128.

42. Engsner, G., Hobte, D., Sjogren, I., and Vahlquist, B. (1974): Brain growth in children with kwashiorkor. *Acta Paediatr. Scand.,* 63:687–694.
43. Enwonwu, C. O., and Worthington, B. S. (1974): Concentrations of histamine in brain of guinea pig and rat during dietary protein malnutrition. *Biochem. J.,* 144:601–603.
44. Enwonwu, C. O., and Worthington, D. S. (1975): Elevation of brain histamine content in protein-deficient rats. *J. Neurochem.,* 24:941–945.
45. Fernstrom, J. D., and Hirsch, M. J. (1975): Rapid repletion of brain serotonin in malnourished corn-fed rats following L-tryptophan injection. *Life Sci.,* 17:455–464.
46. Fish, I., and Winick, M. (1969): Effect of malnutrition on regional growth of the developing rat brain. *Exp. Neurol.,* 25:534–540.
47. Fishman, M. A., Prensky, A. L., and Dodge, P. R. (1969): Low content of cerebral lipids in infants suffering from malnutrition. *Nature (Lond.),* 221:552–553.
48. Fishman, M. A., Prensky, A. L., Tumbleson, M. E., and Daftari, B. (1972): Relative resistance of the later phase of myelination to severe undernutrition in miniature swine. *Am. J. Clin. Nutr.,* 25:7–10.
49. Gaetani, S., Mengheri, E., Spadoni, M., Rossi, A., and Toschi, G. (1975): Effects of litter size on protein, choline acetyltransferase, and dopamine-β-hydroxylase of a mouse sympathetic ganglion. *Brain Res.,* 86:75–84.
50. Gambetti, P., Autilio-Gambetti, L., Gonatas, N., Shafer, B., and Steiber, A. (1972): Synapses and malnutrition: Morphological and biochemical study of synaptosomal fractions from rat cerebral cortex. *Brain Res.,* 47:477–484.
51. Gambetti, P., Autilio-Gambetti, L., Rizzuto, N., Shafer, B., and Pfaff, L. (1974): Synapses and malnutrition: Quantitative ultrastructural study of rat cerebral cortex. *Exp. Neurol.,* 43:464–473.
52. Gourdon, J., Clos, J., Coste, C., Dainat, J., and Legrand, J. (1973): Comparative effects of hypothyroidism, hyperthyroidism, and undernutrition on the protein and nucleic acid content of the cerebellum in the young rat. *J. Neurochem.,* 21:861–871.
53. Griffin, W. S. T., and Woodward, D. J. (1976): Neurological manifestations of undernutrition in rat cerebellum: A Golgi-Cox analysis *(submitted for publication).*
54. Griffin, W. S. T., Woodward, D. J., and Chanda, R. (1976): Malnutrition and brain development: Cerebellar weight, DNA, RNA, protein, and histological correlations *(submitted for publication).*
55. Guthrie, H. A., and Brown, M. L. (1968): Effect of severe undernutrition in early life on growth, brain size, and composition in adult rats. *J. Nutr.,* 94:419–426.
56. Haltia, M. (1970): Postnatal development of spinal anterior horn neurons in normal and undernourished rats. *Acta Physiol. Scand. [Suppl.],* 352.
57. Hatai, S. (1904): The effect of partial starvation on the brain of the white rat. *Am. J. Physiol.,* 12:116.
58. Hatai, S. (1907): Effects of partial starvation followed by a return to normal diet on the growth of the body and central nervous system of albino rats. *Am. J. Physiol.,* 18:309.
59. Hatai, S. (1908): Preliminary note on the size and condition of the central nervous system in albino rats severely stunted. *J. Comp. Neurol.,* 18:151.
60. Heller, I. H., and Elliott, K. A. C. (1954): Desoxyribonucleic acid content and cell density in brain and human brain tumors. *Can. J. Biochem. Physiol.,* 32:584–592.
61. Hernandez, R. J. (1973): Developmental pattern of the serotonin synthesizing enzyme in the brain of postnatally malnourished rats. *Experientia,* 29:1487–1488.
62. Howard, E., and Granoff, D. M. (1968): Effect of neonatal food restriction in mice on brain growth, DNA, and cholesterol, and on adult delayed response learning. *J. Nutr.,* 95:111–121.
63. Im, H. S., Barnes, R. H., and Levitsky, D. A. (1971): Postnatal malnutrition and brain cholinesterase in rats. *Nature (Lond.),* 233:269–270.
64. Im, H. S., Barnes, R. H., Levitsky, D. A., and Pond, W. G. (1973): Postnatal malnutrition and regional cholinesterase activities in brains of pigs. *Brain Res.,* 63:461–465.
65. Jackson, C. M., and Stewart, C. A. (1920): The effects of inanition in the young upon the ultimate size of the body and of the various organs in the albino rat. *J. Exp. Zool.,* 30:97–128.
66. Johnson, J. E., Jr., and Yoesle, R. A. (1975): The effects of malnutrition on the developing brain stem of the rat: A preliminary experiment using the lateral vestibular nucleus. *Brain Res.,* 89:170–174.

67. Kasa, D. (1975): Histochemistry of choline acetyltransferase. In: *Cholinergic Mechanisms,* edited by P. G. Waser, pp. 271–281. Raven Press, New York.
68. Kissane, J. O., and Hawrylewicz, E. J. (1975): Development of Na$^+$-K$^+$-ATPase in neonatal rat brain synaptosomes after perinatal protein malnutrition. *Pediatr. Res.,* 9:146–150.
69. Latham, M. C. (1974): Protein-calorie malnutrition in children and its relation to psychological development and behavior. *Physiol. Rev.,* 54:541–565.
70. Lee, C-J. (1975): Catecholamine-binding brain protein in mice exposed to perinatal malnutrition and neonatal infection. *Pediatr. Res.,* 9:645–652.
71. Lee, C-J. and Dubos, R. (1972): Lasting biological effects of early environmental influences. VIII. Effects of neonatal infection, perinatal malnutrition, and crowding on catecholamine metabolism of brain. *J. Exp. Med.,* 136:1031–1042.
72. Lewis, P. D., Balazs, R., Patel, A. J., and Johnson, A. L. (1975): The effect of undernutrition in early life on cell generation in the rat brain. *Brain Res.,* 83:235–247.
73. Lichtensteiger, W. (1970): Effect of endocrine manipulations on the metabolism of hypothalamic monoamines. In: *Neurochemical Aspects of Hypothalamic Function,* edited by L. Martini and J. Meites, pp. 101–133. Academic Press, New York.
74. Manocha, S. L., and Olkowski, Z. (1972): Cytochemistry of experimental protein malnutrition in primates: Effect on the spinal cord of the squirrel monkey Siamiri sciureus. *Histochem. J.,* 4:531–544.
75. Manocha, S. L., and Olkowski, Z. (1973): Experimental protein malnutrition in primates: Cytochemical studies on the cerebellum of the squirrel monkey Siamiri sciureus. *Histochem. J.,* 5:105–118.
76. Martres, M. P., Bauchy, M., and Schwartz, J. C. (1975): Histamine synthesis in the developing rat brain: Evidence for a multiple compartmentation. *Brain Res.,* 83:261–275.
77. Munro, H. N., and Fleck, A. (1969): Analysis of tissues and body fluids for nitrogenous constituents. In: *Mammalian Protein Metabolism,* Vol. 3, edited by H. N. Munro, p. 424. Academic Press, New York.
78. Newton, G., and Levine, S. (1968): *Early Experience and Behavior.* Charles C Thomas, Springfield, Ill.
79. Ordy, J. M. (1971): Postnatal protein-calorie deficiency effects on learning and neurochemistry of infant rhesus monkeys (abstract). *Trans. Am. Soc. Neurochem.,* 2:99.
80. Paoletti, R., and Galli, C. (1972): Effects of essential fatty acid deficiency on the central nervous system in the growing rat. In: *Lipids, Malnutrition and the Developing Brain,* pp. 121–140. CIBA Foundation Symposium. Elsevier, Amsterdam.
81. Patel, A. J., Balazs, R., and Johnson, A. L. (1973): Effect of undernutrition on cell formation in the rat brain. *J. Neurochem.,* 20:1151–1165.
82. Persson, L., and Sima, A. (1975): The effect of pre- and postnatal undernutrition on the development of the cerebellar cortex in the rat. II. Histochemical observations. *Neurobiology,* 5:151–166.
83. Platt, B. S., Pampiglione, G., and Stewart, R. J. C. (1965): Experimental protein-calorie deficiency, clinical, EEG and neuropathological changes in pigs. *Dev. Med. Child Neurol.,* 7:9.
84. Platt, B. S., and Stewart, R. J. C. (1969): Effects of protein-calorie deficiency on dogs. II. Morphological changes in the nervous system. *Dev. Med. Child Neurol.,* 11:174–192.
85. Plaut, S. M. (1970): Studies of undernutrition in the young rat: Methodological considerations. *Dev. Psychobiol.,* 3:157–167.
86. Prewitt, J. M. S., Reece, D. K., Hutchinson, G., and Jackson, C. K. (1974): *Decide: An Expandable System for Medical Decision-Making,* pp. 153–182. Informatique Medicale, Toulouse.
87. Pysh, J. J., and Perkins, R. E. (1975): Undernutrition and Purkinje cell development. *Neurosci. Abstr.,* 1:756.
88. Rajalakshmi, R., Parameswaran, M., Telang, S. D., and Ramakrishnan, C. V. (1974): Effect of undernutrition and protein deficiency on glutamate dehydrogenase and decarboxylase in rat brain. *J. Neurochem.,* 23:129–133.
89. Reis, D. J., Weinbren, M., and Corvelli, A. (1968): A circadian rhythm of norepinephrine regionally in rat brain: Its relationship to environmental lighting and to regional diurnal variations in brain serotonin. *J. Pharmacol. Exp. Ther.,* 164:135–145.

90. Richter, D., and Crossland, J. (1949): Variation in acetylcholine content of brain with physiological state. *Am. J. Physiol.,* 159:247–255.

91. Roeder, L. M., and Chow, B. F. (1973): Pituitary hormone regulated systems of the progeny of underfed dams. In: *Endocrinology; Proceedings of IV International Congress of Endocrinology* edited by R. O. Scow, pp. 1091–1097. Excerpta Medica, Amsterdam.

92. Rossier, J., Bauman, A., Rieger, F., and Benda, P. (1975): Immunological studies on the enzymes of the cholinergic system. In: *Cholinergic Mechanisms,* edited by D. G. Waser, pp. 283–293. Raven Press, New York.

93. Rozovski, J., Noroa, F., Arbarzua, J., and Monckeberg, F. (1971): Cranial transillumination in early and severe malnutrition. *Br. J. Nutr.,* 25:107–111.

94. Schonback, J., Hu, K. H., and Friede, R. (1968): Cellular and chemical changes during myelination: Histologic, autoradiographic, histochemical, and biochemical data on myelination in the pyramidal tract and corpus callosum of rat. *J. Comp. Neurol.,* 134:21.

95. Schwartz, J. C., Lampart, C., and Rose, C. (1972): Histamine formation in rat brain *in vivo:* Effects of histidine loads. *J. Neurochem.,* 19:801–810.

96. Segal, D. S., Sullivan, J. L., Kuczenski, R. T., and Mandell, A. J. (1971): Effects of long-term reserpine treatment on brain tyrosine hydroxylase and behavioral activity. *Science,* 173:847–849.

97. Selivonchick, D. P., and Johnston, P. V. (1975): Fat deficiency in rats during development of the central nervous system and susceptibility to experimental allergic encephalomyelitis. *J. Nutr.,* 105:288–300.

98. Sereni, F., Principi, N., Perletti, L., and Piceni-Sereni, L. (1966): Undernutrition and developing rat brain. I. Influence on acetylcholinesterase and succinic acid dehydrogenase activities and on norepinephrine and 5-OH-tryptamine tissue concentrations. *Biol. Neonate,* 10:254–265.

99. Shambaugh, G. E., and Wilber, J. F. (1974): The effect of caloric deprivation upon thyroid function in the neonatal rat. *Endocrinology,* 94:1145–1149.

100. Shoemaker, W. J. (1971): The effect of perinatal undernutrition on the metabolism of catecholamines in the rat brain. Doctoral thesis, M.I.T., Cambridge, Mass.

101. Shoemaker, W. J., and Bloom, F. E. (1976): A quantitative electronmicroscopic study of undernourished rat brain utilizing ethanolic phosphotungstic acid *(in preparation).*

102. Shoemaker, W. J., and Dallman, M. F. (1973): Pituitary-adrenal function in perinatally undernourished rats. *Fed. Proc.,* 32:909.

103. Shoemaker, W. J., and Wurtman, R. J. (1971): Perinatal undernutrition: Accumulation of catecholamines in rat brain. *Science,* 171:1017–1019.

104. Shoemaker, W. J., and Wurtman, R. J. (1973): Effect of perinatal undernutrition on the metabolism of catecholamines in the rat brain. *J. Nutr.,* 103:1537–1547.

105. Shoemaker, W. J., Coyle, J. T., Jr., and Bloom, F. E. (1974): Perinatal undernutrition: Effect on neurotransmitters, transmitter synthetic enzymes, and the number of synaptic connections. *Trans. Am. Soc. Neurochem.,* 4:100.

106. Shrader, R. E., and Zeman, F. J. (1969): Effect of maternal protein deprivation on morphological and enzymatic development of neonatal rat tissue. *J. Nutr.,* 99:401–421.

107. Siassi, F., and Siassi, B. (1973): Differential effects of protein-calorie restriction and subsequent repletion on neuronal and nonneuronal components of cerebral cortex in newborn rats. *J. Nutr.,* 103:1625–1633.

108. Sima, A. (1974): Relation between the number of myelin lamellae and axon circumference in fibers of ventral and dorsal roots and optic nerve in normal undernourished and rehabilitated rats. *Acta Physiol. Scand.* [Suppl.], 410.

109. Sima, A., and Persson, L. (1975): The effect of pre- and postnatal undernutrition on the development of the rat cerebellar cortex. I. Morphological observations. *Neurobiology,* 5:23–34.

110. Sobotka, T. J., Cook, M. P., and Brodie, R. E. (1974): Neonatal malnutrition: Neurochemical, hormonal, and behavioral manifestations. *Brain Res.,* 65:443–457.

111. Sourander, P., Sima, A., and Haltia, M. (1974): Malnutrition and morphological development of the nervous system. In: *Early Malnutrition and Mental Development. Symposia of the Swedish Nutrition Foundation XII,* edited by J. Cravioto, L. Hambraeus, and B. Vahlquist, pp. 39–54. Almquist and Wiksell, Stockholm.

112. Stern, W. C., Forbes, W. B., Resnick, O., and Morgane, P. J. (1974): Seizure susceptibility

and brain amine levels following protein malnutrition during development in the rat. *Brain Res.,* 79:375–384.

113. Stern, W. C., Miller, M., Forbes, W. B., Morgane, P. J., and Resnick, O. (1975): Ontogeny of the levels of biogenic amines in various parts of the brain and in peripheral tissues in normal and protein malnourished rats. *Exp. Neurol.,* 49:314–326.

114. Stewart, C. A. (1918): Weights of various parts of the brain in normal and underfed albino rats at different ages. *J. Comp. Neurol.,* 29:511.

115. Stewart, C. A. (1918): Changes in the relative weights of the various parts, systems and organs of young albino rats underfed for various periods. *J. Exp. Zool.,* 25:301.

116. Stewart, R. J. C., Merat, A., and Dickerson, J. W. T. (1974): Effect of a low protein diet in mother rats on the structure of the brains of the offspring. *Biol. Neonate,* 25:125–134.

117. Sugita, N. (1918): Comparative studies on the growth of the cerebral cortex. VII. On the influence of starvation at an early age upon the development of the cerebral cortex: albino rat. *J. Comp. Neurol.,* 29:177–242.

118. Tigner, J. C., and Barnes, R. H. (1975): Effect of postnatal malnutrition on plasma corticosteroid levels in male albino rats. *Proc. Soc. Exp. Biol. Med.,* 149:80–82.

119. Treherne, J. E. (1960): The nutrition of the central nervous system in the cockroach, Periplanta americana L: The exchange and metabolism of sugars. *J. Exp. Biol.,* 37:513–533.

120. Tricklebank, M. D., and Adlard, B. P. F. (1974): Regional brain 5-hydroxytryptamine turnover in adult rats growth retarded in early life. *Biochem. Soc. Trans.,* 2:127–129.

121. Weiner, N. (1970): Regulation of norepinephrine biosynthesis. *Annu. Rev. Pharmacol.,* 10:273.

122. Wiener, S. G. (1972): Post-weaning rehabilitation of catecholamine levels in the rat brain and heart after perinatal undernutrition. Master's thesis, M.I.T., Cambridge, Mass.

123. Wiggins, R. C., Benjamins, J. A., Krigman, M. R., and Morell, P. (1974): Synthesis of myelin proteins during starvation. *Brain Res.,* 80:345–349.

124. Wigglesworth, V. B. (1960): The nutrition of the central nervous system in the cockroach Periplanta americana L: The role of perineurium and glial cells in the mobilization of reserves. *J. Exp. Biol.,* 37:500–512.

125. Winick, M. (1970): Fetal malnutrition and growth process. *Hosp. Pract.,* 5:33.

126. Winick, M., and Noble, A. (1965): Quantitative changes in DNA, RNA, and protein during prenatal and postnatal growth in the rat. *Dev. Biol.,* 12:451.

127. Winick, M., and Noble, A. (1966): Cellular response in rats during malnutrition at various ages. *J. Nutr.,* 89:300–306.

128. Winick, M., and Rosso, P. (1969): The effect of severe early malnutrition on cellular growth of human brain. *Pediatr. Res.,* 3:181.

129. Winick, M., Fish, I., and Rosso, P. (1968): Cellular recovery in rat tissues after a brief period of neonatal malnutrition. *J. Nutr.,* 95:623.

130. Winick, M., Rosso, P., and Waterlow, J. (1970): Cellular growth of cerebrum, cerebellum, and brain stem in normal and marasmic children. *Exp. Neurol.,* 26:393–400.

131. Wood, J. G. (1974): Positive identification of intracellular biogenic amine reaction product with electron microscopic x-ray analysis. *J. Histochem. Cytochem.,* 22:1060–1063.

132. Wood, J. G. (1975): Use of the analytical electron microscope (AEM) in cytochemical studies of the central nervous system. *Histochemistry,* 41:233–240.

133. Wurtman, R. J., and Fernstrom, J. D. (1972): L-Tryptophan, L-tyrosine, and the control of brain monoamine biosynthesis. In: *Perspectives in Neuropharmacology,* edited by S. J. Snyder, pp. 143–193. Oxford University Press, New York.

134. Yu, M. C., Lee, J. C., and Bakay, L. (1974): The ultrastructure of the rat central nervous system in chronic undernutrition. *Acta Neuropathol.,* 30:197–210.

135. Zamenhof, S., van Marthens, E., and Margolis, F. (1968): DNA (cell number) and protein in neonatal brain: Alteration by maternal dietary protein restriction. *Science,* 160:322–323.

136. Salas, M., Diaz, S., and Nieto, A. (1974): Effects of neonatal food deprivation on cortical spines and dendritic development of the rat. *Brain Res.,* 73:139–144.

137. Cordero, M. E., Diaz, G., and Araya, J. (1976): Neocortex development during severe malnutrition in the rat. *Am. J. Clin Nutrition,* 29:358–365.

138. Greenough, W. T., and Volkmar, F. R.: (1973): Pattern of dendritic branching in occipital cortex of rats reared in complex environments. *Exp. Neurol.,* 40:491–504.

139. Greenough, W. T., Volkmar, F. R., and Juraska, J. M. (1973): Effects of rearing complexity on dendritic branching in frontolateral and temporal cortex of the rat. *Exp. Neurol.,* 41:371–378.

*Nutrition and the Brain,* Vol. 2,
edited by R. J. Wurtman and
J. J. Wurtman. Raven Press,
New York © 1977.

# Effects of Protein-Calorie Malnutrition on Biochemical Aspects of Brain Development

Thaddeus S. Nowak, Jr. and Hamish N. Munro

*Physiological Chemistry Laboratories, Department of Nutrition and Food Science,
Massachusetts Institute of Technology, Cambridge, Massachusetts 02139*

## I. INTRODUCTION

Changes in biochemical constituents in the brain of man and experimental animal models caused by protein-calorie malnutrition are described in this chapter. Although an insufficiency of protein and energy in the diet does occur in adults, the major interest in protein-calorie malnutrition and its effects on the brain has focused on the prenatal and early postnatal periods. There is good reason for this. The major period of neuron proliferation occurs in man before birth, and the processes of glial development, myelination, and biochemical maturation of the brain are mostly complete soon after birth. The development of the brain is thus most vulnerable during the perinatal period and shortly thereafter.

As it happens, protein-calorie malnutrition in man expresses itself during pregnancy as underdevelopment of the fetus and placenta, and during the postnatal period as the syndromes of kwashiorkor and marasmus. Thus there are well-recognized conditions of human malnutrition which occur in significant numbers of certain populations at times of life when brain development is actively taking place. Consequently, much clinical study and most of the work on experimental animal models to evaluate the effects of malnutrition on the brain have concentrated on the prenatal and early postnatal periods.

In surveying this evidence, three general points must be made at the outset. First, kwashiorkor (protein deficiency) and marasmus (protein-calorie insufficiency) differ considerably in their clinical and biochemical features, and it is desirable to differentiate between these two syndromes when evaluating the effects of postnatal malnutrition on human brain development. Second, animal models of protein-calorie malnutrition should also differentiate clearly between kwashiorkor and marasmus types. Finally, experimental study of the effects of malnutrition on the brain should recognize that the brains of different species show their maximum rates of development at different times in relation to birth.

In view of these comments, this chapter begins with a description of protein-calorie malnutrition in man and proceeds to consider the validity of animal models proposed for the condition. This is followed by a discussion of several biochemical parameters that can be used as indices of brain development, and then a description of changes observed in these as a result of protein-calorie malnutrition. Alterations in brain and plasma free amino acid pools are then compared with changes observed in conditions of amino acid imbalance that are known to affect brain development. The mechanism of mammalian protein synthesis and its control are reviewed, and the effects of malnutrition on brain protein metabolism and synthesis are finally discussed. Much of the evidence cited in this review relates to brain development in the fetus and in the infant during the early postnatal period, when dramatic responses can be anticipated. It is a generally held dogma that the adult brain is immune to the effects of malnutrition. However, there is abundant evidence (summarized elsewhere in this volume) that amino acid supply to the brain influences neurotransmitter synthesis in the adult, indicating that at least some specialized brain cells are readily responsive to changes in plasma amino acid levels. We should therefore not exclude the possibility that other aspects of metabolism and function in the fully developed brain are influenced (perhaps in a subtle, long-term way) by amino acid supply from the blood, and that this may prove to be a fruitful area for future research.

## II. PROTEIN-CALORIE MALNUTRITION IN MAN AND ANIMALS

### A. Protein-Calorie Malnutrition in Man

Malnutrition during infancy and childhood is classically described in terms of two syndromes: kwashiorkor, associated primarily with protein deficiency in the diet, and marasmus, which is an overall deficit of food intake, notably energy (160). In practice, however, protein-calorie malnutrition is a complex condition of multiple etiology which commonly presents as a spectrum between these two extremes. While primarily due to an inadequate intake of protein and/or calories, the onset of protein-calorie malnutrition is influenced by many other factors, e.g., stage of development, infections, child-rearing practices, and food habits, as well as other cultural factors.

Kwashiorkor occurs classically between the ages of 1 and 3 years in children whose diet is grossly deficient in protein, usually as a result of being transferred from breast milk to a starchy diet, e.g., cassava, plantain, or cereal. The child with kwashiorkor suffers from growth failure, mental apathy, and irritability. Physical examination shows muscle wasting and edema, and there is usually palpable liver enlargement associated with fatty infiltration and tissue damage. Diarrhea and anemia are also common features. In addition, the color and texture of the hair are often altered, with depigmentation of the skin and dermatosis. The most striking biochemical abnormality is the reduced level of plasma albumin, but the fall in serum transferrin content has recently proved to be a more sensitive index of severity (175).

In contrast to kwashiorkor, marasmus occurs most commonly in children under 1 year of age, when it is basically due to insufficient intake of food. Frequently the food supply is also a source of infectious disease which consequently exacerbates the dietary inadequacy. The main clinical features include marked growth failure, the child often being less than 60% of normal weight for age and having a reduced body length. The clinical picture of severe muscle wasting, loss of subcutaneous fat, and wizened facial features contrasts with the characteristic protuberant abdomen. As in kwashiorkor, diarrhea and anemia are common, but serum protein levels are nearly normal and there is no edema.

In practice, many intermediate forms of protein-calorie malnutrition are seen, and these are by far the most common cases encountered. A difficulty in clinical classification is defining the degree of severity of the malnutrition. Biochemical measurements differ in kwashiorkor and marasmus (207), but with the possible exception of serum transferrin levels such biochemical measurements lack adequate precision for classifying severity. Most students of human nutrition generally agree that anthropometric measurements provide the best criteria for diagnosing the degree of malnutrition (107,142,246).

In addition to these classically defined syndromes of postnatal malnutrition, there is now good evidence that maternal malnutrition can be a major factor in the development of the infant. In areas where malnutrition is prevalent in the population, a characteristic finding is an increased frequency of infants of low birth weight, defined as less than 2,500 g body weight. Within the category of low birth weight, several types are recognized, only one of which is of nutritional origin (293,298). In the first place, low birth weight is a signal feature of prematurity. Remaining cases of low birth weight occur after pregnancies of normal duration and represent fetal growth retardation belonging to one of three categories: (a) intrinsic growth failure caused by congenital malformations and genetic diseases, and usually associated with a placenta of normal size; (b) asymmetrical growth failure due to maternal vascular disease, which affects the fetal blood supply and development of the placenta, and reduces liver size but not brain maturation; and (c) symmetrical growth failure due to maternal malnutrition, which reduces the growth of all organs proportionately.

Evidence for the impact of maternal malnutrition on fetal growth comes from observations on populations exposed to short periods of acute food deprivation, as for example during World War II when birth weight was reduced by 200 g during the Dutch famine (257), and in the siege of Leningrad by an average of 500 g (21). Despite this, many years later males from the Dutch study showed no effects on mental or other development at the time of their induction into the army. Birth weight also tends to be below normal in populations chronically exposed to undernutrition; this situation has more serious and permanent consequences for the child, presumably because prolonged malnutrition has more insidious effects on the mother's capacity to reproduce. Among several major studies of this phenomenon, one of the best documented emerged from a comparison of Guatemalan villages in which the native diet was supplemented with energy from a carbohydrate source or from a mixture of protein, fat, and carbohydrate (117). Those mothers consuming 20,000 calories or more of either supplement during their pregnancies showed a significant increase in the birth weight of their children.

## B. Animal Models of Protein-Calorie Malnutrition

In order to assess better the biochemical effects of malnutrition on brain and other tissues, a number of animal models have been employed. Experimental malnutrition has been produced at all stages of development: *in utero,* during the suckling period, and after weaning. The methods used in these studies and the relevance of the experimental conditions to malnutrition in man are now evaluated.

### 1. Prenatal Malnutrition

Fetal malnutrition has been produced in several ways, mostly in rats. Pregnant females have been fed diets deficient in total food intake (45,132), specifically deficient in calories (231,310) or protein (315,317), or lacking a single essential amino acid (309). Severe malnutrition early in pregnancy usually results in failure of implantation of the embryo. Less severe malnutrition, or restriction applied later in pregnancy, allows implantation and delivery to occur, and in these cases the effects of malnutrition on fetal growth can be seen by the beginning of the third trimester. These two effects of malnutrition are considered separately.

Severe deficiency of either protein or calories during early gestation in the rat leads to a reduction in the number of litters produced as well as an increase in the proportion of stillborn offspring. Thus Zamenhof et al.(311) found that when a protein-free diet was fed for the first 10 days of the 21-day gestation 62% of the mated females failed to have a litter. Later periods of severe protein deficiency had less effect on the maintenance of pregnancy but resulted in a relatively higher proportion of stillborns. These results are compatible with earlier studies (201), which showed nearly complete reproductive failure as a result of feeding a protein-free diet from the day of mating, whereas 90% of the litters were delivered when the diet was fed after 7 days of gestation. Recently evidence was presented which suggests that days 7–10 of gestation comprise an especially critical period in the rat during which maternal protein deficiency can affect maintenance of pregnancy (316). This effect of early maternal malnutrition has been related to hormonal deficiencies in the dam which affect implantation and placental development (308). Some investigators therefore artificially maintain pregnancy in severely protein-deficient animals by hormone administration (17,188,202).

Studies summarized by Altman et al. (15) indicate that 5% is the critical level of protein in the diet, at or below which significant fetal resorptions and stillbirths occur. At 10% protein, no effects on offspring were seen. Similarly, reducing caloric intake during later gestation to one-third that given the control mothers, while maintaining adequate protein intake, resulted in failure to litter in approximately 30% of the matings (310). Others reported no statistically significant effects on reproductive performance when food intake was restricted to 50% that of the controls (132). Comparable effects of maternal malnutrition during early gestation have been demonstrated in other species (15). These experimental findings have their counterpart in an observed decrease in human fertility during famine (257), but in man the interpretation is complicated by behavioral factors.

Moderate malnutrition throughout pregnancy or more severe dietary restriction later in gestation are compatible with survival of the fetus, but they lead to changes in growth of both the fetus and placenta, the interrelationships of which are not readily dissociated. The placenta is itself a growing organ, and its cellularity and total mass can be affected by nutritional factors. Consequently the net impact of a period of malnutrition on the fetus is determined by both direct nutrient limitation and the effect this has on placental development. It is of interest in this regard that placental insufficiency leading to impaired fetal development can result from nonnutritional factors (e.g., restricted blood flow); indeed experimental ligation of arteries supplying the placenta has been exploited as a model of intrauterine growth retardation in several species (122,269,288). Placental structure and function are complex, however (for review see 158), and the relevance of these experimental preparations to the problem of placental insufficiency due to malnutrition is uncertain. This question arises specifically with regard to effects on brain growth later in this review. In the rat moderate maternal protein deprivation from the day of mating results in reduced placental DNA by day 13, whereas a reduction in fetal DNA is seen by day 15 (291). Thus it is during the final week of its 3-week gestation that growth of the rat fetus can be influenced by maternal malnutrition of a degree which allows survival of the offspring. Human maternal undernutrition, which leads to low birth weight, is also associated with reduced placental weight and cellularity (293) as well as diminished surface area available for transport (156,157). Evidence from human populations exposed to famine and to less severe malnutrition indicate that, as in the rat, the period of placental and fetal vulnerability is apparently restricted to the third trimester (198,257). Knowledge of the timing of nutritional susceptibility of the growing fetus is particularly relevant in evaluating the impact of prenatal malnutrition on brain growth.

## *2. Malnutrition During the Suckling Period*

While the developing fetus is subject to some degree of growth retardation as a result of inadequate maternal food intake, the neonate is considerably more vulnerable to severe malnutrition. Prior to weaning, the mammalian organism is dependent on the lactation of the mother for its nutrient supply, and most methods of producing experimental undernutrition during this period rely on some means of limiting availability of milk to the young. With regard to both the timing of the nutritional insult and the nature of the deprivation, the experimental state closely resembles the condition of marasmus in man.

There are three methods commonly used to deprive suckling rats. The most widely employed is that of Kennedy (148), in which the size of the litter nursed by a lactating dam is increased. Most often the control litters are adjusted to 8–10 animals, while malnourished litters are increased to 16–20. Although it has been claimed that reduction of litters to 3–4 pups provides superior nutrition, with increased growth of brain and other organs (296), the claim has been challenged (304). Another approach is that of Eayrs and Horn (78), in which the pups are separated from the mother for some part of each day, thereby limiting the time available for feeding. Finally, lactating dams fed a protein-deficient diet or restricted intake of a normal diet produce milk which is reduced in quantity but of normal protein content (190,272). This has been used to advantage by Chow and Lee (45), who fed dams a restricted diet throughout pregnancy and lactation, thereby reducing milk supply and producing malnutrition in the nursing litter. Some workers have used combinations of these methods to produce more severe deprivation (33,116,286). In addition to these commonly used procedures which limit the amount of milk of normal composition available to the pups, a few investigators have replaced milk with tube-fed formulas (180). This technique allows the composition of the diet to be varied and thus makes it possible to identify the impact of individual nutrients.

Altman et al. (16) compared the effectiveness of the deprivation produced by increased litter size with that due to restricted feeding of the mother during the period of lactation. Maternal malnutrition was more reproducible and had a more profound effect on growth of the litter. The variability in response to increasing litter size may be due to the capacity of some mothers to provide for a larger litter with more milk. In addition, it has been pointed out that some pups tend to grow well at the expense of the others, and some workers have selected their experimental animals on the basis of degree of growth retardation to circumvent this problem (72). Of particular importance is the observation that neither of these methods produces significant effects on body growth during the first few days of life (16). At this early stage the milk intake of the young is relatively less than later during the suckling period, and the reserve of mothers that were well fed up to the time of birth is apparently adequate to maintain milk supply through several days of dietary restriction. It would be expected that maternal deprivation during pregnancy and lactation would result in more immediate and severe restriction of milk supply to the young. To distinguish more clearly between the consequences of deprivation during these two periods, the procedure of transferring neonates to a previously malnourished "foster" mother was introduced; this produces malnutrition immediately after birth in offspring of previously well-nourished mothers (31,254).

Although the intended result of these manipulations is production of a nutritional deficiency in the suckling animal, they can influence other factors as well. For example, neonatal rats are usually kept warm during the time they are removed from the mother (78), but they suffer deprivation of maternal influences other than thermal and nutritional. Similarly, differences in the behavior of nutritionally deprived dams or those nursing large litters toward their young have been noted (219,253). While probably of more relevance to behavioral studies than to current biochemical approaches to the brain, these considerations must be included in the total picture of nutritional deprivation. The literature in this area was recently reviewed (164).

### 3. Postweaning Malnutrition

In contrast to malnutrition produced by reducing the total milk supply during the suckling period, malnutrition imposed on experimental animals after weaning usually represents a reduction in the intake either of protein or of energy and protein. The former is analogous to human kwashiorkor, and the latter represents marasmus. Most of the studies attempt to model kwashiorkor, and many of the clinical features of this deficiency state have been successfully produced in the rat (19,82,113,151), guinea pig (81), dog (218), pig (112,218), and certain nonhuman primates (49,60,86,97,150,155,210). Protein-calorie malnutrition resembling marasmus has been produced experimentally not only during lactation as described above but also in postweaning animals by restricting food intake (110,174).

Users of these models of protein-calorie deficiency have not always paid adequate attention to timing. Rats have been fed protein-deficient diets beginning at 28 days (113), but more frequently they are simply young rats of approximately 70 g (19) or 100 g (82,151) body weight. Some primate populations have been of uniform and well-defined age (49,150), whereas in other studies the animals have differed in age by several years (86). As is discussed in detail later, the timing of brain growth in different species determines their value as models for studying the effects of postnatal malnutrition on the brain. To date, most studies of the protein-deficient state in animals have not been concerned with the brain. Exceptions to this include early work in the dog (218), some studies on rats (64,211,226) and monkeys (83–85), and more recent studies combining early weaning and the feeding of low-protein diets as a means of producing malnutrition in miniature swine (28). This study is discussed later in detail.

### III. BIOCHEMICAL PARAMETERS OF BRAIN DEVELOPMENT

The changes in gross brain composition that occur during development are identified in this section. Much of the information relates to the rat, but there is good evidence to show that the sequence of brain development in other species, including man, follows a similar pattern but with an altered schedule that is especially relevant to the impact of malnutrition. Consequently we make cross-species comparisons of changes in brain composition during development. The effects of malnutrition at various stages of brain growth are then presented in the following section.

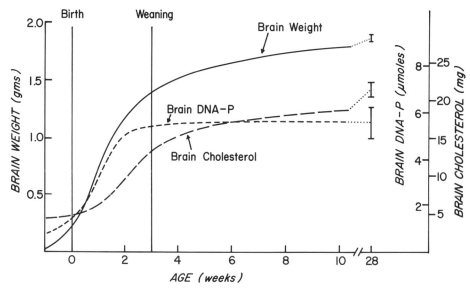

**FIG. 1.** Developmental changes in wet weight, cholesterol, and DNA of rat brain. (Adapted from Dobbing and Sands, ref. 72.)

## A. Gross Components of Brain During Development

As shown in Fig. 1, the weight of the rat brain increases slowly during the 21 days of fetal development to approximately 0.2 g at the time of birth; it then increases rapidly during the suckling period to approximately 1.4 g at weaning (21 days). Subsequent growth slowly increases brain weight to a near-plateau of 1.8 g by 10 weeks, after which a continued slight increase is observed throughout the life of the animal (44,72). Developmental changes in individual major macromolecular components of rat brain are also recorded in Fig. 1. During the first 2 weeks after birth DNA increases with a pattern of increment similar to that of brain weight, indicating that the brain cells proliferate most rapidly during the early postnatal period; this increase in brain cell number therefore accounts for the change in brain weight observed during this time. This period of cellular proliferation is brief, however, and adult DNA content is essentially achieved by the time of weaning (72,91). The increase in the total protein content of the brain (not shown) follows a pattern generally similar to that of brain weight (91).

Cholesterol content begins to accumulate relatively late in postnatal life, reaching a maximum rate of increase at approximately 14 days; it continues to increase in amount more slowly after weaning. Cholesterol content has been used as an index of brain myelination, since although it is not specific to this structure the bulk of brain cholesterol is found in myelin (59). As shown in Table 1, the cerebrosides, which are particularly characteristic of

TABLE 1. *Changes in lipid composition of the developing rat brain*

| Age (days) | Wet wt. (g) | Cholesterol (mmoles) | Phospholipid (mmoles) | Cerebrosides (mmoles) | Molar ratio (cholesterol: phospholipid: cerebrosides) |
|---|---|---|---|---|---|
| Whole brain | | | | | |
| 10 | 1.00 | 16.00 | 33.60 | 0.18 | 100:210:1 |
| 16 | 1.25 | 26.90 | 53.00 | 1.25 | 100:197:4.5 |
| Adult | 1.99 | 96.00 | 119.00 | 22.20 | 100:125:23 |
| Myelin | | | | | |
| 10 | 1.00 | 1.47 | 2.07 | 0.077 | 100:140:5 |
| 16 | — | 3.20 | 4.47 | 0.320 | 100:140:10 |
| Adult | — | 34.0 | 32.0 | 11.8 | 100:95:35 |

From Davison and Dobbing (59).

myelin, show an even more disproportionate increase as the myelin content of the brain increases. In whole rat brain the accumulation of cholesterol uniformly precedes the increase in cerebrosides (59), which would support the validity of using cholesterol as an indicator of some aspect of myelin development. On the other hand, recent work in the developing rabbit shows that, although whole brain and cerebrum show a similar pattern (cholesterol accumulation followed by increases in cerebrosides and sulfatides), the cerebellum shows the opposite sequence and in brainstem the accumulation is essentially simultaneous (119). The use of cholesterol content as more than a crude index of the maturation of brain lipid patterns is thus probably not justified. Recently the whole-brain content of proteolipid protein was shown to increase with a time course similar to that of cholesterol (10).

In Fig. 2 the incremental data shown in Fig. 1 are transformed into velocity curves, in which the rate of addition of each component is plotted. This demonstrates that the maximum velocities of weight and DNA addition occur at 7 days after birth, whereas that of cholesterol occurs at 14 days. In contrast, the peak rate of addition to total body weight is at 6 weeks of age.

This pattern of brain growth relative to birth is considerably different in various species (69). Figure 3 shows that the time of maximum velocity of brain weight change in the rat, which is distinctly postnatal, is not representative of man, in whom the maximal rate of weight increase occurs around the time of birth (73), or the guinea pig, in which brain growth occurs maximally before birth (70). The brain of the pig, like that of man, develops perinatally (63). The timing of the "brain growth spurt" for several other species has been similarly determined. The mouse brain, like that of the rat, develops largely postnatally (59,130). The periods of maximal brain growth of the dog (59) and rabbit (119) fall between those of man and the rat, with that of the rabbit more nearly approximating the perinatal brain growth of man. Brain growth in these species is maximal during the early weeks of life. In contrast, the brain of the

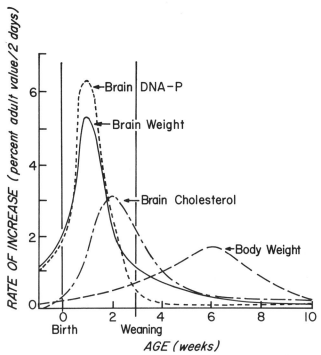

**FIG. 2.** Velocity curves for increases in body weight, brain weight, cholesterol, and DNA in the developing rat. (Adapted from Dobbing and Sands, ref. 72.)

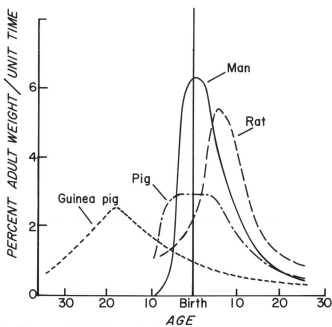

**FIG. 3.** Velocity curves for brain growth in different species. Age is in days for the guinea pig and rat, in weeks for the pig, and in months for man. (From Dobbing, ref. 69.)

rhesus monkey develops largely before birth (43,59). In view of evidence (to be discussed later) that tissues are most susceptible to permanent deficits in cell number owing to restrictions imposed during their period of cell division, these variations in the timing of brain growth must be considered when comparing the effects of nutritional factors on brain development in different species.

### B. Growth of Individual Cells and Regions of the Brain

In the mature rat brain the major cell classes—glia and neurons—occur in the proportion of roughly 2:1 (50), although this ratio varies considerably depending on the method of estimation (38). However, the neuronal population of the mammalian brain is mostly established before the glial cell population begins to develop (69). Consequently the growth spurt in DNA content after birth in the rat represents mainly glial cells and is followed by the synthesis of myelin by the oligodendroglial cells, which accounts for the increments in brain cholesterol content. When we consider the growth spurt in brain cell number for other species, the same sequence of neuronal cell multiplication followed by that of glial cells is also evident. In man the complement of neuronal elements is well established by the beginning of the third trimester of pregnancy (71). This pattern is relevant to the possible impact of maternal malnutrition on neuronal development.

This general picture must be amplified by considering the growth changes in individual regions. In the case of the rat, the cerebrum attains its full cell population (DNA) at approximately 21 days and the brainstem somewhat earlier (Fig. 4), although others have demonstrated a slight increase through 49 days in the cerebrum (110). Protein and lipid continue to expand the average cell size thereafter (not shown). In contrast, the spurt in DNA accumulation in cerebellum between 8 and 17 days postnatally is much greater than in the cerebrum or brainstem. This is accompanied by a disproportionately smaller increase in total protein, resulting in a smaller average cell size in the mature cerebellum (91). By 21 days after birth the rat brain has achieved roughly 75% of its adult weight (Fig. 1). At this age the cerebrum constitutes half of the total brain weight, the brainstem another 30%, and the cerebellum approximately 15% (91). In contrast, the cerebellum accounts for fully 50% of the DNA content of the brain, which at 21 days has achieved adult levels (Fig. 4). Thus brain cellularity is a parameter heavily weighted toward cerebellum in the rat, a fact that must be kept in mind when interpreting data derived from determinations on whole brain. In the case of man, the cerebellum shows a growth pattern relative to other brain regions similar to that of the rat (73). DNA content begins to increase later than in the cerebrum and brainstem, but the increase in the cerebellum proceeds more rapidly and attains adult levels before 2 years of age (Fig. 5). Forebrain and brainstem DNA contents reach 70% of adult levels by 2 years and continue to increase through the first 6 years of life. In contrast, wet weight increases similarly for all regions (data

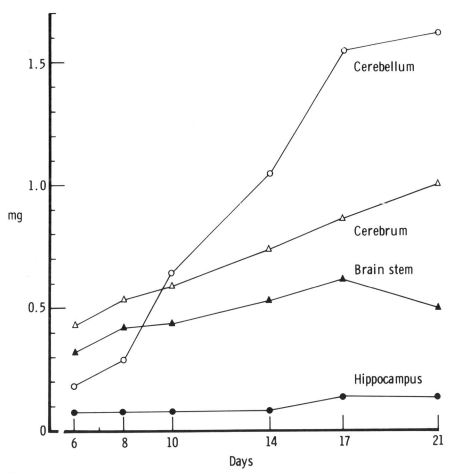

**FIG. 4.** Increase in DNA content of various regions of developing rat brain after birth. (From Winick, ref. 292.)

not shown), reaching adult levels at about 6 years (73). These findings are in contrast to earlier work (290), which suggested that cellular growth (DNA content) of human brain was complete by 5 months of age. Quantitatively, the cerebellum of man, like that of the rat, accounts for a greater proportion of brain DNA (30%) than of total mass (10%) (73). Work in other species indicates a similar regional growth pattern. Thus cerebellar DNA accumulation was complete by 21 days in the miniature swine (28), whereas brainstem DNA continued to increase through 35 days and that of cerebral hemisphere increased throughout the 56-day period studied. In the rabbit, cerebrum and brainstem had not achieved adult DNA levels by 120 days, although the cerebellum showed no increase after 75 days (119).

As an exception to the previously discussed pattern of neuronal followed by glial division, this phase of rapid DNA increase in the cerebellum includes a

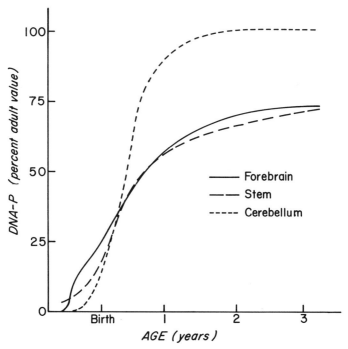

**FIG. 5.** Increases in regional DNA content of human brain during development. (From Dobbing and Sands, ref. 73.)

large increment in the microneuron population (granule, stellate, and basket cells) as well as the glial multiplication common to all regions. In other areas of the brain which also have discrete populations of granule cells (hippocampus, olfactory bulb, cochlear nucleus), the use of tritiated thymidine shows similar extensive microneuron division and migration during the first 2 weeks of postnatal life (13,14). The distinct rise in hippocampal DNA observed between 14 and 17 days postnatally in the rat (Fig. 4) reflects the migration of such neurons into this region (293). Recently Howard (130) showed that the germinal cells of the external granular layer of the cerebellum are mitotically active in the newborn rhesus monkey, which has already attained half of its adult cerebellar DNA content. Neuronal elements of the hippocampus were also shown to undergo division postnatally. The duration of postnatal mitotic activity in the cerebellar microneurons of the rhesus has yet to be determined directly, but the external granule layer reportedly disappears histologically at 2–3 months of age (228). In man this layer is present through roughly the first 20 months of life (224). These observations suggest that extensive microneuron proliferation occurs postnatally in man as well, and would therefore be susceptible to nutritional factors affecting cellular growth. The possibility that microneurons in other brain areas show a similar increase after birth cannot be ruled out. It is only by virtue of their distinct laminated pattern in the regions described above that these cells can be distinguished from histologically similar glial cells.

## IV. IMPACT OF MALNUTRITION ON BRAIN DEVELOPMENT

### A. Malnutrition and Cellular Growth

Tissues respond differently to malnutrition according to whether cell division is still active. Munro and Goldberg (192) demonstrated that adult rats fed a protein-free diet show a reduction in protein per cell for nondividing tissues (liver, kidney), but a reduction in cell number without a change in average cell protein and RNA content for dividing tissues (intestinal mucosa). This principle has been validated for various tissues of the growing rat during their periods of rapid cell division (hyperplasia) followed by an increase in cell size (hypertrophy). Winick and Noble (295) described the impact of a period of dietary restriction imposed at different stages of development on cell number (DNA) and cell size (protein) of several organs immediately after the period of deprivation and again following the refeeding of an adequate diet until adulthood (Fig. 6). When the food intake of the rat was restricted by 50% during the first 21 days of life, all organs examined showed a reduction in growth of cell population (DNA content) without a change in average cell size. In organs other than brain and lung (not shown), this response to dietary insufficiency was again observed when the restriction was imposed between 21 and 42 days. In the case of brain and lung, the cell population was already complete at this time, and a reduced average cell size was observed. Finally, malnutrition applied after 65 days of age did not affect cell number in the tissues examined except for spleen and thymus (not shown), which continue to divide at this stage of development. However, weight and protein content of all tissues were reduced during this later period of restriction. On refeeding the malnourished rats, the effects on cell size were reversed but deficits in cell population were irreversible. Thus for any tissue the time of cell division constitutes a "vulnerable period" during which nutritional deficiency leads to permanently reduced cell number and thus organ size.

With this in mind, the effects of malnutrition on brain growth are now considered in more detail. In view of the sequential pattern of cell population increase in the brain (long-axoned neurons first, followed by microneurons and glial cells), conditions of malnutrition can be chosen so that the impact occurs mainly during periods of neuron increase or of glial cell multiplication. In the case of the rat, this is conveniently demarcated by birth, so that prenatal malnutrition affects the neuron population whereas early postnatal malnutrition affects glial cells. An additional point to remember is that the fetus is relatively more protected from nutritional insult than the neonate, and the effects on it of prenatal malnutrition are generally less severe than those seen postnatally.

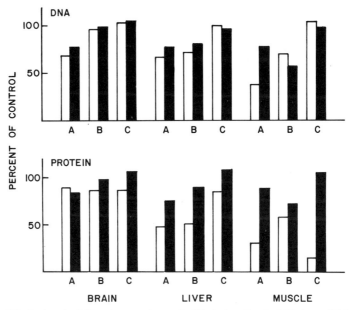

**FIG. 6.** Effect of malnutrition imposed on rats (A) during the first 21 days, (B) between 21 and 42 days, and (C) from 65 through 86 days after birth. During these periods, food intake was reduced to 50% of controls fed *ad libitum.* Some animals from each group were then allowed free access to the diet until 133 days of age. The columns show the percentage of control values for protein and DNA content of brain, liver, and muscle of rats malnourished (open columns) and rehabilitated (filled columns) under these conditions. (Data from Winick and Noble, ref. 295.)

## B. Prenatal Malnutrition and Brain Growth

An interval of prenatal exposure to nutritional deprivation has demonstrable effects on brain growth. Zamenhof et al. (315) observed a 10% reduction in brain DNA, a 20% reduction in brain protein, and a 23% reduction in the brain weight of newborn rats whose mothers were fed an 8% protein diet beginning 1 month before mating. Omission of a single essential amino acid from the diet fed during gestation resulted in similar brain deficits (309), as did severe caloric restriction of the dams (310). Feeding pregnant rats a 6% protein diet throughout gestation resulted in significantly smaller fetal brains beginning on day 18, with a 20% reduction in DNA content evident by 20 days (317). Other organs were similarly affected; but while in other tissues total RNA fell in proportion to cell number, it was not significantly reduced in brain. Winick (291) also reported that, although maternal protein deficiency results in uniformly reduced cell number in brain and other organs, ligation of the uterine artery has no effect on brain DNA content. Other organs show large deficits in cell number. It is suggested from studies in sheep that this sparing of the brain is made possible by increased blood flow to this organ in the deprived fetuses (182).

Relative sparing of the brain has been observed in other species following interference with placental blood supply, but significant deficits in brain cell number are still found. When individual brain regions were examined, the deficits were usually consistent with the timing of regional brain growth in the different species. Thus in the rhesus monkey cerebral weight is slightly reduced by ligating placental blood vessels during the last third of gestation, but DNA and protein content are not affected (122). Cell number and protein content of cerebellum, which begins its growth later in gestation, are significantly reduced. Vascular insult during the third trimester of the rabbit, whose brain develops perinatally like that of man, results in a 12% reduction in cerebral cortex DNA, while cerebellum shows a 20% deficit (269). Spontaneously occurring runt piglets showed reduced weight, DNA, cholesterol, and gangliosides in all regions, although in these studies cerebral cell number was most affected (67). When human infants considered "small for gestational age" were compared with infants of normal birth weight during the first few months of life, the retarded infants showed a 35% reduction in cerebellar weight and DNA content while the rest of the brain showed deficits of 20% (42). Myelin lipids (cerebrosides and sulfatides) were specifically reduced, whereas other lipids were not affected significantly. Thus in all species examined (except perhaps in some models of vascular deficiency), conditions which limit fetal growth result in significantly diminished brain growth as well.

Of particular significance is the impact of prenatal malnutrition on different cell types in the growing brain. Since glial multiplication does not occur significantly before birth in the rat, the deficits in fetal or neonatal brain cell number in this species are neuronal. In contrast, the phase of neuroblast multiplication in man is complete before the nutritionally vulnerable third trimester, and a reduction in brain DNA due to maternal malnutrition therefore reflects a decrease in glial cell population (69). This is consistent with the reduced myelin lipid levels in brains of "small-for-date" infants (42). As discussed previously, microneuron cells, especially in the cerebellum, are exceptions to the generalization that the neuron population is complete before the third trimester. It would be expected that these neurons are susceptible to growth limitation owing to prenatal malnutrition of the human fetus.

It is of interest to determine whether the cellular deficits observed at birth remain evident as a permanent reduction in the cell number of the adult brain. Barnes and Altman (31) observed that restriction of maternal food intake of the rat during pregnancy followed by suckling from well-nourished mothers results in more significant deficits in brain and body weight at 5–10 days postnatally than are observed at birth. However, this carry-over effect is soon lost. Since the bulk of brain cellularity of the rat is acquired after birth, it would be expected that even a 20% reduction in neonatal brain DNA would be obscured by the massive increase that occurs during the first few postnatal weeks. Thus it is not surprising that a period of malnutrition (maternal protein deprivation) during gestation alone has no significant effects on total brain weight, DNA content, or a number of other biochemical parameters when measured at 42 days after birth of the rat (11).

This picture may not be identical for every region of the brain. Zamenhof et al. (314) showed that the deficit in neonatal DNA of the cerebral hemispheres resulting from maternal protein deficiency remains significant at 30 days but is no longer so at 90 days. However, there was still a slight but significant weight reduction of the cerebral hemispheres of the older rats. In contrast, Smart et al. (254) found that a 17% reduction in forebrain DNA remained at 36 weeks after malnutrition imposed during gestation alone; this was more than could be accounted for by the deficits usually seen at birth. In the cerebellum, in which almost all the DNA accumulates postnatally, gestational malnutrition had no significant effect when the offspring were well-nourished during lactation, but the combined effect of undernutrition during pre- and postnatal periods was greater than that observed with malnutrition during lactation alone. This suggests that gestational malnutrition affected the capacity of the cerebellum for cell multiplication after birth. Winick (292) reported a similar synergistic effect of gestational and lactational undernutrition. These results thus indicate some degree of interaction between prenatal malnutrition and postnatal brain growth.

The studies of Zamenhof et al. (312,313) are particularly relevant with regard to persistent effects of prenatal malnutrition. Dams were fed a protein-deficient diet beginning 1 month prior to mating, and at birth the pups showed the expected deficits in body weight and brain parameters. Females of this $F_1$ generation were raised under conditions of adequate nutrition and then mated with normal males. The resulting $F_2$ generation showed significant deficits in body weight, brain weight, and DNA and protein content. This is presumably due to poor performance during pregnancy by the female progeny of the malnourished dams. The consequences of prenatal malnutrition which lead to this later impairment have not yet been elucidated but may be endocrine in nature. Recent studies indicate that rats whose grandmothers were malnourished show learning deficits as adults (37).

### C. Postnatal Malnutrition and Brain Growth

The bulk of experimental evidence regarding the impact of malnutrition on brain growth involves studies in rats during the suckling period. In addition to general growth, which has been given the most attention up to this point, there is considerable information relating to effects of postnatal malnutrition on specific biochemical aspects of brain development. These include myelination and the increase in gangliosides associated with dendritic growth, developmental changes in enzyme activities involved in various aspects of cellular function, and the accumulation and metabolism of various small molecules considered to act as neurotransmitters. The latter is dealt with elsewhere in this volume. Studies of the effects of postnatal malnutrition on each of the other parameters are now summarized; and, where possible, the findings in rats and other species are related to information available from human studies.

## 1. Changes in Cell Population

In accordance with the time of increase in brain cell population, malnutrition before weaning in the rat leads to a reduction in brain weight and DNA content that cannot be restored by nutritional rehabilitation after weaning (Fig. 6) (295). The impact of malnutrition on cell population increase is most severe in the cerebellum, which is consistent with the particularly rapid growth of this region during the suckling period (40). In contrast, protein deficiency or reduced food intake for a period of time after weaning results in decreased brain weight as well as protein and RNA content, but has essentially no effect on brain DNA (11,295); these deficits are reversible with adequate nutrition (295). Similarly, an additional period of malnutrition after weaning in rats undernourished during lactation results in no further deficits in adult brain weight or DNA content after a period of recovery (171). These results suggest that the time of cell division in the brain is very sharply defined, and that deficits in cell number are not restored following the normal period of cell multiplication.

These general observations require some modification in the light of further studies. Thus while Dobbing and Sands (72) demonstrated that the timing of cell division was not substantially altered in malnourished rats, there was an indication that the period of DNA accumulation was somewhat extended. In support of this suggestion, Barnes and Altman (32) found an increase in cerebellar granule cells between 20 and 30 days in malnourished rats, whereas normal cerebellum showed no further increase during this time. This is consistent with recent evidence showing a delayed peak in activity of thymidine kinase (an enzyme associated with actively dividing cells) in the cerebellum of malnourished rats (277). Bass et al. (33) also reported that the germinal zone for cerebral cortex, near the lateral ventricles, was still apparent at 50 days in malnourished rats, whereas it disappears after 20 days in normally nourished animals. In addition, complete recovery of brain cell number has been reported after malnutrition during the first 9 days of life followed by nursing in small litters until weaning (299), but this finding is complicated by the fact that the large increase in DNA later in lactation could obscure a difference of the magnitude that is considered significant at 9 days. These results nevertheless suggest that some degree of compensatory cell division can occur even after the usual period of increase in cell number is over. While cell division in the cerebrum is generally thought to be ended by weaning, there is some evidence that DNA continues to increase in the cerebrum through several weeks after weaning, although the net increase during this period is slight (110). This later phase of DNA accumulation does not occur in rats fed a restricted amount of diet after weaning.

The relative impact of malnutrition on brain and body growth is also of interest. Since all tissues of the body show considerable increases in cell number during the suckling period, it is not surprising that malnutrition at this time severely reduces whole-body and organ DNA content at weaning (294, 295). As shown in one study (Table 2), whole-body DNA content was reduced to 43% of control, while brain, heart, and liver DNA content each showed reductions of 60–70%. In contrast, brain weight and protein content were reduced only to approximately 85% of control, while other organs showed deficits in these parameters which were even greater than that in cell number. Although these data suggest that the relative "sparing" of the brain observed in malnutrition does not apply to cell number as much as cell size, these findings are complicated by the fact that the increase in total brain DNA at this time is largely due to the cerebellum, while the cerebrum provides the greater portion of the increase in weight and protein. Recent studies involving individual brain regions show a more uniform effect on cell number and wet weight within a given region (64a), thus confirming that the contradictions in the picture for the whole brain arise from the disproportionate increase in cell number in different regions.

The brain of the adult rat is preferentially protected from the effects of malnutrition as evidenced by the fact that even prolonged malnutrition of the mature rat has no significant effect on brain weight, protein, or nucleic acid levels (162,173). It has also been reported that keeping body weight constant after 100 days of age in the rat still allowed normal increases in brain weight and cholesterol content to occur (44). However, 8 weeks of protein deficiency beginning at weaning resulted in significantly reduced growth of all brain regions as well as severe stunting of body growth (65). Feeding isocaloric amounts of a diet adequate in protein had no significant effect on brain weight

TABLE 2. *Organ weight and protein and DNA content at weaning of control and malnourished animals*

| Organ | Weight (g) | Protein (mg) | DNA (mg) |
|---|---|---|---|
| Whole animal | | | |
| Control | 59.1 | 5871 | 97.81 |
| Experimental | 28.6 (49%)[a] | 2862 (49%) | 42.21 (43%) |
| Brain | | | |
| Control | 1.49 | 96.14 | 2.18 |
| Experimental | 1.23 (83%) | 84.26 (88%) | 1.48 (68%) |
| Heart | | | |
| Control | 0.36 | 58.08 | 0.622 |
| Experimental | 0.19 (53%) | 27.21 (47%) | 0.377 (60%) |
| Liver | | | |
| Control | 3.14 | 437.5 | 4.96 |
| Experimental | 1.39 (44%) | 200.1 (47%) | 3.28 (66%) |

Data are from Winick and Noble (295).
[a]Numbers in parentheses indicate the percent of the control value.

or protein content; body weight was also less affected, although the deficit remained highly significant. These findings suggest that postweaning protein deficiency has a greater impact than caloric insufficiency on the later growth of the brain.

There is considerably less evidence relating to effects of malnutrition in species other than the rat. In the mouse malnutrition during the suckling period results in deficits similar to those in the rat, with a greater impact on the cerebellum than on the rest of the brain (131). In the rabbit growth restriction during the first 2–3 weeks after birth also led to a somewhat greater reduction in cerebellar weight, DNA, RNA, and protein (242). Monkeys malnourished from 3 to 9 months showed a reduction in brain weight, but other parameters were not measured (209). Early work of Dickerson et al. (66) showed that pigs malnourished from 2 weeks to 1 year had reduced brain weight and cell number. Continued cell division between 1 and 3 years in the brain of this species allowed some degree of recovery of DNA content when an adequate diet was fed during this period. Platt et al. (218) reported reduced brain weight and various histological and neurological anomalies in dogs as a result of protein deficiency imposed after weaning.

There is good evidence that early malnutrition results in reduced brain growth in man. Winick and Rosso (297) found less DNA and proportionately decreased RNA, protein, and wet weight in brains of infants who died of severe malnutrition (marasmus) during the first year of life. Those of particularly low birth weight, indicative of prenatal malnutrition as well, had a lower brain DNA content than malnourished infants of higher birth weight (292,297). Cell number in all brain regions was reduced by early malnutrition (300), which is consistent with the relatively uniform and rapid increase in DNA of all regions of human brain during the first year of life. In contrast, children who died during their second year, particularly those with kwashiorkor, showed little deficit in brain DNA, whereas the dry weight/DNA, protein/ DNA, and lipid/DNA ratios were greatly reduced (292). Thus the principles derived for tissues of the growing rat apparently hold as well for the human brain. The extent to which these deficits can be reversed by adequate nutrition later in life has not been determined in man.

## 2. Myelin and Other Lipid Components

The impact of malnutrition on myelin deposition has been studied extensively, and several points have emerged. First, malnutrition during the suckling period leads to diminished brain myelin content at weaning. If the animals are subsequently allowed access to a better diet, considerable recovery is possible although some permanent deficit in brain lipid often remains. This is usually attributed to a permanent reduction in the population of oligodendroglial cells resulting from the period of malnutrition. Second, myelin isolated from the brains of malnourished animals shows differences in composition indicative of immaturity; this may represent a direct effect of malnutrition in retarding the myelination process in the glial cell. Third, malnutrition shortly after weaning also reduces myelination, and since the cell number is stable by now this also demonstrates a direct effect of malnutrition on the intracellular process of myelin formation. In the case of the older but still growing animal, malnutrition has little effect on continuing brain myelination, thus providing evidence of development of a mechanism protecting the mature brain from nutritional insult. The evidence for these conclusions follows, presented in the sequence just discussed:

1. Evidence for an effect of malnutrition on accumulation of various myelin constituents has been obtained by several workers. Dobbing (68) observed that relatively mild undernutrition during the suckling period produced a greater decrease in brain cholesterol content than in wet weight. Culley and Mertz (52) found that, whereas the smaller brains of malnourished rats had less lipid of all classes at weaning, phospholipids were reduced in proportion to wet weight, although cholesterol and cerebrosides showed relatively greater deficits. Others have also demonstrated particularly large reductions in cerebrosides (35). Plasmalogens, also myelin constituents, were similarly extensively affected (53). Sulfatides are fairly specific constituents of myelin. It has been found that *in vivo* incorporation of $^{35}$S-sulfate into these compounds and the *in vitro* activity of galactocerebroside sulfokinase, which catalyzes the reaction, were lower in the brains of rats malnourished during suckling by raising them in large litters (39). Recent studies demonstrated a specific reduction in the incorporation of labeled amino acids into myelin protein (relative to proteins of other subcellular fractions) in the brains of 20-day-old rats malnourished from birth (286,287). Incorporation of lipid precursors was also reduced (287). All of these observations are consistent with the lower yield of myelin in preparations from the brains of undernourished animals (92,199,287). With regard to man, deficits in myelin lipids and extractable myelin have also been reported in the brains of malnourished infants (93,98).

2. Detailed chemical studies have provided evidence of a subtle effect of malnutrition on myelin composition. The early work of Dobbing and Sands (72) demonstrated that, although malnutrition affected the total amount of lipid deposited in the brain, it did not alter the timing of cholesterol accumulation. Similarly, the time of maximal sulfate incorporation into brain lipid was not found to depend on a schedule of deprivation and refeeding applied during the suckling period (39). These observations suggest that the process of myelination proceeds during a period of malnutrition, but that the magnitude of the deposition is affected. This is supported by studies reporting no gross difference in lipid composition of myelin from rat or human brain due to malnutrition (92,98). Other methods, however, provide direct evidence of altered myelin composition in the brains of malnourished animals. Nakhasi et al. (199) reported a reduction in the specific activity of 2′,3′-cyclic nucleotide-

3'-phosphohydrolase, which is present as a component of myelin, isolated from the brains of weanling rats malnourished during lactation. Similarly, there are reduced proportions of basic and proteolipid protein in the myelin of malnourished rats at 15 or 20 days of age, which nevertheless achieved normal levels by 25 or 30 days of age (287). Cerebroside and sulfatide fatty acid patterns more characteristic of immature brain have also been reported following malnutrition (154).

3. Finally, there is evidence that malnutrition applied after the glial cell population is complete can still affect the process of myelination. Lipid deficits in the brains of animals malnourished during the suckling period can be reversed to some extent by good nutrition immediately after weaning without any increase in glial cell number (35,116). It has also been shown that malnutrition after weaning can cause a deficit in brain lipid content that is completely restored by adequate nutrition (65,74). Thus the major impact of malnutrition at this time appears to be at the level of myelin deposition by existing cells. Permanent deficits which remain in the brains of adult animals severely malnourished during lactation probably reflect a reduction in glial cell number as a result of the early nutritional deprivation (51,102). It is of interest that, while myelin deposition is susceptible to malnutrition shortly after weaning, there is evidence that later periods of brain growth are less vulnerable. Cholesterol deposition in rat brain continues after restriction of the diet at 100 days of age to a level which keeps body weight constant (44). A more detailed study of brain lipids in miniature swine demonstrated that threefold increases in galactosides and proteolipid occurred in animals fed a low-protein diet from 9 to 32 weeks, resulting in only slight and uniform deficits in brain weight and all lipid components (94). In contrast, body weight failed to increase appreciably during the period of deprivation, and attained only 14% of that of control animals at 32 weeks. Thus later phases of myelination appear to be relatively invulnerable to nutritional insult, indicating the establishment of a protective mechanism earlier in brain development.

Another class of lipids, not related to myelination, which shows considerable increases during development is the gangliosides. Studies in both the pig and the rat have shown continued increase in forebrain gangliosides for many months after birth, whereas cerebellum and brainstem tend to reach maximum levels earlier, which thereafter remain stable or decline somewhat (178). It has been suggested that these lipids might be a useful though imperfect marker for dendritic arborization (62,179). Malnutrition during gestation and lactation reduces ganglioside levels in all brain regions later in the suckling period (179). Others found, in addition, that at 17 days brains of malnourished pups show elevated levels of enzymes involved in ganglioside synthesis, indicating a delay in the fall in activity which normally occurs with maturation (187). The role of gangliosides in the brain and the significance of the impact of malnutrition in their accumulation require further investigation.

### 3. Brain Enzymes

As described above, early malnutrition affects enzymes associated with myelin and its synthesis, as well as those involved in the metabolism of gangliosides. The effects of malnutrition on a number of other enzymes have also been studied, and in general the findings can be integrated fairly well into a unified picture of the malnourished brain. It must be kept in mind, however, that enzyme concentrations are regulated by a variety of factors and cannot necessarily be equated with the relative abundance of cells or structures in which they are thought to be localized. This is discussed by Shoemaker and Bloom (*this volume*) with regard to tyrosine hydroxylase, the rate-limiting enzyme of catecholamine synthesis. Interpretations of the results of the various enzyme assays must therefore be regarded as tentative.

Some deficits in total enzyme content in the brain of the malnourished animal can be related to small brain size, and these disappear when expressed per cell (DNA) or per unit of brain protein or weight. Other changes remain after such computations and thus represent a specific loss of an enzyme. Total cerebral levels of lactate dehydrogenase, aldolase, creatine phosphokinase, and isocitrate dehydrogenase were reduced in rats malnourished during the suckling period, whereas enzyme activity expressed per milligram of DNA or of protein were unaltered (261,262). The same relationships held after a period of nutritional rehabilitation from weaning to 110 days (260). It is less clear what occurs to succinate dehydrogenase. Early investigators found that malnutrition had no effect on specific activity of succinate dehydrogenase in brains of suckling rats (247); others reported somewhat reduced succinate dehydrogenase and aldolase activities per gram of brain during the suckling period in rats subjected to combined gestational and lactational undernutrition, although the lysosomal enzyme $\beta$-N-acetylglucosaminidase was not affected (6). Moreover, succinate dehydrogenase and aldolase activities in these studies then returned to control values when deprived animals were well nourished until 16 weeks (5). Oxygen consumption by brain mitochondria of rats malnourished *in utero* was equivalent to that of well-nourished controls per milligram of mitochondrial protein or of brain tissue (197). Whole-brain butyryl cholinesterase, fumarase, and $\beta$-galactosidase showed normal activity when expressed per unit wet weight or protein in weanling rats whose mothers were malnourished from early pregnancy, and 5'-nucleotidase even showed a slight increase (7). Forebrain adenosine triphosphatase and fumarase activities per milligram of protein were equal to those of well-nourished animals at 12 weeks, whether the rats were malnourished throughout life or only until weaning (8). Similarly, concentrations of enzymes involved in fatty acid synthesis were unaffected by malnutrition during lactation (114). These results indicate that for a number of brain enzymes lasting deficits in total brain activity simply reflect a reduction in brain cell number, and therefore brain weight, caused by early malnutrition.

This conclusion contrasts with the effect of malnutrition on enzymes associated with more specialized brain functions. For example, early malnutrition leads to moderately reduced acetylcholinesterase activity per gram (wet weight) in whole brain and in all brain regions at weaning, while reduced brain weight makes the deficit per region or per brain even greater (6,7,255). When malnourished animals are fed a normal diet after weaning, acetylcholinesterase content per brain reaches normal values; because brain weight remains reduced, enzyme activity per gram (wet weight) is increased (5,8,134). A similar result was obtained in malnourished and rehabilitated pigs (135). Early work indicated that acetylcholinesterase was localized in nerve ending particle fractions (61), and in that context these findings suggest that proliferation of nerve terminals is restricted by early malnutrition but that complete recovery is possible with adequate nutrition. The relative invulnerability of neurons to postnatal malnutrition and the relatively large contribution of nonneural elements to the weight of the mature brain are consistent with this hypothesis. However, current data do not support a correlation between acetylcholinesterase and cholinergic nerve terminals (146,239). Furthermore, recent work (79) shows that elevated brainstem acetylcholinesterase of malnourished and then rehabilitated rats is accompanied by decreased choline acetyltransferase, which is a more specific marker for presynaptic cholinergic nerve endings. Others have seen transiently reduced acetylcholinesterase levels in cerebral cortex at 12 days after birth in pups of malnourished mothers. These returned to control values at 24 days even in rats that continued to be malnourished, whereas choline acetyltransferase was not reduced at either age (99). Thus the response of acetylcholinesterase to malnutrition is quite different from that of choline acetyltransferase, and it is not possible to identify changes in either enzyme with specific structural alterations in neurons.

Other studies have dealt with enzymes involved in the metabolism of another neurotransmitter, $\gamma$-aminobutyric acid (GABA). A low-protein diet fed to weanling rats resulted in reduced brain concentrations of glutamate dehydrogenase (which forms glutamate from $\alpha$-ketoglutarate) and reduced glutamate decarboxylase (which synthesizes GABA from glutamate), whereas GABA-transaminase was not affected (227). The deficits in these enzymes following 10 weeks of protein deficiency were reversed by 10 weeks of an adequate diet (225). It has been suggested that glutamate decarboxylase is associated with synaptosomes and is concentrated in brain regions with high levels of GABA, while GABA-transaminase is a more ubiquitous mitochondrial enzyme (48). Other studies show that rats raised in large litters (and thus malnourished prior to weaning) also have reduced concentrations of glutamate dehydrogenase and decarboxylase, which were restored after 5 weeks of *ad libitum* feeding (226). Other workers recently reported a similar reduction in brain glutamate dehydrogenase during lactational undernutrition (41). While protein deficiency during the period after weaning decreased brain enzyme activities of previously well-nourished rats, feeding restricted amounts of an adequate diet affected enzyme activities only if the animals had been malnourished during the suckling period (226). These results suggest that a mechanism which protects the brain of the weanling rat from nutritional deprivation fails to develop adequately in rats malnourished during lactation, and that the brains of even well-nourished weanlings are more susceptible to protein deficiency than to restriction of total food intake.

Another aspect of the biochemical development of the brain that has received some attention is the phenomenon of "metabolic compartmentation," as evidenced by a high specific activity of glutamine relative to glutamate following administration of [14]C-leucine or other precursors. The increase in this ratio during the first several postnatal weeks parallels the appearance of pathways converting glucose to nonessential amino acids (213). Malnutrition during the suckling period impairs the developmental increase in the glutamine/glutamate specific activity ratio, whereas adequate nutrition for several weeks after weaning allows it to regain normal levels for mature brain (214,232).

Of general relevance to the study of the mechanisms by which malnutrition limits cellular growth is the finding of increased alkaline ribonuclease activity in tissues of animals during nutritional deprivation, including placentas subjected to vascular deficiency (240,271,293). In brain *total* ribonuclease activity (per milligram of DNA) does not change in malnutrition during lactation, whereas the proportion of enzyme not bound to the endogenous inhibitor (*free* ribonuclease) increases (240). It has been suggested that reduced inhibitor concentration is responsible for the elevated free ribonuclease activity. Although increased ribonuclease is associated with reduced RNA/DNA ratios in brain and other tissues, the precise functional role of ribonuclease in RNA metabolism has yet to be determined (153,240,271).

## V. FREE AMINO ACID POOLS OF BRAIN

For the purposes of this discussion it is assumed that the intracellular free amino acid pool provides the substrates for protein synthesis in brain. Although several authors studying protein synthesis in surviving pieces of tissue (2,270) interpreted their data to mean that the immediate source of amino acids for protein synthesis is at an extracellular or membranous site, the studies of Fern and Garlick (90) strongly suggest that the proteins of the brain and other tissues are made from amino acids present in the cytosol of the cells. These authors used an ingenious procedure in which injected [14]C-glycine formed [14]C-serine intracellularly, and vice versa. From a study of the relative levels of labeled glycine and serine in the tissue proteins, it was possible to conclude that the specific activities of cytosol glycine and serine gave concordant values for the rate of protein synthesis, whereas the plasma specific activities were not in agreement with the proportion incorporated into tissue proteins.

The interpretation of changes in free amino acid pools of any tissue is a complex problem. The intracellular level of an amino acid depends on its relative rates of influx, efflux, incorporation into and release from cellular protein, degradative metabolism, and *de novo* synthesis. This is further complicated by the existence of functional compartments within cells for which the above rates are not necessarily identical (133,189). Finally, in a tissue as heterogeneous as brain there is the additional complexity of several cell types having different metabolic pools and activities.

With these limitations in mind we can nevertheless demonstrate that free amino acid pools in brain are susceptible to changes in plasma amino acid levels which result from protein deficiency or from various amino acid imbalances. These are also conditions under which brain development can be impaired. In consequence, such changes in the free amino acid pools of the brain may be relevant to the mechanism by which protein-calorie deficiency affects brain development.

## A. Species, Maturational, and Regional Differences in Free Amino Acid Pools of Brain

Five nonessential amino acids (glutamic acid, glutamine, aspartic acid, glycine, and alanine) occur at much higher concentrations in tissues in general than in plasma (191). The brain is no exception. Table 3 displays the free amino acid content of brain at birth and during adulthood for a variety of mammals including man (adult only). Although the data summarized here are derived from species ranging in adult body weight between 30 g (mouse) and 70 kg (man), the concentrations of most amino acids show no trend that can be related in any way to adult body size. There is, however, a reduction in the concentrations of most free amino acids when the brain of the adult is compared with that of the neonate; the exceptions are glutamic and aspartic acids and glutamine, whose concentrations tend to increase with age. During the suckling period of the rat, Miller (180) identified peaks of free amino acid concentration around the 7th and 20th days, and related them causally to increased brain protein synthesis at these times.

Recently Bachmann et al. (25) reported free amino acid concentrations in the cerebrum and cerebellum of macaque monkeys from early fetal development to adulthood. Most amino acids attained peak concentrations during the last third of pregnancy and remained elevated during early postnatal life, declining as the animal attained maturity. However, the acidic amino acids and their amides, as well as cystathionine and GABA, reached maximal values much later, in agreement with data on other species.

The general reduction in free amino acid concentration with age cannot be attributed to any significant extent to a change in water content of the brain with maturation. The water content of the rat brain declines from 88% at birth to 81% at 45 days of age (273), and that of man from 90% at birth to 80% in the

TABLE 3. *Brain amino acid levels$^a$ and water content$^b$ at different ages in various species*

| Amino acid | Mouse Neonate | Mouse Adult | Rat Neonate[c] | Rat Adult[c,d] | Guinea pig Neonate | Guinea pig Adult | Rabbit Neonate | Rabbit Adult |
|---|---|---|---|---|---|---|---|---|
| Taurine | 16.50 | 9.13 | 21.6 | 5.66, 4.84 | 3.42 | 1.61 | 5.94 | 1.04 |
| Glutamic acid | 4.26 | 11.50 | 5.6 | 9.88, 10.1 | 11.14 | 9.51 | 5.21 | 8.53 |
| Aspartic acid | 1.86 | 3.38 | 1.79 | 3.06, 3.02 | 2.79 | 2.36 | 1.23 | 2.05 |
| Glutamine | 3.78 | 4.83 | 4.5 | 5.2 | 4.87 | 3.88 | 3.50 | 3.08 |
| Glycine | 2.72 | 1.61 | 1.50 | 1.00, 1.10 | 2.55 | 0.98 | 3.19 | 0.97 |
| Alanine | 3.26 | 0.66 | 1.16 | 0.63, 0.53 | 0.94 | 0.65 | 0.94 | 0.42 |
| Threonine | 0.68 | 0.39 | 1.19 | 0.64, 1.54 | 0.31 | 0.26 | 0.43 | 0.14 |
| Serine | 1.21 | 0.78 | 1.10 | 1.30, 1.22 | 1.79 | 0.68 | 1.30 | 0.76 |
| Proline | 0.49 | 0.06 | 0.29 | 0.17 | 0.18 | 0.08 | 0.23 | 0.04 |
| Valine | 0.32 | 0.08 | 0.17 | 0.07, 0.09 | 0.10 | 0.06 | 0.21 | 0.08 |
| Leucine | 0.24 | 0.08 | 0.13 | 0.07, 0.05 | 0.08 | 0.07 | 0.15 | 0.06 |
| Isoleucine | 0.14 | 0.04 | 0.05 | 0.03, 0.04 | 0.04 | 0.04 | 0.04 | 0.03 |
| Tyrosine | 0.14 | 0.05 | 0.12 | 0.06, 0.05 | 0.05 | 0.07 | 0.16 | 0.05 |
| Phenylalanine | 0.13 | 0.04 | 0.07 | 0.05, 0.04 | 0.03 | 0.04 | 0.03 | 0.03 |
| Histidine | 0.14 | 0.05 | 0.08 | 0.05, 0.08 | — | — | — | — |
| Arginine | 0.10 | 0.13 | 0.05 | 0.08, 0.07 | — | — | — | — |
| Methionine | 0.02 | 0.03 | 0.065 | 0.064 | 0.02 | 0.10 | 0.02 | 0.01 |
| Lysine | 0.15 | 0.18 | 0.21 | 0.15, 0.21 | 0.02 | 0.07 | 0.06 | 0.04 |
| Tryptophan | 0.07$^h$ | 0.035$^h$ | — | | — | | — | |
| Water (% wet wt.) | 88.4 | 80.3 | 89.5 | 83.2 | 83.5 | 79.5 | 95.0 | 77.0 |

The amino acid levels are expressed as micromoles per gram.
$^a$From Himwich and Agrawal (124) except as noted.
$^b$From Himwich (123) except as noted.
$^c$From Bayer and McMurray (34).
$^d$From Lowden and LaRamée (170).
$^e$From Badger and Tumbleson (28).
$^f$From Enwonwu and Worthington (84).
$^g$From Hansen et al. (118).
$^h$Calculated from data of Hoff et al. (125).

TABLE 3. (continued)

| Amino acid | Cat Neonate | Cat Adult | Dog Neonate | Dog Adult | Miniature swine[e] 5 days | Miniature swine[e] 63 days | Monkey,[f] ~1 year | Baboon,[g] adult | Man,[g] adult |
|---|---|---|---|---|---|---|---|---|---|
| Taurine | 9.20 | 2.30 | 6.82 | 1.28 | 3.21 | 1.50 | 3.10 | 2.01 | 1.25 |
| Glutamic acid | 6.01 | 7.87 | 4.29 | 9.05 | 11.51 | 10.53 | 9.24 | 9.05 | 7.19 |
| Aspartic acid | 1.08 | 1.70 | 1.01 | 3.28 | 2.00 | 2.60 | 2.64 | 2.00 | 1.10 |
| Glutamine | 3.85 | 2.83 | 2.53 | 4.66 | 3.77 | 3.23 | — | 5.27 | 5.33 |
| Glycine | 2.26 | 0.78 | 1.25 | 0.86 | 1.21 | 1.13 | 0.98 | 0.63 | 0.45 |
| Alanine | 2.24 | 0.48 | 0.76 | 0.99 | 0.92 | 0.54 | 0.69 | 0.72 | 0.29 |
| Threonine | 0.58 | 0.17 | 0.86 | 0.29 | 0.58 | 0.62 | 0.46 | 0.27 | 0.28 |
| Serine | 1.08 | 0.48 | 0.79 | 0.58 | 3.00 | 2.30 | 1.07 | 0.81 | 0.44 |
| Proline | 0.22 | 0.03 | 0.17 | 0.06 | — | — | — | 0.19 | 0.08 |
| Valine | 0.21 | 0.06 | 0.09 | 0.17 | 0.24 | 0.14 | 0.15 | 0.14 | 0.14 |
| Leucine | 0.17 | 0.07 | 0.05 | 0.17 | 0.16 | 0.11 | 0.11 | 0.11 | 0.08 |
| Isoleucine | 0.07 | 0.03 | 0.01 | 0.11 | 0.05 | 0.11 | 0.10 | 0.07 | 0.04 |
| Tyrosine | 0.11 | 0.03 | 0.06 | 0.04 | 0.10 | 0.04 | 0.07 | 0.06 | 0.05 |
| Phenylalanine | 0.5 | 0.02 | 0.06 | 0.07 | 0.07 | 0.03 | 0.05 | 0.06 | 0.05 |
| Histidine | 0.02 | 0.02 | — | 0.05 | 0.08 | 0.03 | 0.10 | 0.11 | 0.10 |
| Arginine | — | — | — | — | 0.05 | 0.05 | 0.08 | 0.17 | 0.09 |
| Methionine | 0.01 | 0.02 | — | 0.04 | — | — | — | 0.03 | 0.03 |
| Lysine | 0.07 | 0.08 | 0.19 | 0.23 | 0.09 | 0.09 | 0.18 | 0.27 | 0.12 |
| Tryptophan | — | — | — | — | — | — | — | 0.01 | 0.01 |
| Water (% wet wt.) | 91.8 | 82.3 | 92.1 | 84.6 | — | — | — | — | 80.0 |

adult (73). The brains of other species show comparable changes (Table 3). It is possible that the higher levels of most amino acids in the brain at birth are at least a partial reflection of the high levels of amino acids in fetal plasma relative to maternal plasma, which rapidly fall after birth to adult levels (46). However, the much longer period of time over which the general decrease in brain amino acids occurs suggests that other factors are operating as well (34). Finally, it may be noted that the nonessential amino acids present at higher levels in adult tissues are those which can be synthesized within the tissues, and a number of these have been implicated as neurotransmitters in brain (54).

In addition to maturational changes in amino acid concentration, there are some distinctive regional differences. Glutamic acid concentration is higher in the cerebral cortex and GABA in the hypothalamus and midbrain, while aspartic acid is somewhat elevated in the medulla (54). Again, these may be related to possible localized neurotransmitter roles for these amino acids. Of special interest are maturational and regional changes in the concentration of tryptophan, the precursor of serotonin. Hoff et al. (125) confirmed with mice the finding of Tyce et al. (267) for rats that free tryptophan in brain declines extensively with maturation. Hoff et al. (125) also showed that there are no important regional differences.

### B. Effects of Malnutrition on Brain Amino Acid Levels

Protein deficiency causes changes in plasma amino acids of man, both during infancy and in mature people. Thus studies on human infants suffering from kwashiorkor (36,80,127) show distinctive changes in plasma free amino acid concentrations (Fig. 7). The levels of most essential amino acids, especially the branched-chain amino acids, tend to be depressed, as are those of tyrosine, arginine, and citrulline; in contrast, the concentrations of several nonessential amino acids (glycine, alanine, proline, serine, aspartic acid) and histidine tend to be elevated. Severe malnutrition depresses the levels of all amino acids, but the differential effect on essential versus nonessential amino acids persists. There has been dispute about whether the aminogram in marasmus differs from that in kwashiorkor. In discussing this topic, Waterlow (276) concludes that there is no unanimity about the claim by Whitehead (284,285) that the ratio of essential to nonessential amino acids differs in these two syndromes, marasmus being associated with a normal ratio (even if the amino acid levels are depressed in general). According to Waterlow (276) this ratio can be used legitimately for experimental situations to distinguish between protein deficiency and caloric deficiency; several examples in animal models are described below. Although brain amino acid levels have not been measured in malnourished children, a difference in the impact of kwashiorkor and marasmus on plasma amino acids emphasizes the need to distinguish between these syndromes in evaluating the response of free amino acids in brain to malnutrition.

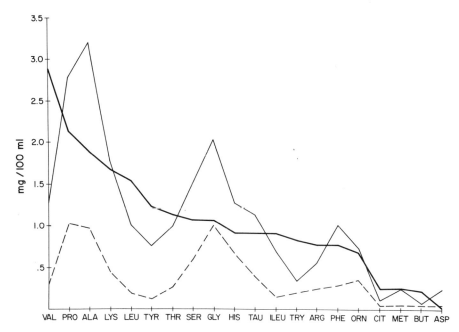

**FIG. 7.** Plasma amino acid changes in kwashiorkor. Bold line indicates normal amino acid levels. Solid and dashed lines designate values in moderate and severe protein deficiency, respectively. (From Holt and Snyderman, ref. 126.)

The effect of a protein-deficient diet on plasma amino acid levels was also examined experimentally in adults. In general, essential amino acids were not markedly affected by 1 or 2 weeks of protein deficiency (4,264), except for some reduction in branched-chain and other large neutral amino acids in one study (283). These findings indicate that the age at which protein deficiency occurs is important in determining changes in plasma amino acids.

These distinctions in type of malnutrition and timing of its onset are supported by studies of experimental malnutrition in miniature swine (26,27), monkeys (83,84), and rats (64,211). The most extensive studies are those of Badger and Tumbleson (26,27), who weaned miniature swine at 5, 21, or 35 days onto either a 20% protein diet, a 5% protein diet (protein deficiency), or the 20% protein diet pair-fed to the malnourished piglets (calorie deficiency). Animals in all groups were killed at 65 days of age. Those fed the protein-deficient diet grew much less than the pair-fed animals (restricted energy intake). The degree of growth failure in the protein-deficient group was equivalent to kwashiorkor in man, whereas the pair-fed group represents mild marasmus, since they gained weight at a rate more nearly comparable to the controls and received a normal level of dietary protein. The most severe effect on weight gain was in the animals weaned at 5 days onto the inadequate diets; in pigs weaned at this age brain growth was reduced by both types of malnutrition. Brain weight was unaffected in animals weaned onto the protein- or calorie-deficient diets at 21 or 35 days of age.

Figure 8 shows plasma aminograms drawn from the data of Badger and Tumbleson (27) on miniature swine malnourished from 21 to 63 days of age. The results are plotted as the percent change from concentrations observed in control animals fed *ad libitum* on the adequate diets containing 20% protein. The data show that the protein-deficient group had very low levels of threonine and the branched-chain amino acids, as well as of phenylalanine and tyrosine, whereas alanine and especially methionine levels were elevated above those of controls fed *ad libitum*. In contrast, the pair-fed (energy-deficient) group showed much less depression of threonine and of the branched-chain amino acids and tyrosine, and there was less elevation of methionine. Pigs malnourished from 5 days of age showed similar patterns, although methionine was not so greatly elevated; those subjected to the same

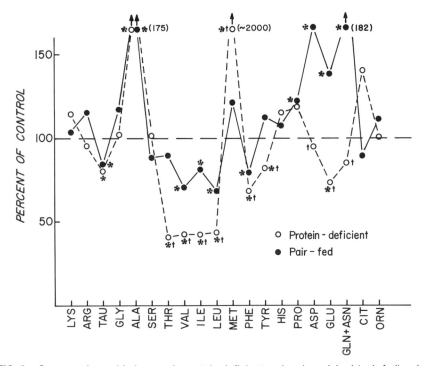

**FIG. 8.** Serum amino acid changes in protein-deficient and malnourished (pair-fed) swine. The swine were weaned onto a 20% protein diet fed *ad libitum* (control group: ---), a 5% protein diet also fed *ad libitum* (protein-deficient group: ○---○), or a 20% protein diet pair-fed with the protein-deficient group (energy-deficient group: ●—●). The diets were fed from 21 to 63 days of age. The amino acid concentrations are expressed as percent of control group values. The asterisk and dagger indicate values significantly different from those of control and pair-fed animals, respectively ($p < 0.05$). (Data from Badger and Tumbleson, ref. 27.)

diets at 35 days of age underwent less characteristic changes, with smaller reductions in most amino acid levels in the plasma.

These authors also measured the free amino acid concentrations in various regions of the brain (26). Recall that brain growth was retarded equally by protein and caloric insufficiencies in the groups weaned at 5 days onto these diets, while no effect on brain weight was produced in animals weaned at 21 or 35 days. Nevertheless, as shown in Fig. 9, protein deficiency from 21 through 65 days severely reduced the cerebral levels of threonine and the branched-chain amino acids, whereas the energy-restricted group showed reductions of a less severe degree in these amino acid levels but not in those of other essential amino acids. Indeed, these patterns reflect the plasma changes in the same animals (Fig. 8). Cystathionine levels, which are particularly high in the brains of protein-deficient animals, may reflect the elevation of plasma methionine, from which cystathionine is then derived (274). A similar picture

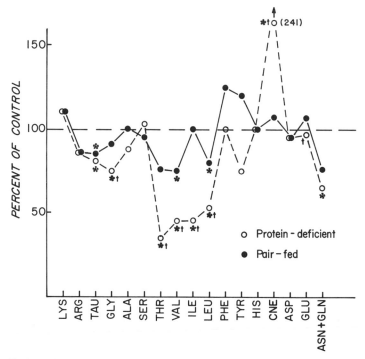

**FIG. 9.** Brain amino acid changes in protein-deficient and malnourished (pair-fed) swine. The groups and treatments are those shown in the legend of Fig. 8. Control (---), protein-deficient (o---o), and pair-fed energy-deficient (•—•) groups are indicated; amino acid concentrations for the latter two groups are shown as percentage values of the controls. The asterisk and dagger indicate values significantly different from those of control and pair-fed animals, respectively ($p < 0.05$). CNE, cystathionine. (Data from Badger and Tumbleson, ref. 26.)

emerges when the data on pigs malnourished from 5 days of age are plotted (not shown). Pigs malnourished from 35 to 65 days of age showed fewer significant alterations in cerebral free amino acid concentrations (not shown). Amino acid concentrations in cerebellum and brainstem were also measured and showed significant effects of both dietary treatments at all ages of weaning, but the patterns of change were not identical in all brain areas. Since brain weight was affected only by feeding the deficient diets to pigs weaned at 5 days (but not at 21 or 35 days), we cannot claim that brain development is inevitably influenced by altered free amino acid levels. More sophisticated tests of brain development and function are needed to answer this question.

Comparable effects of protein deficiency on plasma and brain amino acids have been reported in other species. In young monkeys aged 6 to 9 months fed a low-protein diet *ad libitum,* Enwonwu and Worthington (84) observed low levels of the branched-chain amino acids in all areas of the brain, reflecting the depression of the same amino acids in the plasma. Although no change in plasma histidine was found, 3-methylhistidine, histidine, and homocarnosine ($\gamma$-aminobutyryl-L-histidine) were markedly elevated in brain. Liver showed changes similar to those in brain but of somewhat greater magnitude. In contrast to young animals, older monkeys subjected to protein deficiency showed no reduction in brain amino acid levels, although plasma essential amino acid levels were depressed (83). Increases in brain histidine, 3-methylhistidine, and homocarnosine, as well as lysine, phenylalanine, and tyrosine, were nevertheless seen in these older animals.

Finally, the effects of malnutrition on free amino acid levels in brain were studied in rats. Pao and Dickerson (211) reported that weanling rats given a low-protein diet for 56 days showed depressed plasma levels of valine, isoleucine, and tyrosine, together with elevated levels of aspartic acid, glycine, alanine, and histidine. Histidine and methionine were the only essential amino acids showing consistent changes in brain, and they were uniformly elevated in all regions. In another study the tryptophan level was severely depressed in the plasma of protein-deficient rats, and this was reflected in decreased tryptophan in all brain regions (64). Brain and plasma tryptophan levels returned to control values after 7 days of feeding a diet adequate in protein. Rats fed restricted amounts of a protein-adequate diet showed none of these changes in essential amino acid levels (64,211). With regard to adult rats, early studies (173) showed that prolonged feeding of a protein-free diet resulted in marked depletion of all amino acids except histidine in liver. In brain the only significant differences were elevations in methionine and histidine, a fall in phenylalanine, and increases in serine and arginine levels.

These studies agree in several respects. First, in the young animal (man, swine, monkey, and rat), plasma levels of certain free amino acids, especially the branched-chain amino acids, are severely depressed by protein deficiency and to a lesser extent by caloric deficiency. Second, these changes are also reflected in the free amino acid pools of the brain. Finally, when older animals are subjected to malnutrition the plasma changes due to protein deficiency are less severe and the brain is usually little affected. This is particularly well documented in the swine studies of Badger and Tumbleson (26,27), whose animals were all killed at the same age although malnutrition had been imposed at different times. The persistence of altered amino acid levels in the brains of animals malnourished early in life and killed at a later age suggests that malnutrition applied at this time impairs subsequent development of mechanisms which normally maintain the concentrations of amino acids in the brain later in life even when dietary insufficiency depresses plasma levels.

A few observations on the effects of maternal malnutrition on amino acid levels in the brains of fetal monkeys near the end of pregnancy have been recorded (25). The data are expressed per unit of brain DNA and per unit of wet weight; the former introduces the problem that mean cell size changes could account for differences in free amino acid content per cell. As measured in concentration per gram of wet weight, protein deficiency, calorie deficiency, and a combination of protein and calorie deficiency induced few changes. In the case of the cerebrum, the levels of several amino acids (aspartic and glutamic acids, threonine, and glycine) appeared to be elevated significantly by either protein or calorie deficiency when compared with the response to combined protein-calorie deficiency. The cerebellum behaved differently. Here protein deficiency caused a significant reduction in taurine and lysine levels, while calorie or protein-calorie deficiency reduced the levels of glycine and phenylalanine. The number of animals involved was small, however, and the data must be regarded as preliminary.

## C. Effects of Amino Acid Excess

Excessive blood levels of individual amino acids are known to affect brain function. In infants mental retardation results from high levels of plasma phenylalanine in phenylketonuria, branched-chain amino and keto acids in maple syrup urine disease, and so on for other inborn errors of amino acid metabolism (289). Older children with high plasma levels of phenylalanine appear to be immune to brain damage (128), but this does not necessarily mean that plasma amino acid levels have no effect on brain metabolism after infancy. Neuroendocrine function remains sensitive to dihydroxyphenylalanine (DOPA) administered for Parkinson's disease of adults (177), and the imbalanced plasma amino acid pattern of liver cirrhosis appears to be a significant factor in hepatic coma (194). Experimentally, protein synthesis in the brain of the rat is impaired by administration of large doses of individual amino acids, including phenylalanine (252), methionine (301), and DOPA (279). Finally, enormous doses of glutamic acid and aspartic acid cause necrosis of the hypothalamus of weanling rats and mice (206) but not of other species tested (230).

The effects of excessive plasma levels of single amino acids on brain amino

acid pools have been examined by several authors. In a comprehensive series
of studies, Peng et al. (216) added large amounts of amino acids (methionine,
tryptophan, histidine, leucine, phenylalanine, threonine, lysine, glutamic acid)
singly to a low-protein meal and force-fed each meal to mature rats; control
animals were fed the low-protein meal only. Assays of amino acid concentrations carried out 3 hours later on plasma and brain showed grossly increased
levels of the amino acids added to the diet to create the toxicity, except in the
case of glutamic acid where the elevation in the brain was less than in the
plasma, presumably due to the protective action of the blood-brain barrier. In
contrast, the brain levels of many essential amino acids were depressed more
than in the plasma, the pattern being consistent with competition for entry to
the brain between the amino acid in excess in the plasma and other amino
acids in the same transport class. For example, Fig. 10 shows that feeding
leucine grossly elevated the plasma and brain leucine levels while reducing the
levels of isoleucine and valine to similar extents in the plasma and the brain;
however, the levels of methionine, phenylalanine, tyrosine, and histidine were
much more depressed in brain than in plasma. Following administration of
phenylalanine (Fig. 11), the phenylalanine and tyrosine levels were elevated in

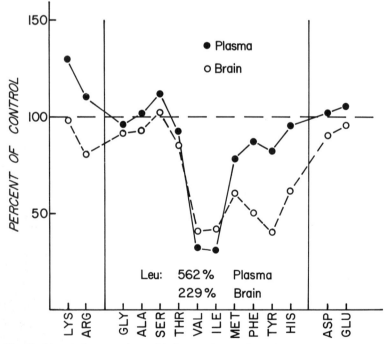

**FIG. 10.** Brain and plasma amino acid changes in rats force-fed a low-protein diet with 5%
leucine added. Amino acid concentrations for animals force-fed the basal low-protein diet
(— —) were assigned values of 100, and rats receiving the high-leucine meal are shown
relative to these values for plasma (•—•) and brain (o---o). (Adapted from Peng et al., ref. 216.)

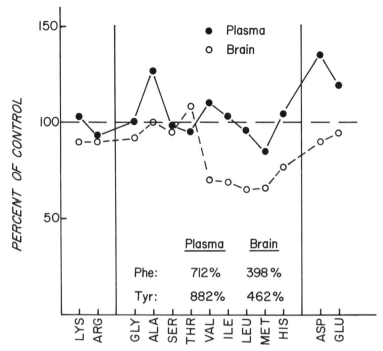

**FIG. 11.** Brain and plasma amino acid changes in rats force-fed a low-protein diet with 5% phenylalanine added. Amino acid concentrations for animals force-fed the basal low-protein diet (——) were assigned values of 100, and rats receiving the high-phenylalanine meal are shown relative to these values for plasma (•—•) and brain (○---○). (From Peng et al., ref. 216.)

plasma and brain. Plasma levels of other amino acids were not appreciably affected, but the brain levels of the branched-chain amino acids and of histidine and methionine were severely depressed. Somewhat similar patterns were found when tryptophan or histidine were fed in excess; lysine administration caused depression only in the brain arginine level, while feeding threonine or glutamic acid had little effect on the brain levels of other amino acids.

Other studies confirm this general picture. Changes similar to those in Fig. 11 were obtained following intravenous (233), intraperitoneal (176), or subcutaneous (170) injection of phenylalanine into adult or infant rats. Intraperitoneal injection or prolonged feeding of excess methionine to weanling rats caused reductions in the brain levels of several nonessential amino acids (57). Administration of histidine intraperitoneally to mature rats depressed brain levels of most neutral essential amino acids (268). Similar changes were induced by feeding 7% histidine in the diet, but 14% histidine raised many brain amino acid levels, possibly by inhibiting brain protein synthesis. Ip and Harper (137) reported a study in which weanling rats were fed a low-protein diet containing 5% tyrosine for 7 days. Food intake was much reduced. Levels of essential amino acids in the brain fell, brain polyribosomes were disaggregated, and incorporation of amino acids into brain protein was inhibited.

Thus both protein deficiency and administration of excessive amounts of single amino acids can produce similar severe reductions in the levels of several brain amino acids, notably the branched-chain and the aromatic amino acids. In the case of protein deficiency, low levels of the corresponding plasma amino acids seem to account for the low brain levels, whereas the same changes in brain amino acid pools following excessive intake of single amino acids can best be attributed to competition for entry into the brain. The question of whether the adverse effects of protein deficiency and amino acid excess on brain function are due to inadequate intracerebral levels of amino acids for brain protein synthesis is considered in the next section.

## VI. BRAIN PROTEIN SYNTHESIS AND THE IMPACT OF MALNUTRITION

An assessment of the impact of malnutrition on brain protein metabolism must include a discussion of the mechanism of mammalian protein synthesis. The mass of information that has now accumulated on this subject is too great to review here in its entirety. However, we begin with a general discussion of mammalian protein synthesis and its regulation. This is followed by a section dealing specifically with studies on protein synthesis in the nervous system, including an evaluation of methods used to measure protein synthetic activity in the brain. Finally, the effects of malnutrition on brain protein synthesis and metabolism are discussed.

### A. Mechanism of Eukaryote Protein Synthesis

Protein synthesis consists of two phases: transcription, in which messenger RNA (mRNA) is made using a DNA template in the nucleus, and translation, in which the mRNA is used by the ribosomes in the cytoplasm to synthesize protein. These steps are followed in many cases by further modification of the newly synthesized peptides. The sequence is summarized in Fig. 12. Each of these processes is subject to regulation, and any studies of perturbations in protein synthesis in the brain must take into account potential changes at each of these sites in brain cells.

### 1. Transcription and Its Control

The first step in protein synthesis is to make the information stored in chromosomes available by transcribing some of the chromosomal DNA into RNA. It is generally accepted that the proteins of chromosomes play a part in regulating which pieces of the encoded information are made available,

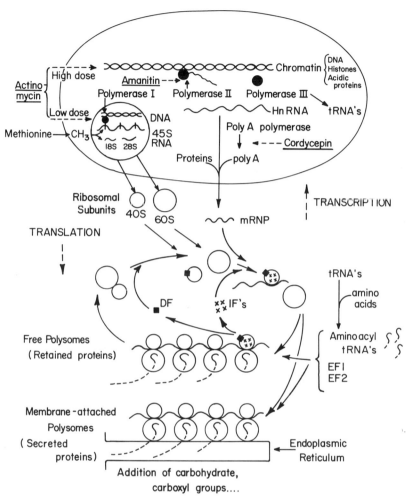

**FIG. 12.** Eukaryote protein synthesis, showing major features of transcription and translation.

although the detailed mechanism of this regulatory function remains uncertain (for review see 256).

The nucleus contains several forms of RNA, separable on sucrose gradients. The nucleolus is the site of ribosomal RNA formation. This is first made as a single strand of 45S RNA, which then undergoes fission into shorter lengths, finally resulting in the 28S and 18S RNAs found in the two ribosomal subunits (rRNA). Cleavage of the 45S RNA (maturation) is regulated by methylation of the ribose residues of certain strategic nucleotides (111). In the nuclear sap (nucleoplasm), RNA of large size (heterogeneous nuclear RNA; HnRNA) is transcribed from the chromosomal DNA; and from this giant RNA, mRNAs with average molecular weights one-fifth that of HnRNA are excised, probably by a mechanism also involving methylation (217). In order to transfer the mRNA from the nucleus to the cytoplasm, it first becomes linked to polyadenylic acid formed by poly A polymerase (3), although some messengers (e.g., those for histones) do not include poly A. Finally, the mRNA becomes associated with protein to produce ribonucleoprotein "informosomes," which then pass to the cytoplasm (244).

The formation of RNA using a template of eukaryotic DNA has long been known to involve the action of DNA-dependent RNA polymerase, and our laboratory (138) and two others (147,236) demonstrated that RNA polymerase activity of whole nuclei can be resolved on DEAE-Sephadex into several species. Polymerase I is found in the nucleolus and is active in transcription of ribosomal RNA. Polymerase II occurs in the nucleoplasm and transcribes HnRNA and thus mRNA. Polymerase III synthesizes tRNA and 5S RNA.

Inhibitors of these processes are important tools for exploring control of protein synthesis. Low doses of actinomycin D inhibit ribosomal RNA synthesis, whereas inhibition of HnRNA (and thus mRNA) synthesis requires a larger amount of actinomycin D, which binds to the DNA template. Formation of mRNA is inhibited by amanitin, which binds specifically to polymerase II rather than the DNA template (140,147), while poly A polymerase is inhibited by cordycepin (58). These inhibitors can therefore be used to block induction of proteins that require additional mRNA synthesis (141).

The response of the RNA-synthesizing system to hormones and other stimuli, including amino acid supply, is an important means for altering protein synthesis, and there are now adequate techniques for exploring how such changes are brought about. For example, liver RNA content increases following administration of corticosteroid hormones to animals (108), mainly reflecting increased rRNA synthesis. A single injection of hydrocortisone into rats is soon followed by an increase in the amount of 45S RNA produced in the liver nucleoli and by a more rapid processing of the 45S RNA into 28S and 18S ribosomal forms (139). This could be due to exposure of more template DNA to nucleolar polymerase by hormone administration, or to an increase in the activity of the nucleolar polymerase I. Indeed Sajdel and Jacob (241) showed that there is a sharp increase in polymerase I (nucleolar enzyme) without any change in the activities of polymerases II and III (nucleoplasmic enzymes). This finding does not exclude changes in the synthesis of specific mRNAs following corticosteroid administration. Indeed corticosteroid administration transiently increases tyrosine aminotransferase and tryptophan oxygenase levels in rat liver by a process that is inhibited by prior administration of actinomycin D (for review see 149). This has been confirmed by extracting more mRNA for tryptophan oxygenase from the liver cytoplasm of steroid-treated rats (245).

Changes in protein synthesis produced by hormones involve specific receptors in the cells of the target organ. The mechanism by which binding of the hormone is followed by increased RNA synthesis has been well worked out in the case of female steroid hormones (for reviews see 143,208). The hormone enters the target cell (e.g., in the uterus) and binds to a specific cytoplasmic. receptor. The receptor undergoes a transformation and enters the nucleus to bind to the chromatin at specific acceptor sites. This is followed by activation of transcription at that site on the chromosome, so that new messenger and other RNA species are made from the underlying DNA. The mRNAs are then transported into the cytoplasm, where they are bound to ribosomes and translated, causing the synthesis of new proteins in the cell or increasing the amount of existing proteins. Some mRNA is also found free in the cytoplasm; a pool of untranslated ferritin mRNA exists, for example, which can be recruited into active translation following iron administration (307).

## 2. *Translation and Its Control*

The process of mRNA translation has been recently reviewed (120). The synthesis of peptide chains on ribosomes can be divided into three phases (Fig. 12). First, there is initiation, in which ribosome subunits, mRNA, initiation factors, and initiator methionyl-tRNA are required. At least three protein initiation factors have been identified in eukaryote cells (1). Initiation is followed by peptide chain elongation, with the addition of successive amino acids to the peptide chain. Some 60 amino-acyl-tRNA species charged with the 20 amino acids of proteins proceed to form complexes with elongation factor 1 (EF 1) and GTP, and then attach to the ribosome to insert the correct amino acid indicated by the codons of the mRNA. This binding of aminoacyl-tRNA is followed by translocation of the growing peptide chain across the ribosome surface under the influence of elongation factor 2 (EF 2) and GTP. During this process of peptide chain elongation, the ribosome undergoes conformational changes as the charged tRNA and elongation factors bind and are released again (258). Finally termination of the peptide chain requires additional protein factors (not shown). The ribosome then separates from the mRNA (run-off ribosome) and dissociates into its two subunits by a mechanism requiring a dissociation factor. As a consequence of repeated initiation of the same mRNA strand, a number of ribosomes become bound to the message, forming a polyribosome (polysome). The proportion of the total ribosome population in the form of polysomes and in the forms of run-off ribosomes and of subunits is determined by the balance between initiation, chain elongation, and the availability of a ribosome dissociation factor. The main changes observed in rate of translation have been traced to effects on rates of chain initiation or elongation. If initiation is reduced, the ribosomes pass along the mRNA strand and accumulate as run-off ribosomes and subunits, the proportion of the latter two forms being dependent on the amount of dissociation factor. The effects of a reduced rate of chain elongation depend on the cause. The antibiotic cycloheximide affects translocation by interfering with EF 2 and GTP binding (29), and in consequence the polysome pattern is not disrupted, although movement in the ribosome cycle slows down. On the other hand, if a single amino acid is not available in adequate amounts, the rate of chain elongation is retarded only at those points where that amino acid must be inserted in the growing peptide chain; beyond that point elongation proceeds at a normal rate. This gives rise to various changes in polyribosome distribution on the messenger, as illustrated by the effects of tryptophan deficiency on globin synthesis in reticulocytes (129) or on rat liver polyribosomes (95,303).

### Posttranslational Events and Their Control

Following formation of the peptide chain, many proteins undergo further change before becoming active structural or enzymic cell components, e.g., hydroxylation of proline in the case of collagen (181). Such posttranslational modifications can provide useful methods of identifying the fate of the peptide chain. Thus for actin and myosin, in which some of the histidine residues become methylated after peptide chain formation, we showed that the 3-methylhistidine so formed is released during intracellular turnover of these proteins and is not further metabolized but is excreted quantitatively in the urine (306). The amount excreted may thus serve as an index of muscle protein turnover.

Some proteins are secreted from cells, many of them being modified by addition of carbohydrates (glycoproteins) after translation (for review see 193). Secreted proteins are made on ribosomes attached to the membranes of the endoplasmic reticulum, which acts as a conducting channel not only for their secretion but also as sites where sugars are added and other changes can also occur—e.g., activation of prothrombin (109), which is due to addition of a calcium-binding carboxyl group to the completed prothrombin chain (200). Some membrane-bound ribosomes appear to belong to a "loosely bound" class that directs its nascent peptide chains into the cytosol and not into the cavity of the endoplasmic reticulum (265). Thus, some subunits of the retained liver protein ferritin are made on membrane-bound ribosomes (152,307).

### B. Protein Synthesis in the Brain

### 1. Components of Brain Protein-Synthesizing Systems

Various components of the protein-synthesis apparatus have been isolated from brain. The earlier work in this area was reviewed by Zomzely-Neurath and Roberts (320) and describes the isolation of ribosomes and ribosomal subunits, free and membrane-bound polyribosomes, mRNA, and the crude pH 5 enzyme fractions and ribosome-associated factors necessary for *in vitro* protein synthesis. The properties of these preparations and conditions for optimal performance are generally similar to those of components derived from other tissues. An earlier claim (319) of a special requirement for unusually high $Mg^{2+}$ in the medium for ribosome isolation has not been substantiated (89). Elongation factors EF 1 and EF 2 have been purified from brain (106,184,185); EF 1 is reported to be in limiting concentrations in brain extracts (106). Gilbert (104) recently observed that an initiation factor fraction from rat brain resulted in translation of brain mRNA to products which differ from those obtained using reticulocyte initiation factors. mRNA has been isolated from rat brain, and two species having sedimentation coefficients of 8S and 16S have been reported (318). Although rapidly labeled RNA (considered to represent mRNA) obtained from polysomes of rat brain is heterogeneous in size, two broad classes of this RNA have been demonstrated in brain cell fractions enriched in both neurons and glia (169).

## 2. Synthesis of Specific Proteins of Brain

The complex cell structure of the brain indicates that a number of proteins specific to individual cells and regions must be synthesized. Interest in marker proteins centers especially around the two major cell types (neurons and glial cells) and the specialized features of the nerve endings. Autoradiographic studies (12) and studies on partially separated brain cell populations (167) in the adult animal show greater protein synthesis in the neurons. Cell-free synthesis of marker proteins specific for each cell type has been demonstrated using polyribosomes or mRNA—in this case the protein designated 14-3-2, representing neurons (gray matter), and S-100 protein for glia (white matter) (321). In the case of nerve endings (synapses), protein synthesis by the abundant mitochondria dominates the picture (121). Synthesis by synaptosome fractions other than mitochondria is difficult to distinguish from ribosomes attached to membranes of cell bodies that have contaminated the preparation (186). Gilbert (103) claimed the presence of a protein-synthesizing system (which can be prepared from membranes of synaptosomes) that makes proteins *in vitro* which differ from those of contaminating neuronal microsomes.

Both membrane-bound and free ribosomes have been recovered from homogenates of brain tissue (18,196), the proportion of those bound being about one-fourth to one-third that of the free ribosomes. The yield of bound ribosomes is probably artificially low, since many are selectively precipitated with the cell debris and mitochondria during initial centrifugation (163). While the membrane-bound ribosomes may secrete some proteins onto the cell surface, some of this polyribosome population seem to discharge their products back into the cell cytosol (18) and thus may belong to the "loosely bound" category of bound ribosomes observed in other cells.

Some specific brain proteins have been associated with membrane-bound or free polyribosomes. Preparations of mRNA made from the bound and free polysomes of rat brain and translated in a cell-free system each synthesize a different spectrum of proteins (103a). The glia-specific protein S100 and the neuron-specific protein 14-3-2 are made exclusively on free ribosomes prepared from rat brain (321). Tubulin is made on both free and membrane-bound ribosomes (96). Finally, Lim et al. (165) extracted mRNA from rat brain that makes myelin peptides *in vitro;* this mRNA is more abundant in membrane-bound polyribosomes.

### 3. Developmental Changes in Brain Protein Synthesis

The intensity of protein synthesis in the brain declines as the animal develops. Suspensions of fetal mouse brain cells are more active than those prepared from neonatal animals (105). Similarly, *in vivo* amino acid incorporation studies (159) and measurement of the *in vitro* activity of brain slices (159) and of cell suspensions (105) show more activity when neonatal mouse or rat brain are used than when the brains of older animals are the source of these preparations. Such changes parallel a reduction in the *in vitro* capacity of brain ribosomes in cell-free systems to synthesize peptide chains (305) which is more marked for membrane-bound than for free ribosomes (18). This may be related to a loss of polyribosome aggregates in the ribosome population (305); it was recently found that highly aggregated polyribosomes prepared from the brains of 9- and 50-day-old rats show similar activities *in vitro* (89). This finding suggests that the reduction in ribosome activity with age is due to a larger proportion of inactive monosomes. The reason for the increased portion of monosomes in the population is unclear. It has been claimed (89) that the pH 5 enzyme fraction (tRNA, tRNA aminoacyl synthetases, and elongation factors) is less active in the brains of older animals. Differences in availability of such soluble factors may also account for the greater incorporating activity of the postmitochondrial supernatant fraction prepared from fetal compared with neonatal rat brains, since polysome aggregation was not greatly dissimilar (105). No differences in tRNA content (145) or in amino acyl-tRNA synthetase activity (144) have been associated with brain development, but it has been claimed (106) that EF 1 is rate-limiting in cell-free systems prepared from brain, and this might prove to be worth investigating.

### C. Protein Turnover in the Brain

Synthesis and turnover of protein in brain cells can be studied in the whole animal by administering labeled amino acids that become incorporated into brain protein or by using tissue slices or homogenates. From the latter can be prepared the individual components of the mechanism of protein synthesis described above and therefore not discussed here. Each of these methods for studying protein synthesis in the brain is now briefly reviewed.

## 1. Whole-Animal Studies of Protein Turnover

The study of protein synthesis and degradation in tissues and organs has been well reviewed by Schimke (243). The estimation of synthetic rate using labeled precursor amino acids requires a knowledge of the specific radioactivity of the labeled amino acid in the precursor pool. Labeling of the free amino acid pools in brain following administration of a radioactive amino acid depends on the route of administration and the individual amino acid. In most tissues, including brain, a single dose of a labeled amino acid given intraperitoneally or intravenously raises the radioactivity in the tissue amino acid pool to peak levels, which then diminish sharply. These kinetic characteristics make it difficult to use the intracellular precursor pool activity to obtain a corrected value for incorporation into the tissue protein, which would reflect the true rate of protein synthesis. This has been overcome in several ways. First, labeled amino acids can be administered by continuous intravenous infusion to achieve a constant plateau of plasma amino acid radioactivity (100,248). The uptake into tissue protein relative to precursor pool of constant specific activity can then be calculated. Second, the body pool of a free amino acid can be flooded with radioactive molecules by gross amounts of the labeled precursor (76). However, administration of excessive amounts of single amino acids can alter the free amino acid pools of the brain (see above). Third, some workers exploited the low solubility of tyrosine to produce a depot of radioactive tyrosine implanted as a pellet and releasing labeled amino acid at a constant rate (159). Finally, labeled glucose can be administered repeatedly, giving rise to labeled glutamic acid and glutamine in the brain (24).

In addition to these maneuvers for maintaining constant tissue levels of radioactivity, there are two additional points to be made with regard to the use of labeled amino acids to measure protein synthesis in the brain of the whole animal. First, the labeled amino acid is often given intracranially (intraventricularly or intracisternally) so that a high level of intracranial activity can be readily achieved. However, intraventricular injections may themselves inhibit brain protein synthesis (77). A further objection is our unpublished observation (238), as well as that of Popov et al. (220), that much of the radioactivity given intracerebrally is deposited intracellularly near the site of injection. Second, the species of labeled amino acid determines its kinetics after intracranial administration (237). Figure 13A shows the percentage of radioactivity as the original amino acid in the acid-soluble pool of rat brain at various times after giving either [14]C-leucine or [14]C-lysine. The former is rapidly metabolized by a branched-chain transaminase in the brain tissue, and consequently the proportion of activity still in leucine quickly declines. On the other hand, after giving [14]C-lysine the proportion remaining as lysine remains elevated because of the relative lack of a metabolizing system in the brain. These differences in precursor specific activity are reflected in the kinetics of incorporation into brain

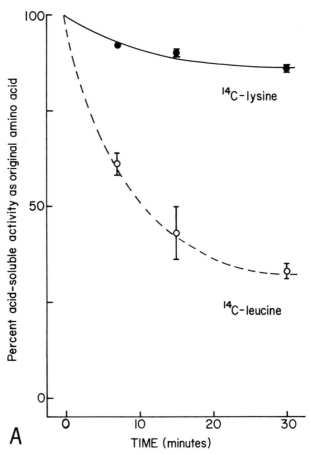

**FIG. 13.** Changes in acid-soluble (free) and protein radioactivity in brain at various times after giving $^{14}C$-leucine or $^{14}C$-lysine intracranially to rats. **A:** Proportion of original injected activity recovered as free amino acid. **B:** Proportion of homogenate radioactivity recovered in brain protein. (Data from Roel et al., ref. 237.)

protein (Fig. 13B). $^{14}C$-Leucine uptake rapidly falls off, whereas $^{14}C$-lysine uptake is linear over the 30-min labeling period. The capacity of brain for branched-chain amino acid oxidation develops after birth (213), so the fate of labeled branched-chain amino acids following injection may well change during early development. This could lead to misinterpretation if it is assumed that the kinetics of labeled leucine removal are the same in animals of all ages.

A second parameter in the protein metabolism of brain is the rate of protein degradation, the measurement of which can be made in several ways (243). The usual procedure is to inject a pulse dose of labeled amino acid, which rapidly results in a peak of incorporation into tissue protein followed by a gradual loss of radioactivity from the protein. This is due to replacement of

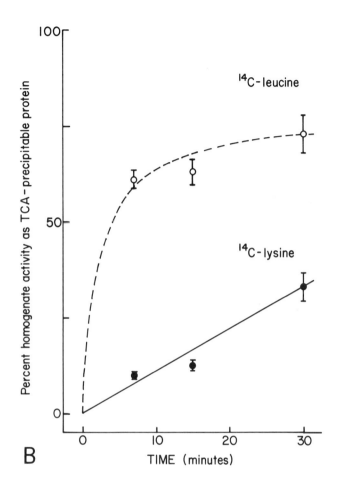

B

labeled protein molecules by unlabeled molecules made after the precursor pool has lost its radioactivity from the initial pulse dose. Obviously, if the labeled amino acids arising from protein breakdown remain in the pool, they are liable to reincorporation, thus sustaining brain protein labeling at an artifactually high level. This phenomenon was particularly apparent in recent studies on the time course of $^3$H-tryptophan incorporation into proteolipid protein of rat brain which accumulates progressively during development (10). Following a single injection of the labeled amino acid, the total radioactivity in proteolipid protein continued to increase for at least 1 week, presumably through reutilization of label from tryptophan in the proteins of other tissues. A similar time course was observed in somewhat older animals for leucine incorporation into S100 protein (47). To obtain accurate estimates of muscle protein turnover, we monitored release of the nonreutilizable amino acid 3-methylhistidine, which is made by methylation of histidine after peptide chain formation and therefore cannot be reincorporated following release from the muscle protein (306).

## 2. Study of Protein Synthesis and Turnover In Vitro

Some of the complexity of whole-animal studies of protein synthesis and turnover can be eliminated by *in vitro* techniques. Protein turnover has been examined *in vitro* using brain slices under optimal conditions (75). Although in neonatal brain the values obtained for slices were comparable to *in vivo* rates of incorporation, slices prepared from older animals underwent a much greater maturational decrease than did the *in vivo* rate (159). This discrepancy may be related to reduced penetration through the increasingly dense neuropil, which is suggested by marked gradients of incorporation between the cut surface and the interior of brain slices incubated with labeled leucine (215). Parks et al. (212) recently described an elegant system for studying protein metabolism in central nervous system tissue. The system employs the isolated rabbit retina and can be maintained for 7 hr without significant loss of retinal protein; moreover, the rate of incorporation is approximately equal to that found *in vivo*. Of particular significance is their observation that the omission of all amino acids from the medium, except for the leucine used as a label, resulted in only a 33% reduction in protein synthesis, indicating the efficiency of amino acid reutilization in the retinal cells.

## D. Impact of Malnutrition on Brain Protein Synthesis

Preceding sections of this chapter recorded how the normal development of the brain can be inhibited by malnutrition. The process of cell multiplication and the development of specialized functions such as myelin formation involve a coordinated series of processes in which programming within the nuclei of the cells determines the timing of events, while transcription and translation of the messages are responsible for relaying the instructions to the cell cytoplasm. Evidence presented elsewhere (195) shows how amino acid supply can influence the process of transcription (RNA synthesis and turnover) and translation (cytoplasmic protein synthesis) in other tissues but throws little light on mechanisms by which developmental processes, including cell multiplication, are affected by nutrient supply. All we can say is that cell division in tissue culture (87) and the intestinal mucosa (192), etc. is dependent on amino acid supply. Similarly, we can offer no substantial evidence regarding the effects of malnutrition on the subtle biochemical control of development programming in the brain and must content ourselves with examining changes in transcription and translation caused by malnutrition, as well as the possible role of amino acid supply to the brain in regulating these.

## 1. Malnutrition and Transcription in the Brain

Only a few studies relate to the effects of malnutrition on events at the transcriptional level in the brain. Lee (161) reported slightly reduced incorporation of radioactivity from labeled orotic acid into RNA of 5-week-old mice malnourished from midgestation. The mice were injected intraperitoneally, and uptake into brain RNA was analyzed 24 hr later. More recently de Guglielmone et al. (115) employed intracerebral injections and a shorter labeling period. They demonstrated reduced incorporation of radioactivity into brain RNA of suckling rats, with RNA in cytoplasmic fractions being more significantly affected than nuclear RNA. Even after 10 days of post-weaning rehabilitation, considerable deficits in labeling of cytoplasmic RNA were evident. In these studies conversion of orotic acid to uridine nucleotides was significantly reduced, and it is possible that a lower specific activity in the precursor pools could account for the reduced incorporation into RNA. However, *in vitro* experiments, allowing better control of precursor pools, demonstrated that nuclei isolated from the brains of 10- and 20-day-old malnourished rats can incorporate less labeled nucleotides into RNA (115). Nuclei from 30-day rehabilitated animals were similar to those of controls, both groups having a lower activity than brain nuclei from the younger animals. It remains to be determined which classes of RNA are affected and which brain cell types are involved.

## 2. Malnutrition and Translation in the Brain

Incorporation of a labeled amino acid into brain proteins following administration is maximal during the first 3 postnatal weeks in the rat—the time when the brain is growing most rapidly (55,214). Dainat (55) reported that the peak in leucine incorporation into cerebellar protein was diminished in malnourished rats. These data were not corrected for differences in leucine uptake or specific activity in the brain. Patel et al. (214) corrected their data for leucine specific activity and showed that incorporation into forebrain protein was indeed reduced in 15- and 21-day-old rats whose mothers had been malnourished from the first week of pregnancy. Adequate feeding for 2 weeks after weaning resulted in normal rates of leucine incorporation in the previously malnourished animals. In contrast, Stern et al. (259) recently found that malnutrition in the lactating mother had no effect on leucine incorporation into brain protein of the offspring, but the values in this study are expressed as percentages of total brain homogenate radioactivity. Since malnutrition retards the development of leucine metabolism via tricarboxylic acid cycle intermediates, the proportion of homogenate activity present as unmetabolized leucine may have been increased (214).

Although the above results provide no information regarding the mechanism of the effect, they indicate that protein and RNA synthesis may indeed be diminished in the brains of young malnourished animals. In contrast, studies of brain protein synthesis in older animals show little effect of malnutrition. Thus 6 days of a protein-free diet given to 150-g rats led to no reduction in the amino acid-incorporating activities of brain slices or the postmitochondrial supernatant fraction (205). Von der Decken and Wronski (275) compared the effect of 4 or 6 days of a protein-free diet on the protein-synthetic activity of microsomes from brain, liver, and muscle of adult rats. The brain microsomes showed no reduction in activity after 4 days and only a slight decrease after 6 days of protein deficiency, whereas liver and muscle showed significant reductions in incorporating capacity at both time points.

### 3. Role of Amino Acid Supply in Regulating Brain Protein Synthesis

In the liver—where much of the evidence on the effects of amino acid availability on protein synthesis has been gathered—the increased supply of amino acids after each meal causes diurnal changes in cytoplasmic protein synthesis that are also coordinated with changes in nucleic acid synthesis and turnover (195). It appears that one essential amino acid in the free amino acid pool of the liver becomes rate-limiting for protein synthesis. This is commonly tryptophan (30,95,222,251), but under conditions of amino acid imbalance other amino acids (e.g., threonine and isoleucine) can be rate-limiting; this is shown by the fact that polysome aggregation and labeled amino acid incorporation into liver protein are dependent on the supply of these amino acids (136,223).

By comparison with studies on the liver, documentation of the role of amino acid supply in brain protein synthesis is fragmentary. One of the most extensively explored examples of how excess amino acid may alter brain amino acid patterns (and concurrently protein synthesis) is phenylalanine (22,252). A single intraperitoneal injection of phenylalanine (1 g/kg) results in increased free phenylalanine and depletion of tryptophan in the brains of 7-day-old rats. This is accompanied by disaggregation of brain polysomes, which follows the same time course as changes in the level of tryptophan but not of phenylalanine, implying that the disaggregation and the accompanying inhibition of *in vitro* protein synthesis are due to changes in tryptophan availability. The reduction of brain tryptophan levels following phenylalanine injection lasts only a few hours, and this may account for the observation of Geison and Siegel (101) that daily injections of phenylalanine during the suckling period failed to depress brain growth.

Many investigators have shown that large doses of amino acids cause decreased incorporation of precursors into brain proteins (for review see 234). Administered amino acids may affect incorporation of precursors into brain proteins in general or into specific proteins, e.g., myelin proteins (9,23,168). Protein synthesis can be altered *in vivo* and *in vitro*. Thus by the above criteria protein synthesis in both cerebral cortex and whole brain decreases *in vivo* after administration of phenylalanine and other amino acids (166,263). *In vitro* protein synthesis systems prepared from brain cells and subcellular preparations are affected (172). Several studies indicate that brain polysomes disaggregate in rats treated with one of several amino acids, and that the ribosomes isolated are defective in protein synthesis *in vitro* (22,301,302). Disaggregation of brain polysomes and decreased protein synthesis occurs after amino acid administration more readily in young animals than adults (22,172,252,279,280,302). Wong and colleagues (301,302) observed that a large dose of phenylalanine or tryptophan given to a pregnant rat can cross the placenta and cause disaggregation of fetal brain polysomes. The reason for developmental differences in the response of rats to excess amino acids has not been elucidated. Young rats may be more susceptible because of the greater vulnerability of their brain free amino acid pools, as indicated above.

These interpretations of the response to hyperphenylalaninemia as an inhibition of brain protein synthesis have not gone unchallenged. The brain polyribosome disaggregation seen soon after administration of phenylalanine has been considered due to a phenylalanine-induced increase in brain ribonuclease breakdown of the polyribosome clusters during their isolation from the homogenate (235). Such a mechanism should result in production of monoribosomes still bearing short fragments of mRNA, whereas true disaggregation produces monosomes without messenger (run-off ribosomes). These two monosome forms can be distinguished by raising the KCl concentration and lowering the $Mg^{2+}$ concentration in the medium, when only the messenger-free monosome separates into its component subunits. Taub and Johnson (266) showed that this is indeed the case for monosomes induced by hyperphenylalaninemia, thus supporting the conclusion that *in vivo* protein synthesis is inhibited.

Yet another criticism has been that the reduced *in vivo* incorporation of labeled amino acids into brain protein following phenylalanine administration is due mainly or exclusively to reduced uptake of the amino acid from the plasma into the brain (presumably as a result of competition for transport). This view is supported by evidence that incorporation of $^{14}C$-leucine and $^{35}S$-methionine into brain protein is inhibited by phenylalanine administration, and that transport of both labeled amino acids into the brain is also reduced, whereas incorporation of $^{14}C$-glycine into brain protein is not affected and its transport across the blood-brain barrier is also unaffected by phenylalanine treatment (9). This picture has been confirmed by Antonas and Coulson (20).

Very recently Hughes and Johnson (132a) described studies on cell suspensions prepared from mouse brain, which they incubated in a medium containing 14 mM phenylalanine. The presence of this large excess of phenylalanine reduced the entry of a majority of the other free amino acids from the medium and increased the exit of amino acids from the cells. In consequence the intracellular levels of many free amino acids were lowered; however, there was little change in the specific activity of labeled amino acids entering the cells from the medium. There was a slight (approximately 10%) reduction in tRNA charging with leucine and isoleucine caused by the excess phenylalanine, and a 30% reduction in the incorporation of these amino acids into mixed brain proteins. When lysine and alanine were the labeled amino acids used, radioactivity in tRNA was not significantly affected by excess phenylalanine, but incorporation of these amino acids into brain proteins was nevertheless reduced by 20%. Thus phenylalanine excess causes a depression in amino acid uptake into brain protein beyond its effects on precursor labeling.

There are other, independent pieces of evidence that brain protein formation is affected by giving excess phenylalanine. Experimental hyperphenylalaninemia in infant rats causes the following changes: reduced thymidine uptake into brain DNA (229); decreased brain succinic dehydrogenase activity (204) and retarded emergence of a divided free glutamate pool (203), each suggestive of delayed brain development (42); a permanently smaller brain weight after rehabilitation of body weight (203); reduced total brain protein, lipid, and DNA, out of proportion to body weight loss (183); a greater change in cerebellar weight, DNA, RNA, and protein than in the corresponding constituents of the cerebral hemispheres (221); a reduction in brain lipid content, especially galactolipids and proteolipids (221,250); and reduced uptake of $^{14}$C-galactose into brain lipids (249). These effects of hyperphenylalaninemia are comparable to the response of the brain of the suckling rat to malnutrition and are thus compatible with the theory of a common mechanism dependent on the inadequacy of free amino acid pools in brain that result from inadequate dietary intake in one case and from competition for entry into the brain in the other.

Exogenously administered amino acids do not necessarily affect brain protein synthesis by limiting uptake and intracerebral availability of amino acids. Our laboratories showed that two amino acids, L-dihydroxyphenylalanine (DOPA) (280) and L-5-hydroxytryptophan (5-HTP) (282) cause disaggregation of whole-brain polysomes through the production of the neurotransmitters dopamine and serotonin, respectively. There is an accompanying reduction in brain protein synthesis rate, as shown by uptake of $^{14}$C-leucine and $^{14}$C-lysine *in vivo* (237). In both cases we demonstrated that, unlike phenylalanine, the amino acid precursors of these biogenic amines do not interfere with protein synthesis through a direct action of the administered amino acids themselves or through an amino acid imbalance; dopamine or serotonin synthesis must occur for the polysome changes to take place. This was demonstrated by showing that an inhibitor of decarboxylation prevents these responses to DOPA and to 5-HTP (280,282). Furthermore, dopamine and serotonin receptor blockers also prevent the effects on protein synthesis (278). The polysome-disaggregating action of phenylalanine is not affected by inhibition of decarboxylation and thus operates by a different mechanism (281).

In the context of malnutrition it would be more satisfying to be able to report direct evidence that protein deficiency or protein-calorie deficiency leads to reduced brain protein synthesis through a reduction in the brain levels of key amino acids. Direct evidence that amino acid supply can influence neuronal protein synthesis is provided by the studies of Parks et al. (212) on rabbit retina. The ability of this tissue to incorporate amino acids *in vitro* at a maximal rate depends on an adequate supply of amino acids in the medium. Miller (180) adduced some indirect evidence for such a relationship at two periods in the development of the rat brain (around the 7th and 20th day postnatally) when an increase in brain protein synthesis is preceded by a rise in brain amino acid pools. Using older rats, Dallman and Spirito (56) showed that brain protein in the well-nourished rat is probably largely maintained by the recycling of amino acids released from within the brain cells, whereas in malnourished animals amino acids from other parts of the body are preferentially incorporated; this may account for the relative immunity of the brain of the mature animal to malnutrition. In man the arteriovenous difference in amino acid concentration across the brain (88) suggests that the human brain takes up approximately 20 g of amino acids daily from the plasma. These pieces of evidence are compatible with a role for amino acid availability in maintaining and regulating brain protein synthesis. What is lacking is direct evidence that protein synthesis at different stages in brain development is reduced by malnutrition in parallel with reductions in brain amino acid levels, and that this impairment is corrected by raising the free amino acid pools. Even if this should be case for the syndrome of kwashiorkor, in which plasma amino acid patterns are severely distorted, it will still be necessary to consider whether the extensive retardation of brain development in marasmus can occur under conditions in which the plasma free amino acid levels are less affected in man (284), swine (27), and the rat (211). This question has not been studied under conditions in which changes in brain amino acid levels due to experimental kwashiorkor and marasmus are correlated with a range of brain parameters sensitive to deficiency.

## VII. CONCLUSIONS AND SUMMARY

Figure 14 summarizes some major features of the maturation of the rat brain and indicates the effects of malnutrition on these developmental events when the malnutrition occurs during pregnancy and postnatally. The events in man differ mainly insofar as the major neuron population is complete before the third trimester of pregnancy and is thus largely immune to malnutrition during pregnancy, which usually has its main impact on fetal development during the

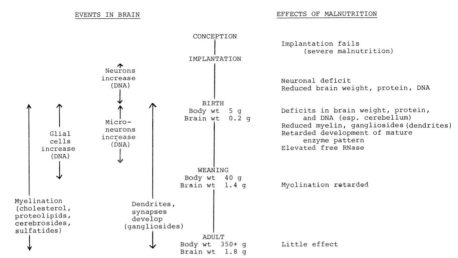

EVENTS IN BRAIN                                    EFFECTS OF MALNUTRITION

**FIG. 14.** Developmental changes in the brain of the rat from conception to adult, and the effects of malnutrition at different stages of growth.

last third of pregnancy. During lactation glial cells and microneurons continue to multiply, myelin is laid down, nerve terminals and dendritic processes ramify, and synaptic connections are established. Malnutrition at this stage thus affects the development of the microneuron population, the formation of dendrites, and the process of myelination. The latter two processes extend into the postweaning period, and thus malnutrition after weaning can still influence the continued development of the brain.

The question of how protein and protein-calorie deficiency exert their actions on brain development remains unanswered. Certainly there are changes in free amino acid levels in the brains of animals with each type of malnutrition, with protein deficiency producing the more severe changes. Alterations in brain amino acid concentrations of a similar pattern occur when excessive amounts of single amino acids (e.g., phenylalanine) are administered to animals. Moreover, chronic excess of phenylalanine results in effects on brain development similar to those caused by protein deficiency. It is thus tempting to conclude that an inadequate concentration of one or more key amino acids is the common factor responsible for limiting brain development in both malnutrition and excess of one amino acid. Even if this proves to be a tenable hypothesis, there is inadequate information about the mechanism by which an insufficient amino acid supply impairs brain development. The rates of synthesis of various brain proteins may indeed be retarded, but when we consider nuclear control of differentiation, the available techniques are still inadequate to explore how free amino acid levels could affect cell division or the expression of genetic information in the orderly unfolding of the developmental process. Future studies can therefore be expected to probe such questions and to correlate the various developmental changes in cell structure and function which parallel the biochemical evidence of brain growth and maturation, and their sensitivity to malnutrition.

## REFERENCES

1. Adams, S. L., Safer, B., Anderson, F. W., and Merrick, W. C. (1975): Eukaryotic initiation complex formation: Evidence for two distinct pathways. *J. Biol. Chem.*, 250:9083–9089.
2. Adamson, L. F., Herington, A. C., and Bornstein, J. (1972): Evidence for the selection by the membrane transport system of intracellular or extracellular amino acids for protein synthesis. *Biochim. Biophys. Acta*, 282:352–365.
3. Adesnik, M., Salditt, M., Thomas, W., and Darnell, J. E. (1972): Evidence that all messenger RNA molecules (except histone messenger RNA) contain poly(A) sequences and that the poly(A) has a nuclear function. *J. Mol. Biol.*, 71:21–30.
4. Adibi, S. A. (1968): Influence of dietary deprivations on plasma concentration of free amino acids of man. *J. Appl. Physiol.*, 25:52–57.
5. Adlard, B. P. F., and Dobbing, J. (1971): Elevated acetylcholinesterase activity in adult rat brain after undernutrition in early life. *Brain Res.*, 30:198–199.
6. Adlard, B. P. F., and Dobbing, J. (1971): Vulnerability of developing brain. III. Development of four enzymes in the brains of normal and undernourished rats. *Brain Res.*, 28:97–107.
7. Adlard, B. P. F., and Dobbing, J. (1972): Vulnerability of developing brain. V. Effects of fetal and postnatal undernutrition on regional brain enzyme activities in three-week-old rats. *Pediatr. Res.*, 6:38–42.
8. Adlard, B. P. F., and Dobbing, J. (1972): Vulnerability of developing brain. 8. Regional acetylcholinesterase activity in the brains of adult rats undernourished in early life. *Br. J. Nutr.*, 28:139–143.
9. Agrawal, H. C., Bone, A. H., and Davison, A. N. (1970): Effect of phenylalanine on protein synthesis in the developing rat brain. *Biochem. J.*, 117:325–331.
10. Agrawal, H. C., Fujimoto, K., and Burton, R. M. (1976): Accumulation and turnover of the classical Folch-Lees proteolipid proteins in developing and adult rat brain. *Biochem. J.*, 154:265–269.
11. Ahmad, G., and Rahman, M. A. (1975): Effects of undernutrition and protein malnutrition on brain chemistry of rats. *J. Nutr.*, 105:1090–1103.
12. Altman, J. (1963): Differences in the utilization of tritiated leucine by single neurons in normal and exercised rats: An autoradiographic investigation with microdensitometry. *Nature (Lond.)*, 199:777–780.
13. Altman, J. (1966): Autoradiographic and histological studies of postnatal neurogenesis. II. A longitudinal investigation of the kinetics, migration and transformation of cells incorporating tritiated thymidine in infant rats, with special reference to postnatal neurogenesis in some brain regions. *J. Comp. Neurol.*, 128:431–474.
14. Altman, J., and Das, G. D. (1966): Autoradiographic and histological studies of postnatal neurogenesis. I. A longitudinal investigation of the kinetics, migration and transformation of cells incorporating tritiated thymidine in neonate rats with special reference to postnatal neurogenesis in some brain regions. *J. Comp. Neurol.*, 126:337–390.
15. Altman, J., Das, G., and Sudarshan, K. (1970): The influence of nutrition on neural and behavioral development. I. Critical review of some data on the growth of the body and the brain following dietary deprivation during gestation and lactation. *Dev. Psychobiol.*, 3:281–301.
16. Altman, J., Das, G. D., Sudarshan, K., and Anderson, J. B. (1970): The influence of nutrition on neural and behavioral development. II. Growth of body and brain in infant rats using different techniques of undernutrition. *Dev. Psychobiol.*, 4:55–70.
17. Anderson, L. L. (1975): Embryonic and placental development during prolonged inanition in the pig. *Am. J. Physiol.*, 229:1687–1694.
18. Andrews, T. M., and Tata, J. R. (1971): Protein synthesis by membrane-bound and free ribosomes of secretory and non-secretory tissues. *Biochem. J.*, 121:683–694.
19. Anthony, L. E., and Edozien, J. C. (1975): Experimental protein and energy deficiencies in the rat. *J. Nutr.*, 105:631–648.

20. Antonas, K. N., and Coulson, W. F. (1975): Brain uptake and protein incorporation of amino acids studied in rats subjected to prolonged hyperphenylalaninaemia. *J. Neurochem.*, 25:309–314.

21. Antonov, A. N. (1947): Children born during the siege of Leningrad in 1942. *J. Pediatr.*, 30:250–259.

22. Aoki, K., and Siegel, F. L. (1970): Hyperphenylalaninemia: Disaggregation of brain polyribosomes in young rats. *Science*, 168:129–130.

23. Appel, S. H. (1966): Inhibition of brain protein synthesis: An approach to the biochemical basis of neurological dysfunction in the amino-acidurias. *Trans. NY Acad. Sci.*, 29:63–70.

24. Austin, L., Lowry, O. H., Brown, J. G., and Carter, J. G. (1972): The turnover of protein in discrete areas of the rat brain. *Biochem. J.*, 126:351–359.

25. Bachmann, C., Nyhan, W. L., Kulovich, S., and Hornbeck, M. E. (1975): Amino acids in the brain during fetal growth and the effects of prenatal hormonal and nutritional imbalance. In: *Fetal and Postnatal Cellular Growth*, edited by D. B. Cheek. Wiley, New York.

26. Badger, T. M., and Tumbleson, M. E. (1974): Protein-calorie malnutrition in young miniature swine: Brain free amino acids. *J. Nutr.*, 104:1329–1338.

27. Badger, T. M., and Tumbleson, M. E. (1974): Protein-calorie malnutrition in young miniature swine: Serum free amino acids. *J. Nutr.*, 104:1339–1347.

28. Badger, T. M., and Tumbleson, M. E. (1975): Postnatal changes in free amino acid, DNA, RNA and protein concentrations of miniature swine brain. *J. Neurochem.*, 24:361–366.

29. Baliga, B. S., and Munro, H. N. (1971): Specificity of mammalian transferase II binding to ribosomes. *Nature [New Biol.]*, 233:257–258.

30. Baliga, B. S., Pronczuk, A. W., and Munro, H. N. (1968): Regulation of polysome aggregation in a cell-free system through amino acid supply. *J. Mol. Biol.*, 34:199–218.

31. Barnes, D., and Altman, J. (1973): Effects of different schedules of early undernutrition on the preweaning growth of the rat cerebellum. *Exp. Neurol.*, 38:406–419.

32. Barnes, D., and Altman, J. (1973): Effects of two levels of gestational-lactational undernutrition on the postweaning growth of the rat cerebellum. *Exp. Neurol.*, 38:420–428.

33. Bass, N. H., Netsky, M. G., and Young, E. (1970): Effect of neonatal malnutrition on developing cerebrum. I. Microchemical and histologic study of cellular differentiation in the rat. *Arch. Neurol.*, 23:289–302.

34. Bayer, S. M., and McMurray, W. C. (1967): The metabolism of amino acids in developing rat brain. *J. Neurochem.*, 14:695–706.

35. Benton, J. W., Moser, H. W., Dodge, P. R., and Carr, S. (1966): Modification of the schedule of myelination in the rat by early nutritional deprivation. *Pediatrics*, 38:801–807.

36. Berry, H. K. (1970): Plasma amino acids. In: *Newer Methods of Nutritional Biochemistry*, Vol. IV, edited by A. A. Albanese. Academic Press, New York.

37. Bresler, D. E., Ellison, G., and Zamenhof, S. (1975): Learning deficits in rats with malnourished grandmothers. *Dev. Psychobiol.*, 8:315–323.

38. Brizzee, K. R., Vogt, J., and Kharetchko, X. (1964): Postnatal changes in glia/neuron index with a comparison of methods of cell enumeration in the white rat. *Prog. Brain Res.*, 4:136–149.

39. Chase, H. P., Dorsey, J., and McKhann, G. M. (1967): The effect of malnutrition on the synthesis of a myelin lipid. *Pediatrics*, 40:551–559.

40. Chase, H. P., Lindsley, W. F. B., Jr., and O'Brien, D. (1969): Undernutrition and cerebellar development. *Nature (Lond.)*, 221:554–555.

41. Chase, H. P., Rodgerson, D. O., Lindsley, W., Jr., Thorne, T., and Cheung, G. (1976): Brain glucose utilization in undernourished rats. *Pediatr. Res.*, 10:102–107.

42. Chase, H. P., Welch, N. N., Dabiere, C. S., Vasan, N. S., and Butterfield, L. J. (1972): Alterations in human brain biochemistry following intrauterine growth retardation. *Pediatrics*, 50:403–411.

43. Cheek, D. B., Mellits, D. E., Hill, D. E., and Holt, A. B. (1975): Mathematical appraisal of biochemical determinants of brain growth. In: *Fetal and Postnatal Cellular Growth*, edited by D. B. Cheek. Wiley, New York.

44. Chevallier, F., Sérougne, C., and Champarnaud, G. (1975): Effect upon brain weight and cholesterol content of maintaining rats of various ages at constant weight. *J. Nutr.*, 105:1003–1011.

45. Chow, B. F., and Lee, C-J. (1964): Effect of dietary restriction of pregnant rats on body weight gain of the offspring. *J. Nutr.*, 82:10–18.
46. Christensen, H. N. (1972): On the development of amino acid transport systems. *Fed. Proc.*, 32:19–28.
47. Cicero, T. J., and Moore, B. W. (1970): Turnover of the brain specific protein, S-100. *Science*, 169:1333–1334.
48. Cooper, J. R., Bloom, F. E., and Roth, R. H. (1974): *The Biochemical Basis of Neuropharmacology.* Oxford University Press, New York.
49. Coward, D. G., and Whitehead, R. G. (1972): Experimental protein-energy malnutrition in baby baboons: Attempts to reproduce the pathological features of kwashiorkor as seen in Uganda. *Br. J. Nutr.*, 28:223–237.
50. Cragg, B. G. (1968): Gross, microscopical and ultramicroscopical anatomy of the adult nervous system. In: *Applied Neurochemistry,* edited by A. N. Davison and J. Dobbing. Davis, Philadelphia.
51. Culley, W. J., and Lineberger, R. O. (1968): Effect of undernutrition on the size and composition of the rat brain. *J. Nutr.*, 96:375–381.
52. Culley, W. J., and Mertz, E. T. (1965): Effect of restricted food intake on growth and composition of preweanling rat brain. *Proc. Soc. Exp. Biol. Med.*, 118:233–235.
53. Culley, W., Yuan, L., and Mertz, E. (1966): Effect of food restriction and age on rat brain phospholipid levels. *Fed. Proc.*, 25:674.
54. Cutler, R. W. P., and Dudzinski, D. S. (1974): Regional changes in amino acid content in developing rat brain. *J. Neurochem.*, 23:1005–1009.
55. Dainat, J. (1974): The incorporation in vivo of L-[$^3$H]leucine into cerebellar proteins in the young normal, underfed, hyperthyroid and hypothyroid rat. *J. Neurochem.*, 23:713–719.
56. Dallman, P. R., and Spirito, R. A. (1972): Brain response to protein undernutrition: Mechanism of preferential protein retention. *J. Clin. Invest.*, 51:2175–2180.
57. Daniel, R. G., and Waisman, H. A. (1969): The influence of excess methionine on the free amino acids of brain and liver of the weanling rat. *J. Neurochem.*, 16:787–795.
58. Darnell, J. E., Philipson, L., Wall, R., and Adesnik, M. (1971): Polyadenylic acid sequences: Role in conversion of nuclear RNA into messenger RNA. *Science*, 174:507–510.
59. Davison, A. N., and Dobbing, J. (1968): The developing brain. In: *Applied Neurochemistry,* edited by A. N. Davison and J. Dobbing. Davis, Philadelphia.
60. Deo, M. G., Sood, S. K., and Ramalingaswami, V. (1965): Experimental protein deficiency: Pathological features in the rhesus monkey. *Arch. Pathol.*, 80:14–23.
61. DeRobertis, E., DeIraldi, A. P., Arnaiz, G. R. L., and Salganicoff, L. (1962): Cholinergic and non-cholinergic nerve endings in the rat brain. I. Isolation and subcellular distribution of acetylcholine and acetylcholinesterase. *J. Neurochem.*, 9:23–35.
62. Derry, D. M., and Wolfe, L. S. (1967): Gangliosides in isolated neurons and glial cells. *Science*, 158:1450–1452.
63. Dickerson, J. W. T., and Dobbing, J. (1967): Prenatal and postnatal growth and development of the central nervous system of the pig. *Proc. R. Soc. Lond. [Biol.]*, 166:384–395.
64. Dickerson, J. W. T., and Pao, S-K. (1975): The effect of a low protein diet and exogenous insulin on brain tryptophan and its metabolites in the weanling rat. *J. Neurochem.*, 25:559–564.
64a. Dickerson, J. W. T., and Pao, S-K. (1975): Effect of pre- and postnatal maternal protein deficiency on free amino acids and amines of rat brain. *Biol. Neonate*, 25:114–124.
65. Dickerson, J. W. T., and Walmsley, A. L. (1967): The effect of undernutrition and subsequent rehabilitation on the growth and composition of the central nervous system of the rat. *Brain*, 90:897–906.
66. Dickerson, J. W. T., Dobbing, J., and McCance, R. A. (1966): The effect of undernutrition on the postnatal development of the brain and cord in pigs. *Proc. R. Soc. Lond. [Biol.]*, 166:396–407.
67. Dickerson, J. W. T., Merat, A., and Widdowson, E. M. (1971): Intrauterine growth retardation in the pig. III. The chemical structure of the brain. *Biol. Neonate*, 19:354–362.
68. Dobbing, J. (1964): The influence of early nutrition on the development and myelination of the brain. *Proc. R. Soc. Lond. [Biol.]*, 159:503–509.

69. Dobbing, J. (1974): The later development of the brain and its vulnerability. In: *Scientific Foundations of Paediatrics,* edited by J. A. Davis and J. Dobbing. Heinemann, London.
70. Dobbing, J., and Sands, J. (1970): Growth and development of the brain and spinal cord of the guinea pig. *Brain Res., 17:*115–123.
71. Dobbing, J., and Sands, J. (1970): Timing of neuroblast multiplication in developing human brain. *Nature (Lond.), 226:*639–640.
72. Dobbing, J., and Sands, J. (1971): Vulnerability of developing brain. IX. The effect of nutritional growth retardation on the timing of the brain growth-spurt. *Biol. Neonate, 19:*363–378.
73. Dobbing, J., and Sands, J. (1973): Quantitative growth and development of human brain. *Arch. Dis. Child., 48:*757–767.
74. Dobbing, J., and Widdowson, E. M. (1965): The effect of undernutrition and subsequent rehabilitation on myelination of rat brain as measured by its composition. *Brain, 88:*357–366.
75. Dunlop, D. S., van Elden, W., and Lajthe, A. (1974): Measurement of rates of protein synthesis in rat brain slices. *J. Neurochem., 22:*821–830.
76. Dunlop, D. S., van Elden, W., and Lajthe, A. (1975): A method for measuring brain protein synthesis rates in young and adult rats. *J. Neurochem., 24:*337–344.
77. Dunn, A. J. (1975): Intracerebral injections inhibit amino acid incorporation into brain protein. *Brain Res., 99:*405–409.
78. Eayrs, J. T., and Horn, G. (1955): The development of cerebral cortex in hypothyroid and starved rats. *Anat. Rec., 121:*53–61.
79. Eckhert, C., Barnes, R. H., and Levitsky, D. A. (1976): The effect of protein-energy undernutrition induced during the period of suckling on cholinergic enzyme activity in the rat brain stem. *Brain Res., 101:*372–377.
80. Edozien, J. C. (1966): The free amino acids of plasma and urine in kwashiorkor. *Clin. Sci., 31:*153–166.
81. Enwonwu, C. O. (1973): Experimental protein-calorie malnutrition in the guinea pig and evaluation of the role of ascorbic acid status. *Lab. Invest., 29:*17–26.
82. Enwonwu, C. O., and Screebny, L. M. (1970): Experimental protein-calorie malnutrition in rats: Biochemical and ultrastructural studies. *Exp. Mol. Pathol., 12:*332–353.
83. Enwonwu, C. O., and Worthington, B. S. (1973): Accumulation of histidine, 3-methylhistidine, and homocarnosine in the brains of protein-calorie deficient monkeys. *J. Neurochem., 21:*799–807.
84. Enwonwu, C. O., and Worthington, B. S. (1974): Regional distribution of homocarnosine and other ninhydrin-positive substances in brains of malnourished monkeys. *J. Neurochem., 22:*1045–1052.
85. Enwonwu, C. O., and Worthington, B. S. (1975): Elevation of brain histamine content in protein-deficient rats. *J. Neurochem., 24:*941–945.
86. Enwonwu, C. O., Stambaugh, R. V., and Jacobson, K. L. (1973): Protein-energy deficiency in non-human primates: Biochemical and morphological alterations. *Am. J. Clin. Nutr., 26:*1287–1302.
87. Everhart, L. P. (1972): Effects of deprivation of two essential amino acids on DNA synthesis in Chinese hamster cells. *Exp. Cell Res., 74:*311–318.
88. Felig, P., Wahren, J., and Ahlborg, G. (1973): Uptake of individual amino acids by the human brain. *Proc. Soc. Exp. Biol. Med., 142:*230–231.
89. Fellous, A., Francon, J., Nunez, J., and Sokolof, L. (1973): Protein synthesis by highly aggregated and purified polysomes from young and adult rat brain. *J. Neurochem., 21:*211–222.
90. Fern, E. B., and Garlick, P. J. (1974): The specific radioactivity of the tissue free amino acid pool as a basis for measuring the rate of protein synthesis in the rat in vivo. *Biochem. J., 142:*413–419.
91. Fish, I., and Winick, M. (1969): Cellular growth in various regions of the developing rat brain. *Pediatr. Res., 3:*407–412.
92. Fishman, M. A., Madyastha, P., and Prensky, A. L. (1971). The effect of undernutrition on the development of myelin in the rat central nervous system. *Lipids, 6:*458–465.
93. Fishman, M. A., Prensky, A. L., and Dodge, P. R. (1969): Low content of cerebral lipids in infants suffering from malnutrition. *Nature (Lond.), 221:*552–553.

94. Fishman, M. A., Prensky, A. L., Tumbleson, M. E., and Daftari, B. (1972): Relative resistance of the later phase of myelination to severe undernutrition in miniature swine. *Am. J. Clin. Nutr.*, 25:7–10.

95. Fleck, A., Shepherd, J., and Munro, H. N. (1965): Protein synthesis in rat liver: Influence of amino acids in diet on microsomes and polysomes. *Science*, 150:628–629.

96. Floor, E. R., Gilbert, J. M., and Nowak, T. S., Jr. (1976): Evidence for the synthesis of tubulin on membrane-bound and free ribosomes from rat forebrain. *Biochim. Biophys. Acta* 442:285–296.

97. Follis, R. H. (1957): A kwashiorkor-like syndrome observed in monkeys fed maize. *Proc. Soc. Exp. Biol. Med.*, 96:523–528.

98. Fox, J. H., Fishman, M. A., Dodge, P. R., and Prensky, A. L. (1972): The effect of malnutrition on human central nervous system myelin. *Neurology (Minneap.)*, 22:1213–1216.

99. Gambetti, P., Autilio-Gambetti, L., Gonatas, N. K., Shafer, B., and Stieber, A. (1972): Synapses and malnutrition: Morphological and biochemical study of synaptosomal fractions from rat cerebral cortex. *Brain Res.*, 47:477–484.

100. Garlick, P. J., and Marshall, I. (1972): A technique for measuring brain protein synthesis. *J. Neurochem.*, 19:577–583.

101. Geison, R. L., and Siegel, F. L. (1975): Tolerance of protein and lipid synthesis to mild hyperphenylalaninemia in developing rat brain. *Brain Res.*, 92:431–441.

102. Geison, R. L., and Waisman, H. A. (1970): Effects of nutritional status on rat brain maturation as measured by lipid composition. *J. Nutr.*, 100:315–324.

103. Gilbert, J. M. (1972): Evidence for protein synthesis in synaptosomal membranes. *J. Biol. Chem.*, 247:6541–6550.

103a. Gilbert, J. M. (1973): Translation of messenger RNA fractions from free and membrane bound rat forebrain ribosomes in a rabbit reticulocyte cell-free system. *Biochem. Biophys. Res. Commun.*, 52:79–87.

104. Gilbert, J. M. (1974): Differences in the translation of rat forebrain messenger RNA dependent on the source of protein synthesis factors. *Biochim. Biophys. Acta*, 340:140–146.

105. Gilbert, B. E., and Johnson, T. C. (1974) Fetal development: The effects of maturation on in vitro protein synthesis by mouse brain tissue. *J. Neurochem.*, 23:811–818.

106. Girgis, G. R., and Nicholls, D. M. (1972): Protein synthesis limited by transferase I. *Biochim. Biophys. Acta*, 269:465–476.

107. Gomez, F., Galvan, R. G., Cravioto, J., and Frenk, S. (1954): Malnutrition in infancy and childhood, with special reference to kwashiorkor. *Adv. Pediatr.*, 7:131–169.

108. Goodlad, G. A. J., and Munro, H. N. (1959): Diet and the action of cortisone on protein metabolism. *Biochem. J.*, 73:343–348.

109. Goswami, P., and Munro, H. N. (1962): The role of ribonucleic acid in the formation of prothrombin activity by rat-liver microsomes. *Biochim. Biophys. Acta*, 55:410–412.

110. Graystone, J. E., and Cheek, D. B. (1969): The effects of reduced calorie intake and increased insulin-induced caloric intake on the cell growth of muscle, liver, and cerebrum and on skeletal collagen in the postweanling rat. *Pediatr. Res.*, 3:66–76.

111. Greenberg, H., and Penman, S. (1966): Methylation and processing of ribosomal RNA in HeLa cells. *J. Mol. Biol.*, 21:527–535.

112. Grimble, R. F., and Whitehead, R. G. (1969): The relationship between an elevated serum amino acid ratio and the development of other biological abnormalities in the experimentally malnourished pig. *Br. J. Nutr.*, 23:791–804.

113. Grimble, R. F., Sawyer, M. B., and Whitehead, R. G. (1969): Time relationships between elevation of the serum amino acid ratio and the changes in liver composition in malnourished rats. *Br. J. Nutr.*, 23:879–888.

114. Gross, I., and Warshaw, J. B. (1975): The influence of dietary deprivation on the enzymes of fatty acid synthesis in rat brain. *J. Neurochem.*, 25:191–192.

115. Guglielmone, A. E. R., de Soto, A. M., and Duvilanski, B. H. (1974): Neonatal undernutrition and RNA synthesis in developing rat brain. *J. Neurochem.*, 22:529–533.

116. Guthrie, H. A., and Brown, M. L. (1968): Effect of severe undernutrition in early life on growth, brain size and composition in adult rats. *J. Nutr.*, 94:419–426.

117. Habicht, J-P., Yarbrough, C., Lechtig, A., and Klein, R. E. (1974): Relation of maternal

supplementary feeding during pregnancy to birth weight and other sociobiological factors. *Curr. Concepts Nutr.*, 1:127–145.

118. Hansen, S., Perry, T. L., Wada, J. A., and Sokol, M. (1973): Brain amino acids in baboons with light-induced epilepsy. *Brain Res.*, 50:480–483.

119. Harel, S., Watanabe, K., Linke, I., and Schain, R. J. (1972): Growth and development of the rabbit brain. *Biol. Neonate*, 21:381–399.

120. Haselkorn, R., and Rothman-Denes, L. B. (1973): Protein synthesis. *Annu. Rev. Biochem.*, 42:397–438.

121. Hernandez, A. G. (1974): Protein synthesis by synaptosomes from rat brain: Contribution by the intraterminal mitochondria. *Biochem. J.*, 142:7–17.

122. Hill, D. E., Myers, R. E., Holt, A. B., Scott, R. E., and Cheek, D. B. (1971): Fetal growth retardation produced by experimental placenta insufficiency in the rhesus monkey. II. Chemical composition of the brain, liver, muscle and carcass. *Biol. Neonate*, 19:68–82.

123. Himwich, W. (1969): Appendix. In: *Handbook of Neurochemistry*, Vol. 1, edited by A. Lajthe. Plenum Press, New York.

124. Himwich, W. A., and Agrawal, H. C. (1969): Amino acids. In: *Handbook of Neurochemistry*, Vol. 1, edited by A. Lajthe. Plenum Press, New York.

125. Hoff, K. M., Baker, P. C., and Buda, R. E. (1974): Free tryptophan levels in regions of the maturing mouse brain. *Brain Res.*, 73:376–379.

126. Holt, L. E., Jr., and Snyderman, S. E. (1964): Anomalies of amino acid metabolism. In: *Mammalian Protein Metabolism*, Vol. 2, edited by H. N. Munro and J. B. Allison. Academic Press, New York.

127. Holt, L. E., Jr., Snyderman, S. E., Norton, P. M., Roitman, E., and Finch, J. (1963). The plasma aminogram in kwashiorkor. *Lancet*, 2:1343–1348.

128. Holtzman, N. A., Welcher, D. W., and Mellits, E. D. (1975): Termination of restricted diet in children with phenylketonuria: A randomized controlled study. *N. Engl. J. Med.*, 293:1121–1124.

129. Hori, M., Fisher, J. M., and Rabinovitz, M. (1967): Tryptophan deficiency in rabbit reticulocytes: Polyribosomes during interrupted growth of hemoglobin chains. *Science*, 155:83–84.

130. Howard, E. (1973): DNA content of rodent brains during maturation and aging, and autoradiography of postnatal DNA synthesis in monkey brain. *Prog. Brain Res.*, 40:91–114.

131. Howard, E., and Granoff, D. M. (1968): Effect of neonatal food restriction in mice on brain growth, DNA and cholesterol, and on adult delayed response learning. *J. Nutr.*, 95:111–121.

132. Hsueh, A. M., Simonson, M., Chow, B. F., and Hanson, H. M. (1974): The importance of the period of dietary restriction of the dam on behavior and growth in the rat. *J. Nutr.*, 104:37–46.

132a. Hughes, J. V., and Johnson, T. C. (1976): The effects of phenylalanine on amino acid metabolism and protein synthesis in brain cells *in vitro*. *J. Neurochem.*, 26:1105–1113.

133. Ilan, J., and Singer, M. (1975): Sampling of the leucine pool from the growing peptide chain: Difference in leucine specific activity of peptidyl-transfer RNA from free and membrane-bound polysomes. *J. Mol. Biol.*, 91:39–51.

134. Im, H. S., Barnes, R. H., and Levitsky, D. A. (1976): Effect of early protein-energy malnutrition and environmental changes on cholinesterase activity of brain and adrenal glands of rats. *J. Nutr.*, 106:342–349.

135. Im, H. S., Barnes, R. H., Levitsky, D. A., and Pond, W. G. (1973): Postnatal malnutrition and regional cholinesterase activities in brain of pigs. *Brain Res.*, 63:461–465.

136. Ip, C. C. Y., and Harper, A. E. (1973): Effect of threonine supplementation on hepatic polysome patterns and protein synthesis of rats fed a threonine-deficient diet. *Biochim. Biophys. Acta*, 331:251–263.

137. Ip, C., and Harper, A. E. (1975): Protein synthesis in liver, muscle, and brain of rats fed a high tyrosine–low protein diet. *J. Nutr.*, 105:885–893.

138. Jacob, S. T., Muecke, W., Sajdel, E. M., and Munro, H. N. (1970): Evidence for extranucleolar control of RNA synthesis in the nucleolus. *Biochem. Biophys. Res. Commun.*, 40:334–342.

139. Jacob, S. T., Sajdel, E. M., and Munro, H. N. (1969): Regulation of nucleolar RNA metabolism by hydrocortisone. *Eur. J. Biochem.,* 7:449–453.
140. Jacob, S. T., Sajdel, E. M., and Munro, H. N. (1970): Different responses of soluble whole nuclear RNA polymerase and soluble nucleolar RNA polymerase to divalent cations and to inhibition by α-amanitin. *Biochem. Biophys. Res. Commun.,* 38:765–770.
141. Jacob, S. T., Scharf, M. B., and Vesell, E. S. (1974): Role of RNA in induction of hepatic microsomal mixed function oxidases. *Proc. Natl. Acad. Sci. USA,* 71:704–707.
142. Jelliffe, D. B. (1966): The assessment of the nutritional status of the community. *WHO Monogr. Ser.,* 53.
143. Jensen, E. V., and DeSombre, E. R. (1973): Estrogen-receptor interaction. *Science,* 182:126–134.
144. Johnson, T. C. (1969): Aminoacyl-RNA synthetase and transfer RNA binding activity during early mammalian brain development. *J. Neurochem.,* 16:1125–1131.
145. Johnson, T. C., and Chou, L. (1973): Level and amino acid acceptor activity of mouse brain tRNA during neural development. *J. Neurochem.,* 20:405–414.
146. Kasa, D. (1975): Histochemistry of choline acetyltransferase. In: *Cholinergic Mechanisms,* edited by P. G. Waser. Raven Press, New York.
147. Kedinger, C., Gniazdowski, M., Mandel, J. L., Gissinger, F., and Chambon, P. (1970): α-Amanitin: A specific inhibitor of one of two DNA-dependent RNA polymerase activities from calf thymus. *Biochem. Biophys. Res. Commun.,* 38:165–171.
148. Kennedy, G. C. (1957): The development with age of hypothalamic restraint upon the appetite of the rat. *J. Endocrinol.,* 16:9–17.
149. Kenney, F. T. (1970): Hormonal regulation of synthesis of liver enzymes. In: *Mammalian Protein Metabolism,* Vol. 4, edited by H. N. Munro. Academic Press, New York.
150. Kerr, G. R., Allen, J. R., Scheffler, G., and Waisman, H. A. (1970): Malnutrition studies in the rhesus monkey. I. Effect on physical growth. *Am. J. Clin. Nutr.,* 23:739–748.
151. Kirsch, R. E., Brock, J. F., and Saunders, S. J. (1968): Experimental protein-calorie malnutrition. *Am. J. Clin. Nutr.,* 21:820–826.
152. Konijn, A. M., Baliga, B. S., and Munro, H. N. (1973): Synthesis of liver ferritin on free and membrane-bound polyribosomes of different sizes. *FEBS Lett.,* 37:249–252.
153. Kraft, N., and Shortman, K. (1970): A suggested control function for the animal tissue ribonuclease-ribonuclease inhibitor system, based on studies of isolated cells and phytohaemagglutinin-transformed lymphocytes. *Biochim. Biophys. Acta,* 217:164–175.
154. Krigman, M. R., and Hogan, E. L. (1976): Undernutrition in the developing rat: Effect upon myelination. *Brain Res.,* 107:239–255.
155. Kumar, V., Chase, H. P., Hammond, K., and O'Brien, D. (1972): Alterations in blood biochemical tests in progressive protein malnutrition. *Pediatrics,* 49:736–743.
156. Laga, E. M., Driscoll, S. G., and Munro, H. N. (1972): Comparison of placentas from two socioeconomic groups. I. Morphometry. *Pediatrics,* 50:24–32.
157. Laga, E. M., Driscoll, S. G., and Munro, H. N. (1972): Comparison of placentas from two socioeconomic groups. II. Biochemical characteristics. *Pediatrics,* 50:33–39.
158. Laga, E. M., Driscoll, S. G., and Munro, H. N. (1974): Human placental structure: relationship to fetal nutrition. In: *Problems of Human Reproduction, Vol. 2: Lactogenic Hormones, Fetal Nutrition and Lactation,* edited by J. B. Josimovich, Jr. Wiley, New York.
159. Lajthe, A., and Dunlop, D. (in press): Protein metabolism in neuroendocrine tissues. In: *Subcellular Mechanisms in Reproductive Neuroendocrinology,* edited by F. Naftolin, K. J. Ryan, and I. J. Davies. Elsevier, New York.
160. Latham, M. C. (1974): Protein-calorie malnutrition in children and its relation to psychological development and behavior. *Physiol. Rev.,* 54:541–565.
161. Lee, C-J. (1970): Biosynthesis and characteristics of brain protein and ribonucleic acid in mice subjected to neonatal infection or undernutrition. *J. Biol. Chem.,* 245:1998–2004.
162. Lehr, P., and Gayet, J. (1963): Response of the cerebral cortex of the rat to prolonged protein depletion. I. Tissue weight, nitrogen, DNA and proteins. *J. Neurochem.,* 10:169–176.
163. Lerner, M. P., Wettstein, F. O., Herschman, H. R., Stevens, J. G., and Fridlender, B. R. (1971): Distribution of polysomes in mouse brain tissue. *J. Neurochem.,* 18:1495–1507.

164. Levine, S., and Wiener, S. (1976): A critical analysis of data on malnutrition and behavioral deficits. *Adv. Pediatr.*, 22:113–130.
165. Lim, L., White, J. O., Hall, C., Berthold, W., and Davison, A. N. (1974): Isolation of microsomal poly(A)-RNA from rat brain directing the synthesis of the myelin encephalitogenic protein in Xenopus oocytes. *Biochim. Biophys. Acta*, 361:241–247.
166. Lindroos, O. F. C., and Oja, S. S. (1971): Hyperphenylalaninaemia and the exchange of tyrosine in adult rat brain. *Exp. Brain Res.*, 14:48–60.
167. Lisy, V., and Lodin, Z. (1973): Incorporation of radioactive leucine into neuronal and glial proteins during postnatal development. *Neurobiology*, 3:320–326.
168. Lo, G. S., Lee, S., Cruz, N. L., and Longenecker, J. B. (1970): Temporary induction of phenylketonuria-like characteristics in infant rats: Effect on brain protein synthesis. *Nutr. Rep. Int.*, 2:59–72.
169. Løvtrup-Rein, H., and Grahn, B. (1974): Polysomes and polysomal RNA from nerve and glial cell fractions. *Brain Res.*, 72:123–136.
170. Lowden, J. A., and LaRamée, M. A. (1969): Hyperphenylalaninemia: the effect on cerebral amino acid levels during development. *Can. J. Biochem.*, 47:883–888.
171. Lynch, A., Smart, J. L., and Dobbing, J. (1975): Motor coordination and cerebellar size in adult rats undernourished in early life. *Brain Res.*, 83:249–259.
172. MacInnes, J. W., and Schlesinger, K. (1971): Effects of excess phenylalanine on in vitro and in vivo RNA and protein synthesis and polyribosome levels in brains of mice. *Brain Res.*, 29:101–110.
173. Mandel, P., and Mark, J. (1965): The influence of nitrogen deprivation on free amino acids in rat brain. *J. Neurochem.*, 12:987–992.
174. McAnulty, P. A., and Dickerson, J. W. T. (1974): The development of the weanling rat during nutritionally-induced growth retardation and during early rehabilitation. *Br. J. Nutr.*, 32:301–312.
175. McFarlane, H., Reddy, S., Adcock, K. J., Adeshina, H., Cooke, A. R., and Akene, J. (1970): Immunity, transferrin, and survival in kwashiorkor. *Br. Med. J.*, 4:268–270.
176. McKean, C. M., Boggs, D. E., and Peterson, N. A. (1968): The influence of high phenylalanine and tyrosine on the concentrations of essential amino acids in brain. *J. Neurochem.*, 15:235–241.
177. Mena, I., and Cotzias, G. C. (1975): Protein intake and treatment of Parkinson's disease with levodopa. *N. Engl. J. Med.*, 292:181–184.
178. Merat, A., and Dickerson, J. W. T. (1973): The effect of development on the gangliosides of rat and pig brain. *J. Neurochem.*, 20:873–880.
179. Merat, A., and Dickerson, J. W. T. (1974): The effect of the severity and timing of malnutrition on brain gangliosides in the rat. *Biol. Neonate*, 25:158–170.
180. Miller, S. A. (1969): Protein metabolism during growth and development. In: *Mammalian Protein Metabolism*, Vol. 3, edited by H. N. Munro. Academic Press, New York.
181. Miller, R. L., and Udenfriend, S. (1970): Hydroxylation of proline residues in collagen nascent chains. *Arch. Biochem. Biophys.*, 139:104–113.
182. Minkowski, A., Roux, J-M., and Tordet-Caridroit, C. (1974): Pathophysiologic changes in intrauterine malnutrition. *Curr. Concepts Nutr.*, 2:45–78.
183. Monckeberg, F. (1975): The effect of malnutrition on physical growth and brain development. In: *Brain Function and Malnutrition*, edited by J. W. Prescott. Wiley, New York.
184. Moon, H. M., and Weissbach, H. (1972): Interaction of brain transferase I with guanosine nucleotides and aminoacyl-tRNA. *Biochem. Biophys. Res. Commun.*, 46:254–262.
185. Moon, H-M., Redfield, B., Millard, S., Vane, F., and Weissbach, H. (1973): Multiple forms of elongation factor 1 from calf brain. *Proc. Natl. Acad. Sci. USA*, 70:3282–3286.
186. Morgan, B. L. G., and Naismith, D. J. (1975): The effect of postnatal undernutrition on the activities of enzymes involved in the synthesis of brain lipids in the rat. *Nutr. Soc. Proc.*, 34:40A–41A.
187. Morgan, I. G. (1970): Protein synthesis in brain mitochondrial and synaptosomal preparations. *FEBS Lett.*, 10:273–275.
188. Morishige, W. K., and Leathem, J. H. (1972): Pregnancy maintenance with corticosterone in protein-depleted rats: A study on fetal protein composition. *Endocrinology*, 90:318–322.
189. Mortimore, G. E., Woodside, K. H., and Henry, J. E. (1972): Compartmentation of free

valine and its relation to protein turnover in perfused rat liver. *J. Biol. Chem.*, 247:2776–2784.

190. Mueller, A. J., and Cox, W. M. (1946): The effect of changes in diet on the volume and composition of rat milk. *J. Nutr.,* 31:249–259.

191. Munro, H. N. (1970): Free amino acid pools and their role in regulation. In: *Mammalian Protein Metabolism,* Vol. 4, edited by H. N. Munro. Academic Press, New York.

192. Munro, H. N., and Goldberg, D. M. (1964): The effect of protein intake on the protein and nucleic acid metabolism of the intestinal mucosa cell. In: *The Role of the Gastrointestinal Tract in Protein Metabolism,* edited by H. N. Munro. Blackwell, Oxford.

193. Munro, H. N., and Steinert, P. M. (1975): The intracellular organisation of protein synthesis. In: *International Review of Science (Biochemistry Series),* Vol. 7, edited by H. R. V. Arnstein. Butterworths, London.

194. Munro, H. N., Fernstrom, J. D., and Wurtman, R. J. (1975): Insulin, plasma amino acid imbalance, and hepatic coma. *Lancet,* 1:722–724.

195. Munro, H. N., Hubert, C., and Baliga, B. S. (1975): Regulation of protein synthesis in relation to amino acid supply—a review. In: *Alcohol and Abnormal Protein Biosynthesis. Biochemical and Clinical,* edited by M. A. Rothschild, M. Oratz, and S. S. Schreiber. Pergamon Press, New York.

196. Murthy, M. R. V. (1972): Free and membrane-bound ribosomes of rat cerebral cortex: Protein synthesis in vivo and in vitro. *J. Biol. Chem.,* 247:1936–1943.

197. Muzzo, S., Gregory, T., and Gardner, L. I. (1973): Oxygen consumption by brain mitochondria of rats malnourished in utero. *J. Nutr.,* 103:314–317.

198. Naeye, R. L., Blanc, W., and Paul, C. (1973): Effects of maternal nutrition on the human fetus. *Pediatrics,* 52:494–503.

199. Nakhasi, H. L., Toews, A. D., and Horrocks, L. A. (1975): Effects of a postnatal protein deficiency on the content and composition of myelin from the brains of weanling rats. *Brain Res.,* 83:176–179.

200. Nelsestuen, G. L., Zytkovicz, T. H., and Howard, J. B. (1974): The mode of action of vitamin K: Identification of γ-carboxyglutamic acid as a component of prothrombin. *J. Biol. Chem.,* 249:6347–6350.

201. Nelson, M. M., and Evans, H. M. (1953): Relation of dietary protein levels to reproduction in the rat. *J. Nutr.,* 51:71–84.

202. Niiyama, Y., Kishi, K., Endo, S., and Inoue, G. (1973): Effect of diets devoid of one essential amino acid on pregnancy in rats maintained by ovarian steroids. *J. Nutr.,* 103:207–212.

203. Nordyke, E. L., and Roach, M. K. (1974): Effect of hyperphenylalaninemia on amino acid metabolism and compartmentation in neonatal rat brain. *Brain Res.,* 67:479–488.

204. Nordyke, E. L., and Roach, M. K. (1974): Effect of hyperphenylalaninemia on succinate dehydrogenase and glutamate dehydrogenase activities in brain regions of developing rats. *Res. Commun. Chem. Pathol. Pharmacol.,* 8:397–400.

205. Ogata, K., Kido, H., Abe, S., Furusawa, Y., and Satake, M. (1967): Activity of protein synthesis of the brain of protein-deficient rats. In: *Malnutrition, Learning and Behavior,* edited by N. S. Scrimshaw and J. E. Gordon. MIT Press, Cambridge.

206. Olney, J. W., and Ho, O. L. (1970): Brain damage in infant mice following oral intake of glutamate, aspartate or cysteine. *Nature (Lond.),* 227:609–611.

207. Olson, R. E. (1975): Introductory remarks: Nutrient, hormone, enzyme interactions. *Am. J. Clin. Nutr.,* 28:626–637.

208. O'Malley, B. W., and Means, A. R. (1974): Female steroid hormones and target cell nuclei. *Science,* 183:610–620.

209. Ordy, J. M., Samorajski, T., and Hershberger, T. J. (1970): Brain vulnerability to postnatal protein calorie deficiency in infant rhesus monkeys. *Proc. Soc. Exp. Biol. Med.,* 135:680–684.

210. Ordy, J. M., Samorajski, T., Zimmerman, R. R., and Rady, P. M. (1966): Effects of postnatal protein deficiency on weight gain, serum proteins, enzymes, cholesterol, and liver ultrastructure in a subhuman primate (Macaca mulatta). *Am. J. Pathol.,* 48:769–791.

211. Pao, S-K., and Dickerson, J. W. T. (1975): Effect of a low protein diet and isoenergetic amounts of high protein diet in the weanling rat on the free amino acids of the brain. *Nutr. Metab.,* 18:204–216.

212. Parks, J. M., Ames, A., III, and Nesbett, F. B. (1976). Protein synthesis in central nervous tissue: Studies on in vitro retina. *J. Neurochem. (in press)*.
213. Patel, A. J., and Balazs, R. (1970). Manifestation of metabolic compartmentation during the maturation of the rat brain. *J. Neurochem.*, 17:955–971.
214. Patel, A. J., Atkinson, D. J., and Balazs, R. (1975): Effect of undernutrition on metabolic compartmentation of glutamate and on the incorporation of [$^{14}$C] leucine into protein in developing rat brain. *Dev. Psychobiol.*, 8:453–464.
215. Pavlik, A., and Jakoubek, B. (1976): Distribution of protein-bound radioactivity in brain slices of the adult rat incubated with labelled leucine. *Brain Res.*, 101:113–128.
216. Peng, Y., Gubin, J., Harper, A. E., Vavich, M. G., and Kemmerer, A. R. (1973): Food intake regulation: Amino acid toxicity and changes in rat brain and plasma amino acids. *J. Nutr.*, 103:608–617.
217. Perry, R. P., and Kelley, D. E. (1974): Existence of methylated messenger RNA in mouse L cells. *Cell*, 1:37–42.
218. Platt, B. S., Heard, C. R. C., and Stewart, R. J. C. (1964): Experimental protein-calorie deficiency. In: *Mammalian Protein Metabolism*, Vol. 2, edited by H. N. Munro and J. B. Allison. Academic Press, New York.
219. Plaut, S. M. (1970): Studies of undernutrition in the young rat: Methodological considerations. *Dev. Psychobiol.*, 3:157–167.
220. Popov, N., Pohle, W., Lössner, B., Schulzeck, S., Schmidt, S., Ott, T., and Matthies, H. (1973): Regional distribution of RNA and protein radioactivity in the rat brain after intraventricular application of labeled precursors. *Acta Biol. Med. Germ.*, 31:51–62.
221. Prensky, A. L., Fishman, M. A., and Daftari, B. (1971): Differential effects of hyperphenyl-alaninemia on the development of the brain in the rat. *Brain Res.*, 33:181–191.
222. Pronczuk, A. W., Baliga, B. S., Triant, J. W., and Munro, H. N. (1968): Comparison of the effect of amino acid supply on hepatic polysome profiles in vivo and in vitro. *Biochim. Biophys. Acta*, 157:204–206.
223. Pronczuk, A., Rogers, Q. R., and Munro, H. N. (1970): Liver polysome patterns of rats fed amino acid imbalanced diets. *J. Nutr.*, 100:1249–1258.
224. Raaf, J., and Kernohan, J. W. (1944): A study of the external granular layer in the cerebellum: The disappearance of the external granular layer and the growth of the molecular and internal granular layers in the cerebellum. *Am. J. Anat.*, 75:151–172.
225. Rajalakshmi, R., Parameswaran, M., and Ramakrishnan, C. V. (1974): Effects of different levels of dietary protein on brain glutamate dehydrogenase and decarboxylase in young albino rats. *J. Neurochem.*, 23:123–127.
226. Rajalakshmi, R., Parameswaran, M., Telang, S. D., and Ramakrishnan, C. V. (1974): Effects of undernutrition and protein deficiency on glutamate dehydrogenase and decarboxylase in rat brain. *J. Neurochem.*, 23:129–133.
227. Rajalakshmi, R., Pillai, K. R., and Ramakrishnan, C. V. (1969): Effects of different supplements to low protein and poor quality protein diets on performance and brain enzymes in the albino rat. *J. Neurochem.*, 16:599–606.
228. Rakic, P. (1971): Neuron-glia relationship during granule cell migration in developing cerebellar cortex: A Golgi and electronmicroscopic study in Macacus rhesus. *J. Comp. Neurol.*, 14:283–312.
229. Reed, P. B., White, M. N., and Longenecker, J. B. (1970): Temporary induction of phenylketonuria-like characteristics in infant rats: Effect on brain DNA synthesis. *Nutr. Rep. Int.*, 2:73–85.
230. Reynolds, W. A., Lemkey-Johnston, N., Filer, L. J., Jr., and Pitkin, R. M. (1971): Monosodium glutamate: Absence of hypothalamic lesions after ingestion by newborn primates. *Science*, 172:1342–1344.
231. Rider, A. A., and Simonson, M. (1973): Effect on rat offspring of maternal diet deficient in calories but not in protein. *Nutr. Rep. Int.*, 7:361–370.
232. Roach, M. K., Corbin, J., and Pennington, W. (1974): Effect of undernutrition on amino acid compartmentation in the developing rat brain. *J. Neurochem.*, 22:521–528.
233. Roberts, S. (1968): Influence of circulating levels of amino acids on cerebral concentrations and utilization of amino acids. *Prog. Brain Res.*, 29:235–243.
234. Roberts, S. (1974): Effects of amino acid imbalance on amino acid utilization, protein synthesis and polyribosome function in cerebral cortex. In: *Aromatic Amino Acids in the*

*Brain*. Ciba Foundation Symposium 22. Associated Scientific Publishers, Amsterdam.

235. Roberts, S., and Morelos, B. S. (1976): Role of ribonuclease action in phenylalanine-induced disaggregation of rat cerebral polyribosomes. *J. Neurochem.*, 26:387–400.

236. Roeder, R. G., and Rutter, W. J. (1969): Multiple forms of DNA-dependent RNA polymerase in eukaryotic organisms. *Nature (Lond.)*, 224:234–237.

237. Roel, L. E., Schwartz, S. A., Weiss, B. F., and Wurtman, R. J. (1974): In vivo inhibition of rat brain protein synthesis by L-DOPA. *J. Neurochem.*, 23:233–239.

238. Roel, L. E., Wurtman, R. J., and Munro, H. N. (1975): Unpublished observation.

239. Rossier, J., Bauman, A., Rieger, F., and Benda, P. (1975): Immunological studies on the enzymes of the cholinergic system. In: *Cholinergic Mechanisms,* edited by P. G. Waser. Raven Press, New York.

240. Rosso, P., and Winick, M. (1975): Effects of early undernutrition and subsequent refeeding on alkaline ribonuclease activity of rat cerebrum and liver. *J. Nutr.*, 105:1104–1110.

241. Sajdel, E. M., and Jacob, S. T. (1971): Mechanism of early effect of hydrocortisone on the transcriptional process: Stimulation of the activities of purified rat liver nucleolar RNA polymerases. *Biochem. Biophys. Res. Commun.*, 45:707–715.

242. Schain, R. J., and Watanabe, K. S. (1973): Effects of undernutrition on early brain growth in the rabbit. *Exp. Neurol.*, 41:366–370.

243. Schimke, R. T. (1970): Regulation of protein degradation in mammalian tissues. In: *Mammalian Protein Metabolism,* Vol. 4, edited by H. N. Munro. Academic Press, New York.

244. Schumm, D. E., and Webb, T. E. (1972). Transport of informosomes from isolated nuclei of regenerating rat liver. *Biochem. Biophys. Res. Commun.*, 48:1259–1265.

245. Schutz, G., Beato, M., and Feigelson, P. (1970): Messenger RNA for hepatic tryptophan oxygenase: Its partial purification, its translation in a heterologous cell-free system, and its control by glucocorticoid hormones. *Proc. Natl. Acad. Sci. USA*, 70:1218–1221.

246. Seoane, N., and Latham, M. C. (1971): Nutritional anthropometry in the identification of malnutrition in childhood. *J. Trop. Pediatr.*, 17:98–104.

247. Sereni, F., Principi, N., Perletti, L., and Sereni, L. P. (1966): Undernutrition and the developing rat brain. I. Influence on acetylcholinesterase and succinic acid dehydrogenase activities and on norepinephrine and 5-OH-tryptamine tissue concentrations. *Biol. Neonate,* 10:254–265.

248. Seta, K., Sansur, M., and Lajtha, A. (1973): The rate of incorporation of amino acids into brain proteins during infusion in the rat. *Biochim. Biophys. Acta*, 294:472–480.

249. Shah, S. N., and McKean, C. M. (1968): Effect of chronic and acute phenylalanine injections on the biosynthesis of glycolipids in the developing rat brain. *Fed. Proc.*, 27:488.

250. Shah, S. N., Peterson, N. A., and McKean, C. M. (1972). Impaired myelin formation in experimental hyperphenylalaninaemia. *J. Neurochem.*, 19:479–485.

251. Sidransky, H., Bongiorno, M., Sarma, D. S. R., and Verney, E. (1967): The influence of tryptophan on hepatic polyribosomes and protein synthesis in fasted mice. *Biochem. Biophys. Res. Commun.*, 27:242–248.

252. Siegel, F. L., Aoki, K., and Colwell, R. E. (1971): Polyribosome disaggregation and cell-free protein synthesis in preparations from cerebral cortex of hyperphenylalaninemic rats. *J. Neurochem.*, 18:537–547.

253. Smart, J. L. (1976): Maternal behavior of undernourished mother rats towards well fed and underfed young. *Physiol. Behav.*, 16:147–149.

254. Smart, J. L., Dobbing, J., Adlard, B. P. F., Lynch, A., and Sands, J. (1973): Vulnerability of developing brain: Relative effects of growth restriction during the fetal and suckling periods on behavior and brain composition of adult rats. *J. Nutr.*, 103:1327–1338.

255. Sobotka, T. J., Cook, M. P., and Brodie, R. E. (1974): Neonatal malnutrition: Neurochemical, hormonal and behavioral manifestations. *Brain Res.*, 65:443–457.

256. Stein, G. S., Spelsberg, T. C., and Kleinsmith, L. J. (1974): Nonhistone chromosomal proteins and gene regulation. *Science,* 183:817–824.

257. Stein, Z., Susser, M., Saenger, G., and Marolla, F. (1975): *Famine and Human Development: The Dutch Hunger Winter of 1944/45.* Oxford University Press, New York.

258. Steinert, P. M., Baliga, B. S., and Munro, H. N. (1974): Available sulphydryl groups of mammalian ribosomes in different functional states. *J. Mol. Biol.*, 88:895–911.

259. Stern, W. C., Miller, M., Forbes, W. B., Leahy, J. P., Morgane, P. J., and Resnick, O.

(1976): Effects of protein malnutrition during development on protein synthesis in brain and peripheral tissues. *Brain Res. Bull.*, 1:27–31.

260. Swaiman, K. F. (1972): The effect of food-deprivation and re-feeding on brain enzyme activity in immature rat brain. *Brain Res.*, 43:296–298.

261. Swaiman, K. F., and Wolfe, R. N. (1970): The effect of food-deprivation and re-feeding on lactic dehydrogenase activity in immature rat brain. *Proc. Soc. Exp. Biol. Med.*, 134:185–187.

262. Swaiman, K. F., Daleiden, J. M., and Wolfe, R. N. (1970): The effect of food deprivation on enzyme activity in developing brain. *J. Neurochem.*, 17:1387–1391.

263. Swaiman, K. F., Hosfield, W. B., and Lemieux, B. (1968): Elevated plasma phenylalanine concentration and lysine incorporation into ribosomal protein of developing brain. *J. Neurochem.*, 15:687–690.

264. Swendseid, M. E., Yamada, C., Vinyard, E., and Figneroa, W. G. (1968): Plasma amino acid levels in young subjects receiving diets containing 14 or 3.5 g nitrogen per day. *Am. J. Clin. Nutr.*, 21:1381–1383.

265. Tanaka, T., and Ogata, K. (1972): Two classes of membrane-bound ribosomes in rat liver cells and their albumin synthesizing activity. *Biochem. Biophys. Res. Commun.*, 49:1069–1074.

266. Taub, F., and Johnson, T. C. (1975): The mechanism of polyribosome disaggregation in brain tissue by phenylalanine. *Biochem. J.*, 151:173–180.

267. Tyce, G. M., Flock, E. V., and Owen, C. A. (1964): Tryptophan metabolism in the brain of the developing rat. *Prog. Brain Res.*, 9:198–203.

268. Tyfield, L. A., and Holton, J. B. (1976): The effect of high concentrations of histidine on the level of other amino acids in plasma and brain of the mature rat. *J. Neurochem.*, 26:101–105.

269. van Marthens, E., Harel, S., and Zamenhof, S. (1975): Experimental intrauterine growth retardation. *Biol. Neonate*, 26:221–231.

270. van Venrooij, W. J., Kuijper-Lenstra, A. H., and Kramer, M. F. (1973): Interrelationship between amino acid pools and protein synthesis in the rat submandibular gland. *Biochim. Biophys. Acta*, 312:392–398.

271. Velasco, E. G., Brasel, J. A., Sigulem, D. M., Rosso, P., and Winick, M. (1973): Effects of vascular insufficiency on placental ribonuclease activity in the rat. *J. Nutr.*, 103:213–217.

272. Venkatachalam, P. S., and Ramanathan, K. S. (1964): Effect of protein deficiency during gestation and lactation on body weight and composition of offspring. *J. Nutr.*, 84:38–42.

273. Vernadakis, A., and Woodbury, D. M. (1962): Electrolyte and amino acid changes in rat brain during maturation. *Am. J. Physiol.*, 203:748–752.

274. Volpe, J. J., and Laster, L. (1972): Transsulfuration in fetal and postnatal mammalian liver and brain: cystathionine synthase, its relation to hormonal influences, and cystathionine. *Biol. Neonate*, 20:385–403.

275. Von der Decken, A., and Wronski, A. (1971): Protein synthesis in vitro in rat brain after short-term protein starvation and refeeding. *J. Neurochem.*, 18:2383–2388.

276. Waterlow, J. C. (1969): The assessment of protein nutrition and metabolism in the whole animal, with special reference to man. In: *Mammalian Protein Metabolism*, Vol. 3, edited by H. N. Munro. Academic Press, New York.

277. Weichsel, M. E., Jr., and Dawson, L. (1976): Effects of hypothyroidism and undernutrition on DNA content and thymidine kinase activity during cerebellar development in the rat. *J. Neurochem.*, 26:675–681.

278. Weiss, B. F., Liebschutz, J. L., Wurtman, R. J., and Munro, H. N. (1975): Pariciption of dopamine and serotonin-receptors in the disaggregation of brain polysomes by L-DOPA and L-5-HTP. *J. Neurochem.*, 24:1191–1195.

279. Weiss, B. F., Munro, H. N., and Wurtman, R. J. (1971): L-DOPA: Disaggregation of brain polysomes and elevation of brain tryptophan. *Science*, 173:833–835.

280. Weiss, B. F., Munro, H. N., Ordonez, L. A., and Wurtman, R. J. (1972): Dopamine: Mediator of brain polysome disaggregation after L-DOPA. *Science*, 177:613–616.

281. Weiss, B. F., Roel, L. E., Munro, H. N., and Wurtman, R. J. (1974): L-Dopa, polysomal aggregation and cerebral synthesis of protein. In: *Aromatic Amino Acids in the Brain*. Ciba Foundation Symposium 22. Associated Scientific Publishers, Amsterdam.

282. Weiss, B. F., Wurtman, R. J., and Munro, H. N. (1973): Disaggregation of brain polysomes by L-5-hydroxytryptophan: Mediation by serotonin. *Life Sci.,* 13:411–416.
283. Weller, L. A., Margen, S., and Calloway, D. H. (1969): Variation in fasting and postprandial amino acids of men fed adequate or protein-free diets. *Am. J. Clin. Nutr.,* 22:1577–1583.
284. Whitehead, R. G. (1964): Rapid determination of some plasma amino acids in subclinical kwashiorkor. *Lancet,* 1:250–252.
285. Whitehead, R. G. (1968): Biochemical changes in kwashiorkor and nutritional marasmus. In: *Calorie Deficiencies and Protein Deficiencies,* edited by R. A. McCance and E. M. Widdowson. Little, Brown, Boston.
286. Wiggins, R. C., Benjamins, J. A., Krigman, M. R., and Morell, P. (1974): Synthesis of myelin proteins during starvation. *Brain Res.,* 80:345–349.
287. Wiggins, R. C., Miller, S. L., Benjamins, J. A., Krigman, M. R., and Morell, P. (1976). Myelin synthesis during postnatal nutritional deprivation and subsequent rehabilitation. *Brain Res.,* 107:257–273.
288. Wigglesworth, J. S. (1966): Foetal growth retardation. *Br. Med. Bull.,* 22:13–15.
289. Wiltse, H. E., and Menkes, J. H. (1972): Brain damage in the aminoacidurias. In: *Handbook of Neurochemistry,* Vol. 7, edited by A. Lajthe. Plenum Press, New York.
290. Winick, M. (1968): Changes in nucleic acid and protein content of the human brain during growth. *Pediatr. Res.,* 2:352–355.
291. Winick, M. (1970): Cellular growth in intrauterine malnutrition. *Pediatr. Clin. North Am.,* 17:69–78.
292. Winick, M. (1970): Nutrition and nerve cell growth. *Fed. Proc.,* 29:1510–1515.
293. Winick, M. (1976): *Malnutrition and Brain Development.* Oxford University Press, New York.
294. Winick, M., and Noble, A. (1965): Quantitative changes in DNA, RNA and protein during prenatal and postnatal growth in the rat. *Dev. Biol.,* 12:451–466.
295. Winick, M., and Noble, A. (1966): Cellular response in rats during malnutrition at various ages. *J. Nutr.,* 89:300–306.
296. Winick, M., and Noble, A. (1967): Cellular response with increased feeding in neonatal rats. *J. Nutr.,* 91:179–182.
297. Winick, M., and Rosso, P. (1969): The effect of severe early malnutrition on cellular growth of human brain. *Pediatr. Res.,* 3:181–184.
298. Winick, M., Brasel, J. A., and Velasco, E. G. (1973): Effects of prenatal nutrition upon pregnancy risk. *Clin. Obstet. Gynecol.,* 16:184–198.
299. Winick, M., Fish, I., and Rosso, P. (1968): Cellular recovery in rat tissues after a brief period of neonatal malnutrition. *J. Nutr.,* 95:623–626.
300. Winick, M., Rosso, P., and Waterlow, J. (1970): Cellular growth of cerebrum, cerebellum, and brain stem in normal and marasmic children. *Exp. Neurol.,* 26:393–400.
301. Wong, P. W. K., and Justice, P. (1972): Effect of amino acid imbalance on polyribosome profiles and protein synthesis in rat cerebral cortex. In: *Sphingolipids, Sphingolipidoses and Allied Disorders,* edited by B. W. Volk and S. M. Aronson. Plenum, New York.
302. Wong, P. W. K., Fresco, R., and Justice, P. (1972): The effect of maternal amino acid imbalance on fetal cerebral polyribosomes. *Metabolism,* 21:875–881.
303. Wunner, W. H., Bell, J., and Munro, H. N. (1966): The effect of feeding with a tryptophan-free amino acid mixture on rat-liver polysomes and ribosomal ribonucleic acid. *Biochem. J.,* 101:417–428.
304. Wurtman, J. J., and Miller, S. A. (1976): Effect of litter size on weight gain in rats. *J. Nutr.,* 106:697–701.
305. Yamagami, S., and Mori, K. (1970): Changes in polysomes of the developing rat brain. *J. Neurochem.,* 17:721–731.
306. Young, V. R., Alexis, S. D., Baliga, B. S., Munro, H. N., and Muecke, W. (1972): Metabolism of administered 3-methylhistidine: Lack of muscle transfer ribonucleic acid charging and quantitative excretion as 3-methylhistidine and its N-acetyl derivative. *J. Biol. Chem.,* 247:3592–3600.
307. Zähringer, J., Baliga, B. S., and Munro, H. N. (1976): Novel mechanism for translational control in regulation of ferritin synthesis by iron. *Proc. Natl. Acad. Sci. USA,* 73:857–861.

308. Zamenhof, S., and van Marthens, E. (1974): Study of factors influencing prenatal brain development. *Mol. Cell. Biochem.*, 4:157–168.
309. Zamenhof, S., Hall, S. M., Grauel, L., van Marthens, E., and Donahue, M. J. (1974): Deprivation of amino acids and prenatal brain development in rats. *J. Nutr.*, 104:1002–1007.
310. Zamenhof, S., van Marthen, E., and Grauel, L. (1971): DNA (cell number) in neonatal brain: Alteration by maternal dietary caloric restriction. *Nutr. Rep. Int.*, 4:269–274.
311. Zamenhof, S., van Marthens, E., and Grauel, L. (1971): DNA (cell number) and protein in neonatal rat brain: Alteration by timing of maternal dietary protein restriction. *J. Nutr.*, 101:1265–1270.
312. Zamenhof, S., van Marthens, E., and Grauel, L. (1971): DNA (cell number) in neonatal brain: Second generation ($F_2$) alteration by maternal ($F_0$) dietary protein restriction. *Science*, 172:850–851.
313. Zamenhof, S., van Marthens, E., and Grauel, L. (1972): DNA (cell number) and protein in rat brain: Second generation ($F_2$) alteration by maternal ($F_0$) dietary protein restriction. *Nutr. Metab.*, 14:262–270.
314. Zamenhof, S., van Marthens, E., and Grauel, L. (1973): Prenatal nutritional factors affecting brain development. *Nutr. Rep. Int.*, 7:371–382.
315. Zamenhof, S., van Marthens, E., and Margolis, F. L. (1968): DNA (cell number) and protein in neonatal brain: Alteration by maternal dietary protein restriction. *Science*, 160:322–323.
316. Zamenhof, S., van Marthens, E., and Shimomaye, S. Y. (1976): The effects of early maternal protein deprivation on fetal development. *Fed. Proc.*, 35:422.
317. Zeman, F. J., and Stanbrough, E. C. (1969): Effect of maternal protein deficiency on cellular development in the fetal rat. *J. Nutr.*, 99:274–282.
318. Zomzely, C. E., Roberts, S., and Peache, S. (1970): Isolation of RNA with properties of messenger RNA from cerebral polyribosomes. *Proc. Natl. Acad. Sci. USA*, 67:644–651.
319. Zomzely, C. E., Roberts, S., Brown, D. M., and Provost, C. (1966): Cerebral protein synthesis. I. Physical properties of cerebral ribosomes and polyribosomes. *J. Mol. Biol.*, 19:455–468.
320. Zomzely-Neurath, C. E., and Roberts, S. (1972): Brain ribosomes. In: *Research Methods in Neurochemistry*, Vol. 1, edited by N. Marks and R. Rodnight. Plenum Press, New York.
321. Zomzely-Neurath, C., York, C., and Moore, B. W. (1973): In vitro synthesis of two brain-specific proteins (S100 and 14-3-2) by polyribosomes from rat brain. I. Site of synthesis and programming by polysome-derived messenger RNA. *Arch. Biochem. Biophys.*, 155:58–69.

*Nutrition and the Brain,* Vol. 2,
edited by R. J. Wurtman and
J. J. Wurtman. Raven Press,
New York © 1977.

# Protein-Calorie Malnutrition and Behavior: A View from Psychology

## Ernesto Pollitt and Carol Thomson

*Department of Nutrition and Food Science, Massachusetts Institute of Technology, Cambridge, Massachusetts 02139*

A naive reader of the literature on protein-calorie malnutrition and intelligence must be cautioned against making erroneous inferences. The state of the art of the disciplines involved permits only approximate measures of the nutritional deficiency and the psychological constructs in question. Data interpretation is also problematic because the social nature of the research problem restricts experimental manipulation of the independent variable. Accordingly, the research designs that can be used are limited. Thus the field today is characterized by a large number of hypotheses and qualified statements; as yet there are no conclusive inferences.

This chapter critically reviews most of the published research studies on the effects of protein-calorie malnutrition on mental development. The focus of the critique is on the research designs, the validity of the psychological tests used, and the treatment validity of intervention programs. Little attention is given to anthropometry as a nutrition variable because its problems of measurement were treated recently in some detail (38,70,79). The chapter is organized into two parts. Some basic concepts of intelligence test theory are discussed briefly in the first. The second part centers on data from studies on the behavioral effects of malnutrition on infants and children. In addition to summarizing main findings we critique the studies in some detail and, whenever possible, attempt to reach some conclusions. A glossary of psychological tests appears at the end of the chapter.

## I. SOME BASIC NOTIONS OF PSYCHOMETRICS

Despite the current considerable interest in Piaget's theory, much of the theoretical and empirical research conducted on intelligence has been based on psychometric theory. The aim of this school has been the measurement of mental abilities and statistical estimation of individual differences. Conversely, Piagetian developmental psychology focuses on the development of structures and processes allegedly universal which underlie man's acquisition of knowledge (31,34). The psychometric approach has guided most of the research conducted on the cognitive function of malnourished children; it is for this reason that it is pertinent to review some of its basic premises.

The psychometric approach is characterized by its pragmatism, in both past and present work. The main impetus in its development can be traced to the work of Charles Spearman in England and Alfred Binet in France during the early part of this century. Spearman generated the concept of a unitary causal factor underlying all cognitive abilities (a "g" factor). It is equated with the capacity for abstract reasoning and problem solving. Common sources of variance among different tests of mental abilities defined the existence of "g." Variance unexplained by this unitary factor was attributed to factors specific (s) to the abilities tested.

In 1904 Alfred Binet, following the request of the Minister of Public Instruction in Paris, developed an intelligence scale for the purpose of identifying intellectually subnormal children attending the Paris schools. Despite the lack of an explicit theory the Binet Intelligence Scale became the root of the individual testing movement in Western Europe and the United States. In its present form it is probably the most widely used intelligence test in the United States (76).

The Stanford-Binet Intelligence Scale Form L-M (1973) and other scales of similar nature such as the Wechsler Intelligence Scale for Children (1949) yield an intelligence quotient (IQ) score which is presumably an expression of the "g" factor. The IQ is a standard score calculated from the total raw score in the scale and the chronological age of the testee. Mental age (MA), usually estimated from the raw score, also reflects the current level of function; it thus differs from the IQ, which tells the rate of mental growth. Accordingly, two children with different chronological ages may have the same MA but different IQs at one point in time.

The existence of "g" is not yet conclusively disproved, but its validity is questioned by studies that fail to find common sources of variance among tests that belong in the intellectual realm (37). Doubt also stems from the poor predictive validity of infant scales or early IQ testing. A correlation coefficient between infant and adolescent mental test scores is not likely to differ from zero. Low correlation cannot be attributed to a lack of test reliability because the test-retest correlations are high if the time interval between tests is short. A better explanation is that substantial developmental changes in the nature of intelligence occur during infancy and the preschool years. Table 1, which presents data from most of the longitudinal studies conducted in the United States, illustrates clearly the low predictive power of early mental testing.

McCall et al. (57) suggested that the stability of performance from infancy or early childhood into adolescence or adulthood is higher in tests of certain specific cognitive abilities than in aggregate measures of intelligence. Similarly, on the basis of some relevant data they suggest that early performance in tests of specific abilities may be better predictors of later IQ than early aggregate measures. For example, timing of early vocalizations among girls

TABLE 1. *Median correlations between infant tests and childhood IQ for normal children*

| Childhood age (years) | Correlation at various ages in infancy | | | |
|---|---|---|---|---|
| | 1–6 months | 7–12 months | 13–18 months | 19–30 months |
| 8–18 | .01 (12/4)[a] | .20 (8/2) | .21 (6/2) | .49 (9/2) |
| 5–7 | .01 (7/5) | .06 (5/4) | .30 (5/4) | .41 (16/4) |
| 3–4 | .23 (7/4) | .33 (5/3) | .47 (6/4) | .54 (16/3) |

[a]Parentheses contain the number of correlations entering into the median/the number of studies included.
From McCall et al., ref. 57.

has an impressive correlation (.74) with IQ data in the mid-20s. While the overall nature of intelligence may change as a function of developmental stage, some specific abilities may be a constant part of intelligence throughout the different developmental levels (57).

In contrast to the above data on normal populations, data on atypical or clinical samples indicate that the predictive power of early testing is greatly enhanced. A series of studies (e.g., 40,49,84) showed that the mental test performance of brain-damaged, "definitely suspect," or mentally retarded children tends to be relatively stable throughout the early and later years of childhood. Nonetheless, the fact remains that, despite a diagnostic validity for true positives, predictive error of infant tests will still be large for false positives. Consider the following example given by McCall (57):

> Suppose a test correctly diagnoses 90% of the infants known to have mental deficiency while incorrectly classifying only 15% of normal infants as being deficient when two groups of 100 definitely abnormals and 100 normals are studied. This would be regarded as an excellent testimony to the validity of the test. However, when a random sample of 1,000 infants is selected, only 50 of whom are truly deficient, while the test correctly identifies 90% or 45 of the abnormals, it also labels 15% or 142 as being deficient

Relevant socioeconomic data collected during early life may be better predictors of childhood IQ than infant intelligence tests. Results from a large collaborative study from the National Institutes of Neurological Diseases and Stroke show, for example, that the 1-year-old IQs of white and black boys and girls were better predicted by either the mother's education or a socioeconomic index than by the scores of a mental scale administered at 8 months of age (12). The predictive power of the social and economic factors is particularly important in connection with samples of young children suspected of having a central nervous system disorder. In these cases prognosis may vary as a function of social-environmental conditions. For example, a well-controlled longitudinal study on the island of Kauai showed that the stability of pediatric neurological signs detected during infancy was related to the social-emotional stability of the home. In stable, organized homes the signs tended to disappear; in unstable, stressful homes the signs remained stable (84). So although the mental test performance of children with very low IQs or neurological damage is relatively stable, it is apparent that in some cases at least it is modifiable by environmental conditions.

Despite atypical examples of dramatic changes in IQ of apparently normal individuals and children exposed to experimental programs of environmental intervention, the test-retest correlations are greatly increased after the age of five. Most relevant studies show correlations on or above .85 when both testings occur during childhood, or even when retesting takes place during the adolescent or adult years (5,9). This stability on test scores indicates that following the preschool years intelligent behavior is dependent on activation of the same types of mental abilities and skills. Accordingly, the notion of a unitary intelligence factor may be meaningful only at approximately age five when an enduring organization of intellectual function is established (4,5,9,57).

Mental tests such as the Stanford-Binet or the Wechsler Scales do not assess innate intellectual potential; instead they tap abilities required by the educational and occupational system in most European and North American countries. These abilities develop as a result of exposure to learning situations modulated by the organization and institutions of those societies. Not surprisingly, therefore, intelligence tests for school-age children have moderately high concurrent or predictive validity in the United States or England in terms of school grades or job achievement (24). Because of cultural fitness serious conceptual and methodological problems arise from the transfer of intelligence tests in whole or in part to societies where the cultural or other ecological factors that contribute to the mental development are different from the countries where the tests were constructed. Evidence now available shows that similar behaviors or activities between culturally different people may not be functionally equivalent, and overtly dissimilar activities may be functionally equivalent (19,27,41).

Despite the widespread recognition of cultural relativism, most researchers on intelligence in developing countries maintain a theoretical position extraneous to the target system. The constructs (i.e., memory, attention, perception) tested are *a priori* defined as universal; moreover, the methodologies used are created by the analyst or adapted from other analysts rather than being discovered in or developed from the system itself. This approach characterizes the studies of malnutrition and mental development. In most cases the methods have been transferred and adapted from the United States or Great Britain to rural or urban slum populations in Latin America or Asia. This transfer rests on the assumption that these methods tap identical psychological constructs regardless of the differences in cultural background, degree of modernization, or ecological conditions.

In some studies on malnutrition discussed in the next section, new norms and standardization procedures have been carefully developed, giving normative validity to the tests. However, normative and construct validity[1] are different issues of test validation (25). Norms bear no overt reference to the nature of the construct behind the test and, most importantly, to the functional significance within the society in question. Within-group differences in the original and new samples may have different significance in terms of an outside criterion. The definition of this criterion in the group to be studied is the key issue.

An approach appropriate or *ad hoc* to the notion of cultural relativism has

---

[1]Construct validation "is evaluated by investigating what psychological qualities a test measures; i.e., by determining the degree to which certain explanatory concepts or constructs account for performance on the test" [American Psychological Association definition adapted by R. Cronbach (25)].

been avoided in most research on intelligence, probably because of its obvious cost and practical complexity. It essentially requires a definition of constructs before test construction. Such definition in turn requires direct observation of culturally representative behaviors and analysis of the processes involved in them. Essentially this is a culturally or ecologically functional approach that calls for the assessment of meaningful behaviors in relation to a particular society. No research published in the area of malnutrition and behavior has used this approach.

In summary, this brief review of psychometric theory and methods suggests that the notion of a unitary intelligence factor is not applicable to infants and children younger than 5 years of age. Early development is characterized by the changing nature and organization of mental abilities. Thus early mental testing may have concurrent but no predictive validity, except for atypical or clinical samples. Socioeconomic status has higher predictive validity than early IQ scores. Accuracy in prediction gradually increases at the beginning of the school-age period.

The review also pointed out that not only the tests but also the constructs behind the tests and their organization probably are culturally dependent. Accordingly, transfer of mental tests from the United States or Great Britain to rural or urban slum populations in Third World countries requires construct validation. Normative validation facilitates statistical comparisons within groups and permits estimate of the relative standing of an individual or a subsample; however, it is not a substitute for construct validity.

## II. MALNUTRITION AND BEHAVIOR: FINDINGS, CRITICISMS, AND CONCLUSION

Protein-calorie malnutrition (PCM)—a condition in which an individual, usually a child, is suffering from an inadequate dietary supply of proteins, calories, or a combination of the two—was first described around the turn of the century. Since that time, the condition has been identified and studied in countries throughout the world. Severe malnutrition is estimated to afflict approximately 0.5–20.0% of the world's population; the prevalence of more moderate PCM ranges from 3.5 to 46.4% (6). Table 2, which presents data on estimated prevalence of moderate and severe degrees of malnutrition in Latin America, Africa, and Asia, clearly identifies moderate malnutrition as a major problem in Third World countries.

This chapter is concerned with the data available on the behavioral effects of both severe and moderate degrees of malnutrition. Discussion of the numerous design and methodological problems associated with these data is interwoven with the review of pertinent studies.

*Marasmus* and *kwashiorkor* are considered the major forms of severe PCM. Generally, marasmus is the result of starvation or semistarvation where intake of both calories and proteins is insufficient. Kwashiorkor is attributed

TABLE 2. *Prevalence of protein-calorie malnutrition in community studies (1963–1972)*

| Region | No. of communities | No. of surveys | No. of children examined | Protein-calorie malnutrition (%) | | |
|---|---|---|---|---|---|---|
| | | | | Severe | Moderate | Severe and moderate |
| Latin America | 20 | 29 | 116,179 | 0–12.0 | 3.5–32.0 | 4.6–37.0 |
| Africa | 16 | 32 | 34,184 | 0–9.8 | 5.6–66.0 | 7.3–73.0 |
| Asia | 10 | 16 | 43,326 | 0–20.0 | 13.0–73.8 | 14.8–80.3 |
| Total | 46 | 77 | 193,689 | 0–20.0 | 3.5–73.8 | 4.6–80.3 |

From Bengoa, ref. 6.

to a lack of proteins relative to the intake of calories. These two conditions, however, are thought to form the extremes of a continuum describing severe PCM. More commonly, severely malnourished children either exhibit signs of both conditions and lie at some point between these two extremes, or alternate between the two (75). *Marasmic-kwashiorkor* is sometimes used to describe a condition where signs of the two syndromes are seen in combination (82).

Figure 1 shows an obtuse triangle which represents the development of the different types of protein malnutrition in children. The side labeled N-M illustrates the starving child, gradually passing through different stages of PCM severity. Line N-K represents the child who receives adequate calories but is deprived of proteins. Finally, the K-M base describes a continuous spectrum between marasmus and kwashiorkor.

Waterlow and Rutishauser (83) believe that marasmus and kwashiorkor have different natural histories, and they described two distinct growth patterns, depicted in Fig. 2. It appears that in kwashiorkor there is a nearly normal growth pattern until around 6–8 months when weight for age begins to decrease sharply to approximately 60–80% of the standard by 14–18 months (Boston Growth Norms) (66). With marasmus, on the other hand, poor growth is seen from birth and a large deficit in weight for age (<60% of standard) is apparent during the first few months of life. These chronological differences

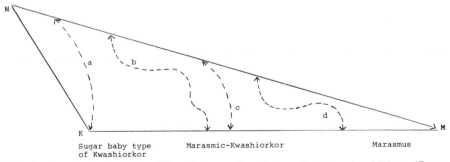

FIG. 1. Development of the different types of protein malnutrition in children. (From Scrimshaw and Behar, ref. 75.)

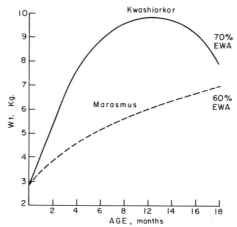

**FIG. 2.** Hypothetical natural histories of kwashiorkor and marasmus, showing percent of expected weight for age (EWA) for each syndrome. (From Cravioto et al., ref. 23*a*.)

between the two syndromes were also explicated by McLaren (59) in Lebanon through the identification of different events that precipitate the development of marasmus and kwashiorkor. Figure 3 illustrates the progression of these events. Marasmus is preceded by early abrupt weaning, which leads to the intake of diluted dirty formula, resulting in repeated infections (especially

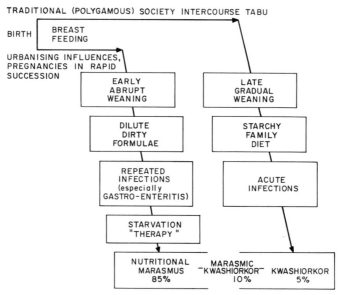

**FIG. 3.** Paths leading from early weaning to nutritional marasmus and from protracted breast feeding to kwashiorkor. Percentages of types of malnutrition are based on figures for Jordan but are typical for many other countries. (From McLaren, ref. 59.)

gastroenteritis). These recurrent infections are treated by fasting the child, a procedure that eventually results in full-blown marasmus. The pathway leading to kwashiorkor is identified by a later, more gradual (6–8 months) weaning that is subsequently followed by intake of the family diet, largely consisting of carbohydrates. This high-carbohydrate, low-protein diet increases the susceptibility of the child to acute infections. Physiological stress from illness coupled with the low-protein diet often results in kwashiorkor.

Lack of data on the premorbid development of marasmic and kwashiorkor children makes it difficult to validate the diagnostic assertions on the different forms of PCM. Probably large variations exist among the etiological factors coming into play in both syndromes. This variability may be a function of geographical area, sociocultural (including dietary) practices, and rate of infection. Nonetheless, available cross-sectional, postmorbid data make feasible some conclusions relevant to an assessment of the effects of PCM on behavior: (a) Kwashiorkor is more likely to be an acute rather than a chronic condition; marasmus, by definition, is chronic. (b) Kwashiorkor is more likely to appear after the first year of life, whereas marasmus usually develops throughout the early months of life. (c) Kwashiorkor is largely the result of a dietary deficiency, whereas marasmus is likely to have multiple causes.

Behavioral symptoms associated with acute kwashiorkor have been well documented in clinical reports (2,33,42). Anorexia, apathy, withdrawal, and irritability often accompanied by a whimpering, monotonous cry are commonly observed. In some extreme cases the child becomes immobile, lying "absolutely quiet in a fetal position with open eyes staring at nothing" (42). These behavioral changes have been attributed to a variety of alterations in the organism which Jelliffe (42) classifies into four areas: biochemical, biophysical, anatomical, and psychological. Biochemical changes include low values for plasma proteins (2), an imbalance between essential and nonessential amino acids, reduced enzyme secretions, and edema appearing in various areas of the body (2,82). Biophysical changes include electroencephalographic (EEG) abnormalities, hypothermia (10,42), alterations in the mucous membranes, and dyspigmentation of the skin (2). Anatomical changes which include cortical and subcortical atrophy (56), hypotonia, and poorly developed motor skills are almost always present. In some extreme cases affected children give no measurable responses to items on mental development scales (33).

Reduced brain weight, cortical atrophy, hypotonia, and reduced activity have also been associated with the marasmic condition (56,85). In contrast to kwashiorkor, however, the marasmic infant or child is often hungry (58). Arrest or severe growth retardation with marked loss of subcutaneous fat are pathognomonic signs of the marasmic condition.

Of all the behavioral symptoms associated with kwashiorkor or marasmus, that of reduced activity, or lethargy, is the most commonly observed. While no empirical evidence exists to correlate this lethargy with psychological depression, the association is a likely possibility. If the malnourished child were depressed, a number of cognitive and motivational alterations would be expected. Among these alterations would be irritability, easy frustration, some delayed speech, and short attention span (67).

Empirical evidence of specific alterations in attention have been reported by Lester and co-investigators in Guatemala (52,53). Two experiments were conducted with male infants approximately 1 year of age, who were suffering from second- and third-degree malnutrition, using the Gomez classification. The control group had average expected weights for age. Attentional processes were assessed by measuring heart rate deceleration to novel auditory stimuli. Heart rate deceleration has been found to correlate with the orienting reflex to a novel stimulus. When the individual becomes accustomed to the stimulus, habituation occurs and cardiac deceleration decreases. These physiological responses measure responsivity to the environment and attention (48).

In the second and more rigorous experiment, the responses of 20 malnourished male infants to 750 and 400 Hz at 90 db showed *no cardiac orienting* to the onset or change of the stimuli tones. Conversely, well-nourished children evidenced cardiac orienting response to both onset and change of tone, and subsequent habituation to repeated stimuli. Figure 4 shows the percentage of well- and malnourished infants who displayed the behavior orienting response (BOR) to the tones. Well-nourished infants showed a gradual decrease in BOR with a small recovery on trials 11 and 16. Malnourished infants failed to display the BOR above the 10% level on any trial.

These cardiac habituation data suggest that a state of severe protein and energy deficiency includes a diminished responsivity to environmental signals and therefore a reduction in the organism's capacity for information processing. As becomes evident later, it is probable that following nutritional rehabilitation the attentional deficit may persist. Klein et al. (48) suggest that an attentional deficit may lie behind the often-reported poor performance of severely malnourished children on psychological tests.

Graves (36) investigated the social dimension of lethargic behavior in the malnourished child in Nepal, India. Twenty-three index children suffering from second-degree malnutrition at the time of testing were studied. The focus of the study was on exploratory behavior and mother-child interaction. Developmental test performance and socioeconomic and nutritional-developmental status of each child were also assessed. A salient finding in this novel study was that older (13–18 months) malnourished children displayed significantly less vigor in their exploratory behavior and less social interaction with their mothers. However, maternal responsiveness was reduced toward the malnourished as compared to the well-nourished children. These behavioral differences were not significant for the younger groups. Also, no differences between groups were found on developmental test performance.

Although the two studies just discussed (36,52) fail to specify the type of

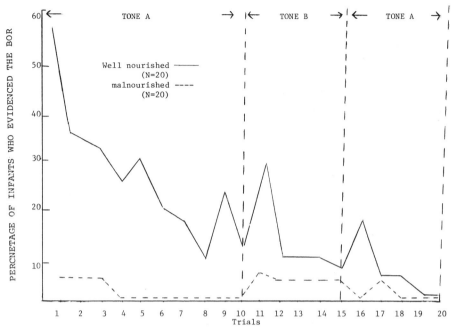

**FIG. 4.** Percentage of well-nourished and malnourished infants in experiment 2 who showed the behavioral orienting response (BOR). With the infant seated in his mother's lap, 3 tones (750 Hz, 400 Hz and 750 Hz) were presented for a total of 20 trials for 5 sec. each at 90 db. Measures of heart rate and BOR (movement of head or eyes in the direction of the sound speaker) were obtained for each trial. Approximately 58% of the well-nourished infants displayed BOR on trial 1 and showed some recovery on trials 11 and 16; whereas, the BOR of malnourished infants did not rise above 10% on any trial. (From Lester, ref. 52.)

childhood malnutrition studied (i.e., marasmus, kwashiorkor, or marasmic-kwashiorkor), they provide excellent quantitative data that make clinical observations on children with severe protein-calorie deficiency more meaningful.

The anecdotal and experimental data reviewed justify the conclusion that in conditions of severe protein and energy deficiency the child exhibits a low responsivity to environmental stimuli and poor attention maintenance. Inferentially, it can also be concluded that the child's monotonous behavior ensures that he will function as a low-key stimulus in competing for the attention of others in the environment.

A corollary to these conclusions is that severe malnutrition places the child in double jeopardy in regard to his intellectual growth. There is an impoverishment in learning experiences secondary to the reductions in the reciprocal mother–child interaction, as well as a limitation of the organism's capabilities to act on his environment. The former may obviously limit the accumulation of useful information for subsequent developmental adaptation. The latter, perhaps even more importantly, indicates that protein-calorie deficiency inter-feres with the very axis of intellectual development. According to Piaget's theory (31) of intelligence, the organism and the environment act as an interlocking system. Progressive developmental changes leading toward successful adaptation are partly dependent on the child's active *search* for solutions of internal disequilibrium. This latter state results from discrepancies between the changing level of competence of the organism and the increasing demands of the environment. Search implies a dynamic process, an action on the environment. Thus in Piagetian terms, under conditions of severe and chronic deprivations of energy and proteins where organism and environment do not function as interlocking systems, it is understandable that developmental retardation may result.

In contrast to the severe forms of PCM, there is no clearly distinct set of behavioral symptoms or other clinical signs associated with mild-to-moderate malnutrition except for some degree of retarded physical growth. In effect, the latter feature alone is often used as a selection criterion in distinguishing malnourished from adequately or well-nourished children. Other alleged characteristics of chronic mild-to-moderate PCM (i.e., reduced head circumference and retardation of intellectual functions) are not well substantiated and cannot be regarded as definitive factors.

The literature review that follows is divided into two main sections. The first focuses on severe PCM; it includes studies on marasmus, kwashiorkor, and undifferentiated or mixed types. It also includes a brief review on secondary malnutrition, or malnutrition stemming from neonatal disorders. The second section looks at the literature on mild-to-moderate malnutrition and includes a study on the effects of famine in an industrialized country.

### A. Marasmus, Kwashiorkor, and Undifferentiated or Mixed Studies

Tables 3 through 5 summarize the research that has been done on severe malnutrition. Most of these data have been reviewed in detail elsewhere (68) and are presented here in tabular form to facilitate discussion.

Except for one study—that of Cravioto and DeLicardie (21), depicted in Table 5—all studies on severe PCM have used retrospective research designs and so no data exist on the children's developmental characteristics prior to the onset of malnutrition. Birth weights, morbidity, and data on achievements of developmental landmarks are generally lacking. The chronology of events and evidence on whether the signs of intellectual impairment preceded or followed the episode of postnatal malnutrition remain unknown.

Matching index and control children for demographic, social, and economic correlates of intelligence has been a strategy used to cope with the flaws inherent in the *ex post facto* design. This approach is salient in the study by Champakam et al. (15) (Table 4), who matched the children in both groups for age, sex, birth order, family size, caste, religion, socioeconomic status, and educational background of the parents. Despite such thorough research, it is likely that matching underestimates the number of variables that really differentiate malnourished and well-nourished children. Natural exposure to an independent variable such as undernutrition must represent what has been described in connection with other research endeavors as the "lawful product of numerous antecedents" (14). For example, there must be differences in child care practices leading to substantially different states of nutrition.

A few studies have used siblings of the index children as controls, as in that of Pollitt and Granoff (69) in Table 3 and of Birch et al. (8) in Table 4. Rationale for this approach is that the environmental correlates of malnutrition which influence intellectual development remain constant if the household is the same for both index and controls. However, such an approach may well have resulted in selective unmatching. Development of undernutrition in one child in an environment where a sibling is well nourished indicates either differential treatment, differential response to the treatment, or a combination of both conditions. Thus the apparent control is deceptive.

*Ex post facto* designs used in the studies of severe protein-calorie malnutrition make it impossible to determine whether index and control children would have been equivalent had it not been for the nutritional conditions. Actually, data on the developmental characteristics and social-familial background of children who become severely malnourished suggest that an assumption of equivalence is likely to be incorrect. Evidence to this effect is found among studies on the behavioral effects of PCM and on so-called social-ecological studies of malnutrition. In the former group the best illustration is the work by Richardson and co-workers (39,72,73,74) (Table 5). These studies were based on a sample of Jamaican malnourished children whose intellectual performance was found to be below that of their siblings and peers (39) (Table 5).

With the mental test data at hand, Richardson and co-investigators researched the social and biological background of the index versus the comparison groups (72). Interviews were conducted with the child's principal caretaker (mother or guardian) in which questions on caretaking capability, mother's health and pregnancy, economic and housing conditions, mortality, and social and educational experiences of the target child were asked. Results indicated that index children differed significantly ($p = 0.05$ or better) from comparison children on a number of important environmental factors. The index child had poorer housing (structure, furnishings, and crowding), a more disadvantaged caretaker (availability of human resources, poorer caretaker upbringing and education), less intellectual stimulation, and less schooling in addition to higher mortality among siblings.

Studies in Latin American (35,87), Asia (54,71), and Africa (44) corroborate Richardson's findings (72) on social-environmental idiosyncrasies among families of malnourished children which jeopardize cognitive growth. These data show that families of children with third-degree malnutrition are often unstable, live under extremely crowded conditions, or are more financially disad-

TABLE 3. Summary of behavioral studies of children with nutritional marasmus

| Study | Experimental subjects | | No. and description of control Ss (if any) | Age of experimental and control Ss at evaluation | Test used and type of measure obtained | Results |
|---|---|---|---|---|---|---|
| | No. and description of nutritional condition | Age at time of hospital admission | | | | |
| Brockman and Ricciuti (11) | N = 20 Diagnosed as marasmus; body weight less than 50% of expected for age; free of apparent edema; normal serum albumin | Mean of 10 younger children: 9.2 mo Mean of 10 older children: 16.2 mo | N = 19 Matched for sex and age with patients; attended regularly day care centers of Lima slums; body length at or above 10th percentile of Boston growth curves | Experimental: mean of 10 younger children: 17.9 mo; mean of 10 older children: 34.9 mo Controls: mean of 9 younger children: 18.7 mo; mean of 10 older children: 33.8 mo | Categorization behavior through 10 sorting of 8 objects each | Average test scores:<br>       < 24 mo  > 24 mo<br>Exp.    9.2       20.0<br>Cont.  21.0     40.0 |
| Cabak and Najdanvic (13) | N = 36 Marasmus; slight edema present in a few; 27% or below the correct weight for their age; no TB or CNS diseases | 4–24 mo; most were below 12 mo | | 7–14 yr | Adaptation of the Binet-Simon Scale: IQ | Mean IQ 88; IQ frequency distribution:<br>N  IQ range<br>18  91–110<br>12  71–90<br>6   ≤70<br>Mean IQs of children from two nearby communities: 101 and 109 |
| McLaren et al. (60) | N = 30 Groups Us and S: same children as in | | N = 15 Healthy; matched for age and | Means: Group Us 42 mo Group S 49 mo | Stanford-Binet Intelligence Scale: IQ | Mean IQ: Group S 78.9 Sibs 92.2 |

| Reference | Subjects | Age at onset | Comparison group | Age at testing | Test | Results |
|---|---|---|---|---|---|---|
| Yaktin and McLaren (88) | N = 15 Group U: moderately undernourished for ca. 3 yr no hospitalization | | socioeconomic status N = 14 Healthy sibs of group S N = 15 Healthy sibs of group Us N = 15 Healthy sibs of group U | Group U 62 mo Group C 37 mo | | Group Us 86.1 Sibs 94.9 Group U 87.7 Sibs 94.9 Control 98.7 |
| Monckeberg (64) | N = 14 Severe marasmic malnutrition | 3–11 mo (mean 6.2 mo) | | 3–6 years | "Binet Method:" Intelligence Quotient | Mean IQ 62: no child with IQ above 76 |
| Pollitt and Granoff (69) | N = 19 Weight deficit of 40% or more for age; free from edema; normal serum albumin | 6–8 mo (mean 16 mo) | N = 28 Sibs of patients; no history of malnutrition | Experimental: 11–32 mo (mean 22 mo) Control: 3–30 mo (mean 9 mo) | Bayley Scales of mental and motor development: mental DQ, motor DQ | Results reported on mean sigma scores. Mental scale Motor scale. Exp: −4.05 −3.76; Cont: −0.70 −5.50 |
| Yaktin and McLaren (88) | N = 30 Acute, severe marasmus; 53% of 50th percentile Boston standard for weight | 2.5–16 mo (mean 8 mo) | | Tested on admission and subsequently every 2 weeks for 14 weeks | Griffiths Mental Development Scale: DQ | Mean DQ on admission: stimulated 51, unstimulated 46 DQ at end of 14 weeks: stimulated ≅ 79, unstimulated ≅ 68 |

TABLE 4. *Summary of behavioral studies of children with kwashiorkor*

| Study | Experimental subjects | | | No. and description of control Ss (if any) | Age of experimental and control Ss at evaluation | Test used and type of measure obtained | Results |
|---|---|---|---|---|---|---|---|
| | No. and description of nutritional condition | Age at time of hospital admission | | | | | |
| Barreda-Moncada (3) | N = 60 Growth retardation; skin change; edema; psychic changes; hair changes; liver hypertrophy | 15.7–71.0 mo | | | 60 cases tested 7–12 wk after hospital admission; 75% of cases evaluated 2 yr later | Gesell Schedules: DQ | After 7–12 weeks of hospitalization: DQ 65 (expected 100) Marked retardation in language (DQ 50–60); most improvements in motor development (DQ 74); after 2 yr DQ 61–88 |
| Birch et al. (8) | N = 37 Edema; skin lesions; evidence of fewer dietary proteins than calories | 6–30 mo | | N = 37 Healthy sibs | Experimental: 5–13 yr Control: 5–12 yr | Wechsler Intelligence Scale for Children: IQ | Mean IQ index 68.5 Control 81.5 |
| Champakam et al. (15) | N = 19 "Classic signs of kwashiorkor" | 18–36 mo (mean 27.1 mo) | | N = 50 Control matched for: age, sex, religion, caste, SES, family size | Experimental: 8–11 yr (mean 9.2 yr) Control: 8–11 yr (mean 10.1 yr) | Intelligence test; subscales in four areas: memory, perception, abstraction, verbal Intersensory development: | Performance of experimental Ss on IQ test expressed as % of the controls: *Age (yr)*    *Mean %* 8–9      31.30 9–10     54.45 10–11    52.44 Greatest difference in |

| Reference | Subjects (N / Criteria) | Age | Testing | Measures | Results |
|---|---|---|---|---|---|
| | | | | visual-haptic, visual-kinesthetic, haptic-kinesthetic | abstract and perceptual abilities; Intersensory organization poorer in experimentals than controls; Difference between groups decreased as age increased |
| Cravioto and Robles (22) | N = 20; Third-degree protein-calorie malnutrition; presence of edema | 6–30 mo | 1 yr after hospitalization | Gesell Schedules: DQ | Younger (<6 mo): Ss performance decreased with increased hospitalization; Older Ss (>6 mo): performance improved to nearly normal with hospitalization |
| Evans et al. (29) | N = 40; Documented history of kwashiorkor; N = 40 Sibs of experimental Ss matched for age | 10–48 mo (mean 19.6 mo) | Experimental: mean 11.5 yr; Control: mean 11 yr | New S. African Individual Scale: intelligence score; Goodenough-Harris Drawing Test: drawing score | Intelligence score / Drawing score: Exp. 77 / 76; Cont. 78 / 80; Av. normal 83 |
| Gerber and Dean (33) | N = 25; Conformed to description of kwashiorkor | 23 Ss: 1–3 yr | Tested during hospitalization | Gesell Developmental Schedules | All Ss scored moderately at hospital release |

TABLE 5. Summary of behavioral studies dealing with mixed or undifferentiated protein-calorie malnutrition

| Study | Experimental subjects | | No. and description of control Ss (if any) | Age of experimental and control Ss at evaluation | Test used and type of measure obtained | Results |
|---|---|---|---|---|---|---|
| | No. and description of nutritional condition | Age at time of hospital admission | | | | |
| Chase and Martin (16) | N = 19 Diagnosed as undernourished: weight-age/height-age ratio < 1 | 1.5–10.0 mo (2 Ss readmitted at 18 and 24 mo) | N = 19 Matched for: birth date, place of birth, weight, sex, race | Experimental: 24–41 mo; Control: 24–41 mo | Yale Revised Developmental Examination: DQ | Mean DQ: index 82, control 99. Lowest score of index group was in language area; index children admitted >4 mo of age show lower scores than those admitted <4 mo |
| Cravioto and DeLicardie (21) | N = 22 Clinical kwashiorkor and marasmus (10 treated at home, 12 hospitalized) | 4–53 mo | Healthy; matched at birth for gestational age, body length, and weight | Experimental and control: birth to 58 mo | Gesell Developmental Schedule: language development score; Bipolar concept test: bipolar concept score; Bettye Caldwell Inventory: home stimulation score | Index had lower language development score than controls from ca. 1 to 3 yr. Index had lower bipolar concept scores from 26 to 58 mo. Index scored lower on home stimulation score at 6 and 48 mo |
| DeLicardie and Cravioto (26) | N = 14 Subset of above children | 4–38 mo | Group CB: Subset of children in above group (ref. 21); Group CIQS: Children matched at age 5 for IQ and sex | Experimental and control: 5 yr | Adaptation of Wechsler Preschool and Primary Scale; Behavioral response to cognitive demands | Index gave smaller proportion of work responses to cognitive demands than either group CB or CIQS. Index gave fewer verbal responses than |

| Study | Malnourished sample | Age | Control | Age at testing | Method | Findings |
|---|---|---|---|---|---|---|
| Fisher et al. (30) | N = 72<br>Kwashiorkor 44<br>Marasmus 12<br>Marasmic-kwashiorkor 13<br>Unclassified 3 | Mean 1.6 yr | N = 143 | Index: 9.6–16.5 yr<br>Control: 10.2–15.2 yr | Derivation of Koh's Blocks and a test requiring completion of two matrices | Experimental group did "consistently" poorer than control; no statistics available |
| Hertzig et al. (39) | N = 71<br>Diagnosed as having marasmus, kwashiorkor, or marasmic-kwashiorkor | < 2 yr | N = 71 Classmates of same sex and similar age<br>N = 38 Healthy, male sibs | Experimental: 5 yr 11 mo to 10 yr<br>Sibs: 6 yr to 12 yr 11 mo<br>Control: 5 yr to 10 yr 11 mo | Wechsler Intelligence Scale for children: IQ | Mean IQ:<br>Index 57.7<br>Siblings 61.8<br>Control 66.0 |
| Klein et al. (48) | N = 8<br>Severely malnourished | | N = 8 Adequately nourished | Experimental: 14 mo | Cardiac habituation | Index required more trials to respond to a novel auditory stimulus |
| | N = 17 Malnourished | | N = 11 Adequately nourished | Experimental: 5–6 yr | Eleven psychological tests | Index performed more poorly on tests requiring high level of attention |
| Richardson (72) | N = 71 Same children as Hertzig et al. (39) | | Control group not investigated | | Home interviews with mothers or guardians: socioeconomic and environmental data | Index had poorer housing and more disadvantaged caretaker, less schooling, and higher sibling mortality |
| Richardson et al. (73) | Same index group as above except N reduced to 62 | | Same as above plus sib control group (N = 31) | Same as above (ref. 72) | Wide Range Achievement Test: reading spelling, arithmetic | Index averaged 7–9 points lower on WRAT than controls; index and sibs obtain nearly identical scores |

TABLE 5. (continued)

| | Experimental subjects | | No. and description of control Ss (if any) | Age of experimental and control Ss at evaluation | Test used and type of measure obtained | Results |
|---|---|---|---|---|---|---|
| Study | No. and description of nutritional condition | Age at time of hospital admission | | | | |
| | | | | | Teacher evaluation | Teacher evaluations lower for index than controls; no difference between sibs and their comparison groups |
| | | | | | Median school grade | Index had lower median grade than controls; no differences between sibs and their comparisons |
| Richardson et al. (74) | Same as above (ref. 73) | | Healthy; same sex sibs  Classmates of same sex and similar age | | Home interviews with mothers or guardians; behavioral data | Index Ss were less liked by sibs, more unhappy in school, and behaved more immaturely, clumsily, and unsociably than controls; sibs did not differ from their comparisons |

280

vantaged than the average family from the same locality. The mothers are more likely to be illiterate or have fewer years of education and have more health problems than mothers of well-nourished children. Moreover, although some studies (21) (Table 5) failed to find differences in graduated parameters of social structure between families of well-nourished and malnourished children, they did find differences in specific behaviors of maternal care in the expected direction. Thus socioeconomic and behavioral distinctions made *between* populations with and without prevalent problems of malnutrition may also be applied *within* a population where malnutrition is endemic in order to differentiate those families which have children with severe malnutrition from those families that do not.

Among the studies on severe malnutrition, the research design in the work of Cravioto and DeLicardie (20,21,26) (Table 5) in Mexico stands alone. Their longitudinal approach allows collection of extensive postnatal developmental data beginning at birth. Thus antecedents of children who became malnourished before the age of five are identified. Within this context the importance of the specific timing of onset of the nutritional deprivation, its clinical nature, and its final course are emphasized. Such data are simply unavailable elsewhere. It is unfortunate, however, that among the reports we reviewed on this Mexican study there are no data on the duration of deficiency for each of the index children.

In addition to the flaws inherent in the research design, there are also serious limitations associated with the measurement of the dependent variable among the studies on PCM. Except in two cases—studies by Brockman and Ricciuti (11) (Table 3) and by Cravioto and DeLicardie (20,21,26) (Table 5)— all research on primary malnutrition focused on mental tests of global intelligence such as the Wechsler or Bayley Scales. Researchers made between-group statistical comparisons of mean IQs or development quotients (DQs) in order to infer differences in levels of intellectual function. Discrimination in the test scores was taken as indicative of substantive differences between the index and control children in competence of the alleged test construct. In this conceptual leap the investigators implicitly assumed that if the normative validity of the test is transferable from one culture to another then the construct validity can also be immediately transferred. However, this assumption disregards indications from test data that the tests do not behave in the same manner as in the culture in which the test was developed. This point is made more clear in the example discussed below.

Hertzig et al. (39) (Table 5) reported that the control group ($N = 71$) in their study on severely malnourished Jamaican children had a mean Wechsler Full Scale IQ of 65.99 (SD 13.59); the IQs of the index ($N = 71$) and sibling ($N = 83$) groups were 57.72 (SD 10.75) and 61.84 (SD 10.82), respectively. All between-group comparisons among the three groups studied were statistically significant at the 0.10 level or better. Still, the controls' IQ, the highest of the three groups, is approximately four points below the IQ level used as the cutoff point between the retardate and nonretardate level in the United States. However, 41% of the controls were rated by their teachers as having outstanding, good, or above-average school work; only 28% of this sample were rated as doing poor or severely backward work (73). A significant relationship was found ($X^2 = 6.74$; $p < 0.025$) between the overall evaluation of school performance and the Full Scale IQ among the control children. In spite of this latter evidence of concurrent validity, there is a conceptual discrepancy in terms of intellectual behavior between a mean IQ of 65.99 and the school performance of the children. This discrepancy perhaps could be reconciled if these children were in special education programs. Under such conditions the IQ and rating criteria may have convergent meanings. However, no reported data support such a possibility. Thus one must accept these data *prima facie* and assume that unidentified cultural and social idiosyncracies of the populations from which the samples were selected could explain such discrepancies. Otherwise, one must question the meaning attributed to the test IQ scores; this is particularly true when the between-group differences, although statistically significant at some arbitrarily set probability level, are relatively small and do not convey specific behavioral significance.

The two studies—those of Brockman and Ricciuti (11) in Table 3 and Cravioto and DeLicardie (21) in Table 5—that used tests for specific cognitive processes (categorization and bipolar concepts) do not give any rationale for their selection. Evidently the assumption behind the choice is that the specific cognitive construct allegedly tested is central to overall cognitive development. However, in both conditions some immediate problems are apparent. Cravioto and DeLicardie's task is heavily dependent on language skills, which are likely to be particularly sensitive to social-environmental influences. In connection with the task selected by Brockman and Ricciuti, it should be indicated that there is no work yet done on the predictive, concurrent, or construct validity of the test.

Aside from the problematic research issues discussed, an analysis of the findings from the studies summarized in Tables 3–5 provides a basis for a few inferences. For this purpose the following observations are pertinent. First, the set of studies on marasmic children is the only one that reports uniform findings. By contrast, there are both negative and positive findings among the kwashiorkor studies. Secondly, the magnitude of the cognitive deficits observed among some of the marasmic children is much higher than among any of the children included in all the remaining studies on severe malnutrition. Among the studies of marasmus there is a performance pattern of approximately 1–2 SD below that of the control groups. Third, except for one study that included an intervention program—that of Yaktin and McLaren (88), none of the studies on marasmic children report any amelioration with age. Conversely, in addition to two reports of negative findings, the studies of children with kwashiorkor yielding positive results show that either the magnitude of the deficit is relatively small or that such deficits ameliorate with age.

Differential patterns of development in nutritional marasmus and kwashiorkor (Fig. 2) may lie behind the differences in the magnitude of the deficits observed in the two syndromes. Kwashiorkor is likely to be an acute condition with onset during the second year of life, whereas marasmus is a chronic condition with possible prenatal or early postnatal onset. Thus differences in clinical signs and biochemical profiles between the two syndromes are combined with differences in timing, history, and duration.

The importance of chronology in nutritional marasmus to explain its behavioral sequelae is based on two reasons. First, it occurs during a period of peak velocity in brain growth. Second, it produces a lengthy deterioration in child-environment interaction. In the case of severe but acute malnutrition occurring during the second year of life, the chances of mental rehabilitation are enhanced. In addition to lessened brain vulnerability, the child's contact with the environment is only temporarily interrupted.

In connection with relationships between timing of onset and vulnerability, note that a few studies included in Tables 3–5 tried to establish the covariation between age at hospitalization and magnitude of subsequent intellectual deficit; see, for example, the studies of Cravioto and Robles (22) in Table 4 and Chase and Martin (16) in Table 5. However, most studies have no data on the nutritional status and developmental characteristics of the target children before hospitalization. Therefore there is likely to be a large error in the estimated time of onset, and it is not surprising that there is no uniformity in the findings regarding periods of larger or smaller vulnerability. Our impression of the data now available is that they do not lend themselves to the formation of valid inferences regarding the degree of vulnerability of intellectual function as a function of relatively small ($\pm 6$ months) age periods during the first 2 years of life. Valid comparisons in this regard are limited to gross time periods such as those comparing the first with the second year of life.

The following conclusions can now be advanced:

1. Severe protein-calorie deficiency occurring throughout most of the first 12 months of life among populations where malnutrition is endemic results in a severe deficit (1–2 SD below the average of 100) in intellectual function (DQ) as compared to standards from the same population.

2. Severe but acute protein-calorie deficiency occurring during the second year of life among populations where malnutrition is endemic may, but generally does not, leave measurable retardation in intellectual function (DQ) as compared to standards from the same population.

3. There are no available current data to determine whether severe but acute episodes of protein-calorie malnutrition with an onset during the second year of life result in any impairment of intellectual function.

## B. Secondary Malnutrition

The studies available on malnutrition secondary to neonatal disorders such as cystic fibrosis, pyloric stenosis, and other gastrointestinal disorders appear in Table 6. In all cases malnutrition results from interference with digestion of food and absorption of nutrients. A rationale for the conduct of these studies has been that since these disorders are not limited to the lower socioeconomic strata, assessment of the nutritional variable out of the context of poverty is feasible.

Studies on secondary malnutrition also have used retrospective research designs and are therefore subject to criticisms similar to those formulated in connection with research on marasmus, kwashiorkor, and severe undifferentiated PCM. A major additional problem with these studies arises from the very fact that the malnutrition variable is divorced from the poverty variable; i.e., conclusions from them may not be generalizable to situations where the two factors coexist. Both variables may have interactive rather than independent effects, so that the effects of malnutrition may be modified by the socioeconomic context in which malnutrition occurs. (For an excellent discussion of the importance of *context* on behavioral research see Kruglanski, ref. 51). This consideration is especially important if the studies on secondary malnutrition yield negative findings; adverse nutritional effects may ameliorate or disappear if the child is raised in a protected and educationally oriented environment. Conceptual and empirical data on interactions between biological stress factors and social-environmental variables were discussed in Section I of this chapter.

Furthermore, results from the studies on secondary malnutrition are not uniform. Concurrence of findings would have heightened their significance since they were based only on tentative assumptions and hypotheses given the retrospective nature of the study design.

## C. Mild-to-Moderate PCM

1. Field studies

Comparatively little work has been done on the moderately or mildly malnourished child. Nonetheless, excellent recent attempts at description of intellectual functioning and physical growth associated with mild-to-moderate PCM have been and are being completed by researchers in Colombia, Guatemala, and Mexico. As in the studies on severe PCM, the effects of mild-to-moderate malnutrition on mental development are intimately interwoven with the effects of genetic and social environmental factors. The state of the art still does not allow causal statements regarding the unique effects of nutritional insult on human intelligence. However, considerable progress has been made toward understanding the nature of the relationships between the variables involved.

Among the reasons for the difference between the large number of studies on severe PCM and the relatively small number of reports on mild-to-moderate PCM have been the costs involved and the availability of samples. The samples of children with third-degree malnutrition are small. Also (except for Cravioto's sample in Mexico) they are, at one time or another, a captive population available to the researchers through hospitals or nutrition research facilities. The studies on mild-to-moderate malnutrition are field studies in rural villages or urban slums. They necessitate building institutional facilities in order to deal with large study samples. Furthermore, while most retrospective studies on severe malnutrition were limited to a cross-sectional approach, most research on mild-to-moderate malnutrition employed a longitudinal design.

The field studies on mild-to-moderate malnutrition are here classified into two main groups according to their treatment of the independent variable and their research designs. The first group includes three studies (23,47,86) in which there was no experimental manipulation; the nutritional variable was defined only by anthropometric measures, and the study was retrospective. The second set includes studies from four research projects (18,46,62,65) where there is controlled nutritional—and in one case psychoeducational—intervention, and the study designs are prospective. Additionally, one study (78), on the effects of short-term famine in an industrialized country, is treated separately. In this case malnutrition does not coexist with poverty as is the case with the studies included in the two main groups.

Table 7 summarizes the three studies in group I. These studies are retrospective and use height and weight data to define the nutrition variable. It is now recognized that the use of nutritional anthropometry as the only definition of the nutrition variable introduces a large error in studies on the behavioral effects of malnutrition (38,70). Thus the contributions that these studies make to the understanding of the malnutrition-behavior relationship is limited indeed. Consequently the following critical review focuses only on the work that includes an intervention component. This experimental approach represents a significant advancement in the field; and the data, which are still far from complete, represent a contribution not only to the malnutrition literature but also to our understanding of child development in general. Substantive information from these four studies is not yet available in published form, and much of what is to come will probably answer some of the critical questions raised in the remaining part of this chapter.

The work of Mora and colleagues in Bogotá, Colombia, on children living in urban poverty provides an example of a study, which, given the current limitations in the definition and measurement of mild-to-moderate malnutrition, attempts to assess the ecology of malnutrition. Data available to date are based on a pilot study which preceded the ongoing project study.

In the pilot study (65) pairs of siblings of the same sex and similar parentage and nutritional status were placed in malnourished and well-nourished groups

TABLE 6. *Summary of behavioral studies dealing with malnutrition secondary to neonatal disorders*

| Study | Experimental subjects | | Age of experimental and control Ss at evaluation | No. and description of control Ss (if any) | Test used and type of measure obtained | Results |
|---|---|---|---|---|---|---|
| | No. and description of nutritional condition | Age at time of hospital admission | | | | |
| Berglund and Rabo (7) | *N* = 202 Hypertrophic pyloric stenosis; divided into four groups of severity based on weight and duration | | | | Intelligence test used at induction for military service: score Adaptation test: score | No relationship found between degree of severity and level of test scores |
| Ellis and Hill (28) | *N* = 22 Diagnosis of cystic fibrosis in infancy; 19 cases had 20–40% weight deficit during first year; 3 cases had >40% weight deficit during first year | | Index and control: 7–19 yr | *N* = 16 Diagnosis of cystic fibrosis in infancy; weight deficit <20% during first year of life | Wechsler Intelligence Scale for Children: IQ Wide Range Achievement Test: score Parental interview: socioeconomic data | Full-scale WISC IQ and WRAT scores: no significant differences between groups No differences between groups on socioeconomic data |
| Klein et al. (45) | *N* = 50 Hypertrophic pyloric stenosis at 0–3 mo; no neurological damage; divided into high (21–42%), moderate (11–20%), | 1–60 days | Experimental: 5–14 yr (mean 9 yr 2 mo) Sib: 5–15 yr (mean 10 yr 1 mo) | *N* = 44 Siblings nearest in age *N* = 50 Matched for age, sex, and father's education | Numerous tests including: Peabody Picture Vocabulary Test: score; Wechsler Intelligence Scale for children: | Lowest weight deficit associated with lower test scores Index have lowest scores on coding, digit span No consistent differences between groups on PPVT or |

| | | | | |
|---|---|---|---|---|
| | and low (0–10%) severity of starvation based on weight at admission | | vocabulary score, coding score, digit span<br>Raven Progressive Matrices: score<br>Parental estimate development scale<br><br>Ottawa school behavior checklist: score | Raven<br>Significant correlation between severity of starvation and parental estimate development scale<br>Onset between 21 and 30 days related to more school problems measured by OSBCL |
| Lloyd-Still et al. (55) | N = 41<br>34 had cystic fibrosis, 11 meconium ileus, 4 protracted diarrhea, 3 ileal atresia; weight <3rd percentile for first 4 mo; edema, neurological abnormalities, and biochemical disturbances present in some cases | N = 41<br>Siblings not malnourished | Index: 2–21 yr<br>Control: 2–19 yr | 18–72 mo: Merrill-Palmer Scale: score<br>5–15 yr: Wechsler Intelligence Scale for children: IQ<br>14–21 yr: Wechsler Adult Intelligence Scale: IQ<br>5–15 yr: Lincoln-Oseretsky<br>Vineland Scale of Social Maturity | Significant difference: index 40th %tile, control 70th %tile<br>WISC + WAIS IQ: no significant differences<br><br>No significant differences<br>No significant differences |
| Valman (80) | N = 20<br>Group 1 (N = 7) had resection of ileum; group 3 (N = 13) had cystic fibrosis of pancreas | N = 26<br>A class of schoolchildren | Index: group 1, 5–14 yr; group 3, 6–12 yr<br>Control: 6.5–7 yr | Goodenough-Harris drawing test: score<br>Teacher assessment for group 1 | Group 1, 106.3; group 3, 98.4; control 99.9<br>All progressing normally |

TABLE 7. Summary of mild-to-moderate studies: field studies

| Study | Experimental subjects[a] No. and description of nutritional condition | No. and description of control Ss (if any) | Age of experimental and control Ss at evaluation | Test used and type of measure obtained | Results |
|---|---|---|---|---|---|
| Cravioto et al. (23) | N = 143 Upper and lower height quartiles of presumably mildly to moderately malnourished children living in a rural environment | N = 120 Upper and lower height quartiles of well-nourished children living in upper-class, urban environments | 6–11 yr | Tests of intersensory organization: visual kinesthetic, visual-haptic, haptic-kinesthetic: total error scores | Urban group had fewer errors on all tests than rural group; total X errors score of rural lower quartile higher than upper quartile For urban group few differences seen in lower vs. upper quartiles Highest X error score for both urban and rural was in youngest age group (6 yr); no statistical significance provided |
| Klein et al. (47) | Mildly to moderately malnourished children living in four isolated Guatemalan villages | | 3–6 yr | Language Facility: score Short Term Memory for Numbers: score Perceptual Analysis: score | Nutritional and social variables are correlated to psychological test performance Magnitude of correlation of social or nutrition variables varies with type of test and child's sex |
| Winick et al. (86) | N = 41 Group 1: severely malnourished; height and weight 3rd %tile N = 51 Group 2: moderately malnourished; height and weight >3rd <25th %tile | N = 47 Height and weight >25th %tile | 7–15 yr | Information on IQ scores and achievement scores obtained | Mean IQ: Group I 103.46 Group II 104.81 Controls 113.4 X̄ %tile achievement scores: Group I 5.07 Group II 5.79 Controls 6.48 |

[a]The ages of the experimental subjects in these studies were not available.

based on weight and height percentages. A well-nourished child had a height equal to or greater than 95%, and a weight equal to or greater than 90%, of the same standard. Height and weight criteria of the malnourished children correspond to approximately the third percentile of the Boston Growth Curves. Half of the well-nourished and half of the malnourished groups received weekly food supplements. Home visits, 24-hr recall surveys, and food-purchasing questionnaires were used to monitor dietary intake.

Nutritional and health status was assessed approximately six times during the year using standardized anthropometric measures (height and weight, skinfold thickness, and head and arm circumference), as well as biochemical analyses of blood (hematocrit, hemoglobin, total protein, albumin, and globulins) and of urine (urea nitrogen and creatinine in casual samples). Also, visits to the childrens' homes provided weekly records of morbidity.

Control of socioeconomic-environmental factors known to correlate with intellectual development was achieved via maternal interviews. In addition to a detailed medical history which provided data on maternal health during pregnancy, multiple-item scales were used to gather information on socioeconomic status; parents' reading habits, age, and education; family possessions; social contact and emotional status of the mother; and the mother's teaching of children.

Intellectual status was assessed both before and after 1 year of supplementation. Several tests were used, including the Griffiths Test of Mental Abilities, as well as a battery of Piagetian-based instruments and tests adopted from the INCAP project in Guatemala. This report (65) provides information on the results of the Griffiths test only. For the initial measures, the well-nourished and malnourished children were subclassified into younger and older groups. Griffiths scale mean score comparisons between the young-well-nourished ($\overline{m}$ 100.91, SD 13.17) and young-malnourished ($\overline{m}$ 86.25, SD 14.74) children as well as between the older-well-nourished ($\overline{m}$ 95.07, SD 12.79) and the older-malnourished ($\overline{m}$ 80.88, SD 15.10) children were statistically significant and in the expected direction ($p < 0.01$). In both comparisons the differences in scores amounted to more than 14 points. Also, younger siblings performed significantly better than older siblings regardless of nutritional status ($t = 2.32$; $p < 0.025$).

The well-nourished sibling families had higher scores on all major indicators of socioeconomic status than did malnourished families. For example, family income, size of dwelling, and possession of a radio all differed between groups at a statistically significant level ($p < 0.025$, one-tailed test). The mothers of malnourished children spent significantly less time with their children, including less time devoted to direct teaching than did the mothers of the well-nourished children ($p < 0.025$). On measures of childhood morbidity and mother's health during pregnancy, both adverse pregnancy factors and health of the child (newborn and current status) were found to be positively associated with nutritional status ($p < 0.001$).

Multiple regression analyses using social-environmental factors and nutritional status (height and weight) as predictors of Griffiths scores demonstrated that both sets of independent variables, either combined or independently, were significantly related to IQ. The combination of both sets of variables accounted for 35% of the Griffiths test score variance for younger children ($p < 0.01$) and 31% for that of the older siblings ($p < 0.05$). When the variance of the social factors and the covariance between the two sets of variables were controlled, nutritional status no longer explained a significant percent of the Griffiths score variance.

To examine the effects of food supplementation, one-half of the sets in each group were randomly assigned to a supplemented or nonsupplemented subgroup. Mental growth measures were obtained at the end of 1 year and compared to those obtained at the beginning of the study. The supplemented malnourished children raised their IQ from 82.8 to 89.3 (nonsignificant) points while the nonsupplemented malnourished gained only 2.1 points, from 85.72 to 87.81 (nonsignificant). The well-nourished group, on the other hand, not only showed no increase in IQ but for both subgroups showed a nonsignificant slight decrease (supplemented from 98.02 to 96.46; nonsupplemented from 97.95 to 95.76). The authors argue that while regression effects may explain the increase and decrease in scores of the malnourished and well-nourished children, respectively, the difference in mean score increments between supplemented and nonsupplemented malnourished children cannot be explained by these same effects. Results showed that Griffiths scores of the malnourished groups (supplemented and nonsupplemented) increased over time whereas that of the well-nourished groups (supplemented and nonsupplemented) decreased slightly over the same time period ($p < 0.01$).

The above findings formed the basis for a larger longitudinal study now in progress in Bogotá, Colombia. The new study no longer uses siblings; instead children are assigned randomly to supplemented and control groups. In addition, each child is studied beginning at 6 months' gestation. Supplemental food to the mother also begins at that time and continues until the child reaches 6 months or 3 years of age. A third group receives no supplemental food, and a fourth is supplemented from 6 months to 3 years. All four groups are given the same health care and periodic anthropometric measurements. Results from this longitudinal study will provide more conclusive answers on the relative effects of malnutrition on intellectual functioning.

Klein and colleagues focused on four isolated villages in rural Guatemala. These villages were matched for biological, psychological, and sociocultural variables; they allegedly differed only in type of imposed experimental treatment (i.e., medical and nutritional supplementation in combination or singly, or no treatment conditions).

From 1969 to 1973 the entire birth cohort in all four villages was studied extensively (46). Pregnant mothers and their offspring were supplemented with either a protein-calorie food (atole) or a calorie beverage (fresco) to the degree they participated in the study (i.e., high, moderate, or low intake). Numerous social-environmental variables were assessed, and developmental measures (both neonatal and preschool) taken.

Consistent and significant findings to date show that high-supplemented mothers (> 20,000 calories), regardless of whether they received atole or fresco, had fewer low-birth-weight (< 2,500 g) babies. Moreover, these babies showed a significantly smaller percentage ($p < 0.01$) of growth retardation at 36 months of age than offspring of either middle- or low-supplemented mothers. That this finding was not an artifact of some uncontrolled maternal variable was demonstrated by examining birth weights of siblings—one the product of high supplementation, the other of low. The relationship between supplementation and birth weight was maintained.

Total amount of calorie supplementation regardless of type was also associated with psychological test performance. The high-, middle-, and low-supplemented groups at 15 months of age had means of 72.3, 67.8, and 62.9 ($F = 4.65$; $p < 0.01$), respectively, on the mental subscale of the infant test, and means of 82.6, 77.2, and 73.8 ($F = 6.25$; $p < 0.01$), respectively, on the motor subscale. Thus by 15 months of age high-supplemented (a summation of mother plus child total supplemental calories up to time of testing) children performed significantly better on an infant scale than low- or middle-supplemented children. This relationship between supplement ingestion and test performance was also maintained at 24 months of age (mental, $F = 8.45$, $p < 0.01$; motor, $F = 11.61$, $p < 0.01$). Item analyses of the infant scale indicated that motor, in contrast to more linguistic or cognitive, items were more closely associated with supplementation effects. This finding was consistent with that of the Colombian group, who found an association between nutritional status and the motor-oriented Griffiths test (65).

At 36 and 48 months of age all children again were tested using a battery of Piagetian-based tests. Four of the 13 tests given at age 36 months showed significant differences between groups ($p < 0.05$). However, the high-supplemented children performed significantly better than the middle- or low-supplemented groups on only two of these tests (Reversal Discrimination Learning Time and Verbal Inferences). Similarly, four of the 13 tests given at 48 months showed significant differences between groups ($p < 0.05$), but of these the high-supplemented group scored significantly higher than the other two groups in only two tests (Reversal Discrimination Learning Sum and Vocabulary Naming) plus a composite test score category.

Thus caloric supplementation was found to be significantly related to growth up to 36 months of age, and to performance on psychological tests at 15–48 months of age. Those children receiving high levels of supplementation, either in the atole or fresco villages, in general showed superior results.

The importance of the supplementation timing on test performance was also examined. Essentially, when gestational supplementation was controlled, the relationship between caloric supplementation and test performance disappeared. Conversely, when postnatal supplementation was controlled, the calorie-test performance relationship remained unchanged. Gestational supplementation then appears to be the critical time period for future effects on psychological test performances.

Finally, results from this study have considerably clarified the interaction between nutritional, socioeconomic (SES), and test performance variables. After 36 months of age, a poorly supplemented, low-SES child is three times more likely to score in the lowest pentile of test performance than in the high pentile. A poorly supplemented, high-SES child, on the other hand, has an approximately equal probability of scoring in the high as in the low pentile of test performance. The authors consider the latter finding an important element in interpretation of the effect of nutritional supplementation and malnutrition on mental test performance.

Chavez and colleagues (17,18) researched the effects of supplementation through the study of two groups of 17 mother-child units. One group received supplementation beginning the 45th day of pregnancy and were followed up to 6 years of age. The other group was used for control. Both groups resided in a small, rural, Mexican community and were of the same socioeconomic status. The unsupplemented group of mothers, between 18 and 36 years of age, all had healthy, normal babies and represented the healthy norm of the village. The supplemented mothers, similar to the first in selection criteria, were given powdered milk, vitamins, and iron supplements beginning in the sixth week of pregnancy and continuing through lactation. Offspring of the supplemented mothers received measured quantities of milk and baby food beginning the third month of life. The data on mother-child and family interaction were gathered by means of a 72-hr direct observation in the home using time sampling and scaling techniques. In addition, each child was given the Gesell Developmental Schedules test.

The results showed differences in anthropometry and activity between the two groups from birth; however, no statistical evidence was provided for any finding. Babies born to the supplemented mothers were heavier and larger. This difference in growth in terms of both height and weight became more marked at approximately 11 months and continued through 3 years of age. From 24 weeks onward, the supplemented children were more physically active, slept less, and spent more time out of the crib than the contrast children. Play activity at first increased for the supplemented group over contrast, then decreased at approximately 49 months, increasing again at around 56 months. At that time (56 months) the supplemented children were also more talkative and cried less.

In terms of mother and family-child interaction, supplemented children smiled at their mothers more, were spoken to more frequently, and were cleaned and bathed more often than contrast children. Fathers of supplemented children more frequently participated in the care of the child than fathers of the unsupplemented group. While some of these results were presented graphically, none was accompanied by statistical confirmation.

Gesell Developmental scores showed consistent differences in all areas in favor of the supplemented child. These differences between groups (presented graphically) were apparent by 2 months of age. In sum, the supplemented child was characterized as an active playful youngster who frequently verbalized and demanded. This behavior, according to the investigators, stimulates the parent's behavior, resulting in more frequent and varied interactions between parent and child.

A study by McKay et al. (61,62) focused on the effects of psychoeducational intervention, nutrition, and health care on the mental development of mild-to-moderately malnourished, low-SES children living in Cali, Colombia. The study design involved 360 children who were placed into six groups. Groups 1 through 4 and 6 were all low-SES, preschool children, mild-to-moderately malnourished. Group 5 was a reference group composed of upper-income, well-grown children living in Cali. Each of the six groups, with the exception of groups 4 and 5, received either comprehensive treatment including psychoeducation, health and nutritional intervention, or a combination of nutrition and health care only. Groups 4 and 5 were no-treatment control groups. The comprehensive treatment groups (1–3) began treatment in successive years to control for time effects. Subclassification of group 6, the nutrition and health care group, into three smaller groups allowed for the same time-effect control. All groups received anthropometric examinations and psychological tests (unspecified) at approximately the same time.

Unfortunately, available results presented graphically are not substantiated with statistical tests. The authors report that after 1.5 years of treatment, group 1 (comprehensive treatment for 3 years) was superior to groups 4 and 6 but below the upper-income reference group 5 on five subtests of the Wechsler Preschool and Primary Test. On a test of verbal reasoning, on the other hand, the mean score of group 1 was approximately the same as the mean of group 5. Those groups which received no treatment or else nutrition and health care only (groups 4 and 6, respectively) not only showed appreciably lower scores than groups 1 and 5, but the mean of group 4 decreased from the beginning of the study while that of group 6 remained the same. The authors interpret this finding as evidence that a combination intervention program can raise the level of verbal reasoning in malnourished, low-income children to that of normal children. Nutrition and health care alone, however, apparently did not effect a change in any of the results of the tests used in the study. Similar results were obtained on two recognition tests (unspecified): the mean score of group 1 was superior to the means of groups 4 and 6, but below that of group 5. While it is difficult to assess these findings in the absence of statistical validation, perhaps the most important result concerns short-term memory as measured by the children's performance on a test of memory for sentences and on Knox

Cubes. After 1.5 years of treatment there were no appreciable differences on these tests among the malnourished groups; and the results in all of these groups were apparently below those of group 5. It is interesting to note that Klein et al. (48) reported poor performance on short-term memory tests among 5- to 6-year-old malnourished children, a finding they attributed to an attentional deficit. In sum, the work of McKay et al. suggests that poor IQ and psychological performance demonstrated by mild-to-moderately malnourished children (with the exception of short-term memory) are amenable to improvement in an enriched environment which includes cognitive stimulation as well as nutritional and medical care.

2. Exposure to famine conditions

While the longitudinal studies reviewed above attempted to estimate and control for the role of social-environmental factors in determining the nature of the relation between malnutrition and mental development, the study discussed below was based on a situation in which the malnutrition variable presumably equally affected individuals of all socioeconomic levels. The Dutch famine of 1944–1945 caused by a transport embargo by the Nazis on western Holland resulted in widespread, severe malnutrition in the entire western part of the country. Stein and co-workers (77,78) undertook a retrospective cohort study using data from the famine and from later military induction examinations. The available information on birth place and date made the construction of two birth cohorts feasible: those subjected and those not subjected to the famine. These cohorts were further subclassified into those conceived and those born before, during, or after the famine. With prenatal exposure to famine as the independent variable, a number of variables related to mental competence and health were examined as dependent variables. Our review is limited to a discussion of those variables related to mental performance, i.e., incidence of both mild and severe mental retardation, and IQ scores from the Raven Progressive Matrices Test.

Data analysis showed that the frequency of neither mild nor severe mental retardation was related to conception or birth during famine. The authors state that multiple regression analysis of exposure to famine and rates of retardation yielded negligible results (no statistics presented). Nonsignificant correlations were also obtained for total Raven Matrices scores and maternal caloric rations received during the first, second, and third trimesters of pregnancy. Thus no association between Raven Matrices scores and period of famine was found. The possibility that socioenvironmental factors were confounding this association was dismissed because none of the social variables yielded significant correlations with either caloric rations during trimesters or Raven scores. For example, birth order correlated 0, .00, and .01 with the first, second, and third trimesters of pregnancy and .10 with Raven Matrices. Similarly, correlations of family size with pregnancy trimesters and Raven scores ranged from .02 to .19. While social status (manual versus nonmanual work) showed trivial correlations with pregnancy trimesters (highest $r = .01$), it yielded the highest correlation among the social variables with Raven scores ($r = .24$). Considering this correlation, it is noteworthy that the manual-working groups had consistently higher rates of mild retardation and lower Raven scores than the nonmanual-working group despite lack of detectable effects due to famine. These latter findings, however, were not statistically supported. In assessing the results of this study, it is important to note that infant (<1 year of age) diets during the famine were not inadequate—assessed as well over 100% adequacy (Oxford Nutrition Survey standard allowances) in both calories and protein—while those of pregnant mothers varied in adequacy ranging from 64% to 29% adequate in calories and 73% to 41% adequate in protein (78). Thus although infants in this birth cohort may have been exposed to malnutrition prenatally, it appears that postnatally they received ample food during the first year of life for nourishment and growth.

With the completion of this brief report on studies of mild-to-moderate malnutrition, we now begin appraisal of their scientific merit. As was the case with the studies on severe PCM, we focus on methods and design.

By controlling dietary intake, intervention studies have removed many problems associated with the use of anthropometry as the only criterion for the nutritional variable. Consumption of the food supplement at the research post provides a unique opportunity to measure intake accurately. However, this approach is not free of methodological problems. Probably the most important is determination of the nature of the intervention. Labeling a treatment does not define its true dimensions. Among the field research conditions that seriously threaten treatment validity are two of particular import in connection with the studies reviewed. One is the plausible effects of treatment covariants. For example, distribution of food supplements in the Chavez et al. (18) and Klein et al. (48) studies may have broadened the social contacts of the tested subjects (mothers and/or children) and heightened the chance for verbal interactions. This by-product of the implementation of nutritional treatment may be having an effect on the behavioral variable measured.

The psychoeducational intervention used in the McKay et al. (61,62) study also faces a serious challenge in demonstrating that intervention was limited to the defined variable. This study is an excellent illustration of how a research program, which defines its independent variables as psychoeducational, nutritional, and health inputs, can best be conceptualized as *life intervention*. The description of psychoeducational and nutritional inputs in the Second Progress Report (61) of the Cali project illustrates that the comprehensive treatment includes far more than what was originally intended. Definition of the psychoeducational treatment in terms of five specific intellectual tasks (verbal production, understanding of elementary spatial relations, manual skills, maintenance of attention and concentration, and independent decision-making) is incomplete. These tasks are only a part of the intellectual treatment package, which presented under multiple conditions of social interaction include not only adult-child relations but also child-child and adult-adult relations. Furthermore, the social-emotional and the intellectual portions of the treatment cannot be entirely separated. Thus it is clear that the investigators' conceptual breakdown of the input into three discrete segments *is* artificial. It is reasonable, for example, to argue that an additional strong component of the intervention is emotional support. Here it is pertinent to add that the nutritional treatment includes not only food but also a regimen of intake in pleasant physical and social surroundings. This nutritional treatment as part of the comprehensive condition has little in common with the nutritional treatment that provides only food supplements at home.

The other problem connected with treatment validity is a reactive effect to a treatment-context interaction. The treatment may activate nontarget behaviors, which in turn may modulate the relationship of the independent-dependent variable which the experimenter tries to establish. In the case of the McKay et al. or Chavez et al. study, selection of subjects for special treatment may have encouraged the mother's attention on those children, resulting in particular treatment at home.

It must be noted that the study in Guatemala originally intended to control for the effects of treatment covariants and treatment-context interaction by having a treatment group (given atole: high-protein, high-calorie) and a control group (given fresco: high-calorie only). Subsequently when the researchers found no differences between groups, they decided to analyze the relation between calories and performance, combining data from the atole and fresco groups. They then found a relation between amount of caloric intake (or rate of attendance) and test performance, which they interpreted as a nutritional effect. However, no evidence exists to discard the possibility that such an effect was not codetermined by uncontrolled variables.

If the nature of the comprehensive treatment remains unknown, both the possibility of treatment replication and the implications of the treatment for social policy are negligible. Evidently there is need for further work on experimental validation of the treatment variable. A very recent publication on the specific behavioral effects of environmental intervention during the preschool years (63) is an excellent illustration of the feasibility of assessing treatment validation in large-scale programs. In this study the specific dimensions of treatment were carefully described and then analyzed in connection with the observed effects. As may be expected, there were more effects than could be predicted from the nature of the treatment itself.

Recognizing the multivariate dimension of the treatment, it must be concluded that although the experimental intervention approach may be taken as a methodological improvement over the correlational *ex post facto* design it is not free of confounding variables. Currently it is difficult and sometimes impossible to estimate the contribution of the nutrition variable alone.

The measurement of the behavioral variable has also received more attention and greater care in the studies on mild-to-moderate malnutrition than in those on severe malnutrition. Klein et al. (47) (Table 7) standardized, on the native Guatemalan population, the battery of tests constructed for their study. Mora and colleagues reordered the test items of the Griffiths Scale according to levels of difficulty for their target population in Bogotá, Colombia (81). This move away from aggregate measures of intelligence (IQ) as the sole dependent variable has resulted in an increased understanding of the possible mechanisms underlying the effects of malnutrition.

Improvements in the methodology of dependent variable measurement, however, have not been accompanied by persistent efforts to define the constructs underlying the tests or by attempts to estimate test construct validity (see first part of this chapter for a discussion of construct validity). One attempt in this regard is a study on the performance of Guatemalan rural and Colombian urban children in tests selected from the battery constructed by Klein et al. (Vuori and Engle, *unpublished observations*). These investigators established some similarity in test score patterns in the two cultures. The finding was interpreted by Vuori and Engle as evidence that the same nomological networks were tapped in both situations. However, this interpretation must be questioned on the basis of the correlation coefficients they report for males and females in both country samples. For example, for both sexes there are four pairs of correlations (between different tests) that reach statistical significance for the females but not for the males. In addition, although the authors do not report statistical comparisons between correlation coefficients, it is apparent that there are many pairs of coefficients that differ substantially from each other. Consequently it is not clear, as the authors claim, whether the test tapped the same constructs in all subjects tested. No final conclusions can be made, however, in the absence of factor analysis data.

Further study of dependent variable measurement among studies reviewed shows that except for a few instances (23) (Table 7) the choice of tests was not preceded by specific consideration of the determinants behind the test constructs. Support for this inference is found in the total absence of theorizing in all reports regarding the sensitivity of any one particular measure to the specific effects of the nutrition variable. Differential sensitivity among tests is, however, well demonstrated in data reported by Klein et al. (47) (Table 7) on multiple correlations of physical and social measures with psychological measures, and independent contributions of physical measures to the multiple R.

Data on intertest relationship (Vuori and Engle, *unpublished data*) and on differences in language and perception variance explained by the physical growth measures (47) (Table 7) indicate the considerable risk of error in cross-cultural comparability of findings from these studies. As discussed above, the errors may stem from cultural differences in the nomological networks behind the dependent variables and from differences in measure sensitivity. Thus there seems to be little justification for making inferences from results obtained with different measures (e.g., intersensory organization and Griffiths Scales) and in different communities having dissimilar histories and cultural backgrounds (e.g., Colombian urban slums and Mexican rural villages).

Almost all studies on the effects of mild-to-moderate malnutrition with or without an intervention component indicate the researchers' concern with possible confounding effects of social-environmental variables. This concern results in a more cautious interpretation of the published data. Analysis of the environmental variables used in investigations indicates that variable selection follows no overt theoretical rationale that would propose an order in social factor interaction or identification of variable position within a causality tree. Thus whereas some researchers limit their study of the social environment to direct (i.e., income) or indirect (i.e., mother's dress) measures of graduated parameters of social structure, others include behavioral process variables of diverse nature (i.e., mother took child out of neighborhood last month). This empirical approach creates serious problems for interpretation of regression coefficients between nutritional status and mental test scores, regardless of their statistical significance. These coefficients change as a function of the number of relevant social variables entering into the equation. Therefore the significance of the nutrition variable may diminish from one study to the next depending on the number of social factors covarying with the nutrition variable that explain part of the variance in the dependent variable.

The Dutch epidemiological study would seem to cope with confounding effects of social variables given the conditions in which the undernutrition occurred. However, the difficulties of generalization mentioned in connection with the studies on secondary malnutrition also exist in this large and well-designed study. Mild-to-moderate malnutrition in low-income countries is an intergenerational endemic condition, whereas the Dutch famine had epidemic-like characteristics. Also, it has been pointed out that the effects of the social and nutritional variables may not be independent of each other; consequently the effects of malnutrition may be modified by the socioeconomic context in which it occurs. With the exclusion of this study because of irrelevancy, we now turn to the issue of data handling and analysis before reaching some specific conclusions.

Mora et al. (65) and Klein et al. (48) used multivariate statistics to estimate the variance of the dependent variable that can be attributed to nutrition intervention. Conversely, most of the data reported by McKay et al. and by Chavez et al. lack statistical analyses and instead are presented graphically. Chavez presents some results from between-group statistical comparisons, but it is apparent that the data collected would yield more useful information if it were treated with refined multivariable statistics now available. For example, in 1972 he reported on effects of the supplement on physical activity (17); between-group differences on physical activity were calculated at nine points in time using $t$-tests. Correlation coefficients within groups between physical activity and chronological age were then calculated independently. This simple approach missed the opportunity of estimating time effects (not obtained by Pearson coefficients) or group-by-time interactions. Further analysis also would have yielded the shape of the time response for both groups (50).

The report by Mora et al. (65) of a beneficial effect of the nutrition variable on the Griffiths IQ is indeed impressive. However, it is apparent that the observed effects may still be, in part, a statistical artifact—a possibility the researchers have not dismissed. The authors report (65):

> The changes in Griffiths scores between the initial and final observations are compatible with regression effects that may have raised the scores of the malnourished and lowered the scores of the well nourished children. However, the difference in mean score increments between supplemented and nonsupplemented malnourished children cannot be explained by regression effects and appears to be associated with the supplementation program.

Even if the authors' interpretation of the between-group differences cannot totally be attributed to regression, there still may be a contribution from regression. Regression effects are not exclusive of other random effects. Thus what the authors report as significant treatment effects may be simply the contribution of regression and a small but nonsignificant treatment effect. The significant finding resulted from the combined effect of the two factors.

It is premature to make a critical appraisal of recently available findings from the Guatemalan study (48). Klein's report at the Cornell Conference on Malnutrition and Behavior (46) is evidently incomplete, as there is not much information on possible interactions between social-environmental variables and caloric intake. However, it seems pertinent to mention at this time that although the impact of the treatment is statistically significant it is numerically small and there are yet no data to show its daily-life behavioral significance.

Despite the numerous critical comments and observations already made, a few general conclusions can now be drawn. The paucity of conclusions perhaps does not justify the effort invested in the data review but may represent a significant step in understanding such a complex problem.

1. Among populations where malnutrition in endemic, infants and young children of comparatively low stature are likely to perform less well than average-size children from the same community on aggregate tests of intelligence or on tests of specific cognitive process (e.g., language or perception).

2. Among populations where malnutrition is endemic, infants and young children of comparatively short stature are more likely to come from families found in the lowest strata of the socioeconomic structure of that population than children of similar age but of average size.

3. Stature and graduated parameters of social structure (i.e., income, maternal education) explain significant parts of cognitive development test variance among infants and preschool children of populations where malnutrition is endemic. Their independent contributions to test variance depend on

the nature of the test construct in question. It is not currently possible to determine the constructs that are more amenable to the effects of one or the other set of factors.

4. Upgrading the quality of life through infancy and the preschool years improves the performance of children on aggregate scales of intelligence or on tests of specific cognitive factors as compared to their original performance before the change in life took place.

All told, we can now evaluate the significance of endemic protein-calorie malnutrition on the development of children and the extent to which it affects their potential to function as instruments of social and economic change. Despite a lack of specific information on the nature of the nutrition-intelligence relationship, available evidence indicates that protein-calorie malnutrition has an adverse effect on the ontogenetic process, retarding the rate of developmental change. However, except for those cases of severe and chronic undernutrition with an onset during the prenatal period or early postnatal life, protein-calorie deficiency does not *arrest* development. Indeed, among the populations that have been investigated there is no reason to believe that older children and early adolescents fail to acquire the cognitive structures necessary to attain the level of logicomathematical operations (43). Conversely, these populations lack to a large extent the ontogenetic learning experiences and accumulation of information necessary for modernization and industrialization.

Identification of the role of nutrition will bring useful additional information to our understanding of human development, and solution of the nutritional problems in the Third World will surely upgrade the quality of life. However, the role of nutrition in societal growth must be placed in proper perspective. Current evidence does not support the notion that better nutrition *ipso facto* increases intelligence, which in turn leads to betterment of people. It is apparent that intelligence can work only with information, and it is useful only if applied. Information and the opportunity to use it are obviously not dependent on nutrition. Living conditions of the populations where malnutrition is endemic generally must be improved. This means solving undernutrition, decreasing morbidity, increasing educational facilities, providing well-remunerated jobs, and facilitating individual participation in the economic and political development of the society.

## ACKNOWLEDGMENT

Supported in part by research grants 1 R22 HDO9228-01 and 1 RO1 HD08109-01A1 from the National Institute of Child Health and Human Development, US Public Health Service.

## REFERENCES

1. Anastasi, A. (1968): *Psychological Testing,* 3rd ed. Macmillan, London.
2. Autret, M., and Behar, M. (1954): *Sindrome Pluricarencial Infantil (Kwashiorkor) and Its Prevention in Central America,* Food and Agricultural Organization of The United Nations, Rome.
3. Barreda-Moncada, G. (1963): *Estudios Sobre Alteraciones del Crecimiento y del Desarrollo Psicologico del Sindrome Pluricarencial (Kwashiorkor).* Editora Grafas, Caracas, Venezuela.
4. Bayley, N. (1955): On the growth of intelligence. *Am. Psychol.,* 10:805–818.
5. Bayley, N. (1970): Development of mental abilities. In: *Carmichael's Manual of Child Psychology,* Vol. 1, 3rd ed., edited by P. H. Mussen. Wiley, New York.
6. Bengoa, J. M. (1974): The problem of malnutrition. *WHO Chron.,* 28:3–7.
7. Berglund, G., and Rabo, E. (1973): A long-term follow-up investigation of patients with hypertrophic pyloric stenosis—with special reference to the physical and mental development. *Acta Paediatr. Scand.,* 62:125–129.
8. Birch, H. E., Pineiro, C., Alcalde, E., Toca, T., and Cravioto, J. (1971): Relation of kwashiorkor in early childhood and intelligence at school age. *Pediatr. Res.,* 5:579–585.
9. Bloom, B. S. (1964): *Stability and Change in Human Characteristics.* Wiley, New York.
10. Botha-Antoun, E., Babayan, S., and Harfouche, J. K. (1968): Intellectual development related to nutritional status. *J. Trop. Pediatr.,* 14:112–115.
11. Brockman, L., and Ricciuti, H. (1971): Severe protein-calorie malnutrition and cognitive development in infancy and early childhood. *Dev. Psychol.,* 4:312–319.
12. Broman, S. H., Nichols, P. L., and Kennedy, W. A. (1975): *Preschool IQ: Prenatal and Early Developmental Correlates.* Wiley, New York.
13. Cabak, V., and Najdanvic, R. (1965): Effect of undernutrition in early life on physical and mental development. *Arch. Dis. Child.,* 40:523–534.
14. Campbell, D. T., and Stanley, J. C. (1972): *Experimental and Quasi-Experimental Designs for Research,* 9th ed. Rand McNally, Chicago.
15. Champakam, S., Srikantia, S., and Gopalan, C. (1968): Kwashiorkor and mental development. *Am. J. Clin. Nutr.,* 21:844–852.
16. Chase, H. P., and Martin, H. P. (1970): Undernutrition and child development. *N. Engl. J. Med.,* 282:933–939.
17. Chavez, A., Martinez, C., and Bourges, H. (1972): Nutrition and development of infants from poor rural areas; nutrition level and physical activity. *Nutr. Rep. Int.,* 5:139–144.
18. Chavez, A., Martinez, C., and Yaschine, T. (1974): The importance of nutrition and stimuli on child mental and social development. In: *Early Malnutrition and Mental Development,* edited by J. Cravioto, L. Hambraeus, and B. Vahlquist. Almqvist & Wiksell, Uppsala.
19. Cole, M., and Scribner, S. (1974): *Culture and Thought.* Wiley, New York.
20. Cravioto, J., and DeLicardie, E. (1972): Environmental correlates of severe clinical malnutrition and language development in survivors from kwashiorkor or marasmus. In: *Nutrition, the Nervous System and Behavior.* Pan American Health Organization, Washington, D.C.
21. Cravioto, J., and DeLicardie, E. (1973): Longitudinal study of language development in severely malnourished children. In: *Nutrition and Mental Functions,* edited by G. Serban. Plenum Press, New York.
22. Cravioto, J., and Robles, B. (1965): Evolution of adaptive and motor behavior during rehabilitation from kwashiorkor. *Am. J. Orthopsychiatry,* 35:449–464.
23. Cravioto, J., DeLicardie, E., and Birch, H. (1966): Nutrition, growth and neurointegrative development: An experimental and ecological study. *Pediatrics (Suppl.),* 38:part II.
23a. Cravioto, J., Hambraeus, L., and Vahlquist, B., editors (1974): *Early Malnutrition and Mental Development,* p. 15. Almquist & Wiksell, Uppsala.
24. Cronbach, L. J. (1960): *Essentials of Psychological Testing.* Harper & Row, New York.
25. Cronbach, L. J. (1971): Test validation. In: *Educational Measurement,* 2nd ed., edited by R. L. Thorndike. American Council on Education, Washington, D.C.
26. DeLicardie, E. R., and Cravioto, J. (1974): Behavioral responsiveness of survivors of clinically severe malnutrition to cognitive demands. In: *Early Malnutrition and Mental*

*Development,* edited by J. Cravioto, L. Hambraeus, and B. Vahlquist. Almqvist & Wiksell, Uppsala.

27. Echensberger, L. H. (1973): Methodological issues of cross-cultural research in developmental psychology. In: *Life Span Developmental Psychology: Methodological Issues,* edited by J. R. Nesselroade and H. W. Reese. Academic Press, New York.

28. Ellis, C. E., and Hill, D. E. (1975): Growth, intelligence and school performance in children with cystic fibrosis who have had an episode of malnutrition during infancy. *J. Pediatr.,* 87:565–568.

29. Evans, D., Moodie, A., and Hansen, J. (1971): Kwashiorkor and intellectual development. *S. Afr. Med. J.,* 45:1413–1426.

30. Fisher, M. M., Killcross, M. C., Simonsson, M., and Elgie, K. A. (1972): Malnutrition and reasoning ability in Zambian school children. *Trans. R. Soc. Trop. Med. Hyg.,* 66:471–478.

31. Flavell, J. H. (1963): *The Developmental Psychology of Jean Piaget.* Van Nostrand, Princeton.

32. Freeman, F. S. (1962): *Theory and Practice of Psychological Testing,* 3rd ed. Holt, Rinehart and Winston, New York.

33. Gerber, M., and Dean, R. F. A. (1956): The psychological changes accompanying kwashiorkor. *Courrier,* 6:3–14.

34. Ginsburg, H., and Opper, S. (1969): *Piaget's Theory of Intellectual Development: An Introduction.* Prentice Hall, Englewood Cliffs, N. J.

35. Graham, G. C., and Morales, E. (1963): Studies in infantile malnutrition. I. Nature of the problem in Peru. *J. Nutr.,* 79:479–487.

36. Graves, P. L. (1976): Nutrition, infant behavior and maternal characteristics: A pilot study in West Bengal, India. *Am. J. Clin. Nutr.,* 29:305–319.

37. Guilford, J. P. (1967): *The Nature of Human Intelligence.* McGraw-Hill, New York.

38. Habicht, J. P., Yarbrough, C., and Klein, R. E. (1974): Assessing nutritional status in a field study of malnutrition and mental development: Specificity, sensitivity and congruity of indices of nutritional status. In: *Early Malnutrition and Mental Development,* edited by J. Cravioto, L. Hambraeus, and B. Vahlquist. Almqvist & Wiksell, Uppsala.

39. Hertzig, M. E., Birch, H. G., Richardson, S. A., and Tizard, J. (1972): Intellectual levels of school children severely malnourished during the first two years of life. *Pediatrics,* 49:814–823.

40. Honzik, M. P., Hutchings, J. J., and Burnip, S. R. (1965): Birth record assessments and test performance at eight months. *Am. J. Dis. Child.,* 109:416–426.

41. Irvine, S. H. (1974): Contributions of ability and attainment testing in Africa to a general theory of intellect. In: *Culture and Cognition: Readings in Cross-Cultural Psychology,* edited by J. W. Berry and P. R. Dasen. Methuen, London.

42. Jelliffe, D. B. (1965): Effect of malnutrition on behavioral and social development. In: *Proceedings of Western Hemisphere Nutrition Congress,* pp. 24–27. American Medical Association, Chicago.

43. Kagan, J., and Klein, R. E. (1973): Cross-cultural perspectives on early development. *Am. Psychol.,* 28:947–961.

44. Kanawati, A., Darwish, O., and McLaren, D. (1974): Failure to thrive in Lebanon. III. Family income, expenditure and possessions. *Acta Paediatr. Scand.,* 63:108–112.

45. Klein, P. S., Forbes, G. B., and Nader, P. R. (1975): Effects of starvation in infancy (pyloric stenosis) on subsequent learning abilities. *J. Pediatr.,* 87:8–15.

46. Klein, R., Arenales, P., Arevalo, S., Delgado, H., Engle, P., Guzman, G., Irwin, M., Lechtin, A., Martorell, R., Pivaral, V., Teller, C., and Yarbrough, C. (1975): Malnutrition and human behavior: a backward glance at an ongoing longitudinal study. Presented at the Cornell Conference on Malnutrition and Behavior, November 1975.

47. Klein, R., Freeman, H., Kagan, J., Yarbrough, C., and Habicht, J. P. (1972): Is big smart? The relation of growth to cognition. *J. Health Behav.,* 13:219–225.

48. Klein, R., Lester, B., Yarbrough, C., and Habicht, J. (1975): On malnutrition and mental development: some preliminary findings. In: *International Conference on Nutrition,* edited by A. Chavez. Karger, New York.

49. Knobloch, H., and Pasamanick, B. (1967): Prediction from the assessment of neuromotor and intellectual status in infancy. In: *Psychopathology of Mental Development.* Grune & Stratton, New York.

50. Kowalski, C. J., and Guire, K. E. (1974): Longitudinal data analysis. *Growth,* 38:131–169.

51. Kruglanski, A. W. (1975): Context, meaning and the validity of results in psychological research. *Br. J. Psychol.,* 66:373–382.
52. Lester, B. M. (1975): Cardiac habituation of the orienting response to an auditory signal in infants of varying nutritional status. *Dev. Psychol.,* 11:432–442.
53. Lester, B. M., Klein, R. E., and Martinez, S. J. (1975): The use of habituation in the study of the effects of infantile malnutrition. *Dev. Psychobiol.,* 8:541–546.
54. Levinson, F. J. (1974): *Morinda: An Economic Analysis of Malnutrition Among Young Children in Rural India.* Cornell/MIT International Nutrition Policy Series, Cambridge, Mass.
55. Lloyd-Still, J. D., Hurwitz, I., Wolff, P., and Shwachman, H. (1974): Intellectual development after severe malnutrition in infancy. *Pediatrics,* 54:306–311.
56. Marcondes, E., Lefevre, A., Machado, D., Garcia de Barros, N., Vacallo, A., Gazal, S., Quarentei, G., Setian, N., Valente, M., and Barbieri, D. (1973): Neuropsychomotor development and pneumoencephalographic changes in children with severe malnutrition. *Environ. Child Health,* 19:135–139.
57. McCall, R. B., Hogarty, P. S., and Hurlburt, N. (1972): Transitions in infant sensorimotor development and the prediction of childhood IQ. *Am. Psychol.,* 27:728–748.
58. McCance, R. A., and Widdowson, E. M. (1966): Protein deficiencies and caloric deficiencies. *Lancet,* 2:158–159.
59. McLaren, D. S. (1966): A fresh look at protein-calorie malnutrition. *Lancet,* 2:485–488.
60. McLaren, D. S., Yaktin, U. S., Kanawati, A., Sabbagh, S., and Kadi, Z. (1973): The subsequent mental and physical development of rehabilitated marasmic infants. *J. Ment. Defic. Res.,* 17:273–281.
61. McKay, H., McKay, A., and Sinisterra, L. (1973): Second progress report: Stimulation of intellectual and social competence in Colombian preschool age affected by the multiple deprivations of depressed urban environments. Human Ecology Research Station, Cali, Colombia.
62. McKay, H., McKay, A., and Sinisterra, L. (1974): Intellectual development of malnourished preschool children in programs of stimulation and nutritional supplementation. In: *Early Malnutrition and Mental Development,* edited by J. Cravioto, L. Hambraeus, and B. Vahlquist. Almqvist & Wiksell, Uppsala.
63. Miller, L. B., and Dyer, J. L. (1975): Four preschool programs: Their dimensions and effects. *Monogr. Soc. Res. Child Dev.,* 40(5–6), Serial No. 162.
64. Monckeberg, F. (1968): Effect of early marasmic malnutrition on subsequent physical and psychological development. In: *Malnutrition, Learning and Behavior,* edited by N. Scrimshaw and J. Gordon. MIT Press, Cambridge, Mass.
65. Mora, J. O., Amezquita, A., Castro, L., Christiansen, N., Clement-Murphy, J., Cobos, L., Cremer, H., Dragastin, S., Elias, M., Franklin, D., Herrera, M., Ortiz, N., Pardo, R., de Paredes, B., Ramos, C., Riley, R., Rodriguez, H., Vuori-Christiansen, L., Wagner, M., and Stare, F. J. (1974): Nutrition, health and social factors related to intellectual performance. *World Rev. Nutr. Diet.,* 19:205–236.
66. Nelson, W. E., Vaughan, V. C., and McKay, R. J. (1969): *Textbook of Pediatrics,* 9th ed. Saunders, Philadelphia.
67. Ossofsky, H. (1974): Endogenous depression in infancy and childhood. *Compr. Psychiatry,* 15:19–25.
68. Pollitt, E. (1973): Behavioral correlates of severe malnutrition in man. In: *Nutrition, Growth and Development of North American Indian Children,* edited by W. Moore, M. Silverberg, and M. Read. DHEW Publication No. (NIH)72-26.
69. Pollitt, E., and Granoff, D. (1967): Mental and motor development of Peruvian children treated for severe malnutrition. *Rev. Interam. Psycol.,* 1:93–102.
70. Pollitt, E., and Ricciuti, H. (1969): Biological and social correlates of stature among children in the slums of Lima, Peru. *Am. J. Orthopsychiatry,* 39:735–747.
71. Rao, N., Pralhad, D. S., and Swaminathan, M. C. (1969): Nutritional status of pre-school children of rural communities near Hyderabad city. *Indian J. Med. Res.,* 57:2132–2346.
72. Richardson, S. A. (1974): The background histories of schoolchildren severely malnourished in infancy. *Adv. Pediatr.,* 21:167–195.
73. Richardson, S. A., Birch, H. G., and Hertzig, M. E. (1973): School performance of children who were severely malnourished in infancy. *Am. J. Ment. Defic.,* 77:623–632.
74. Richardson, S., Birch, H., and Ragbeer, C. (1975): The behavior of children at home who

were severely malnourished in the first two years of life. *J. Biosoc. Sci.,* 7:255–267.

75. Scrimshaw, N. S., and Behar, M. (1961): Protein malnutrition in young children. *Science,* 133:2039–2047.
76. Silverstein, A. B. (1971): The measurement of intelligence. In: *International Review of Research in Mental Retardation, Volume 4,* edited by N. R. Ellis. Academic Press, New York.
77. Stein, Z., Susser, M., Saenger, G., and Marolla, F. (1972): Nutrition and mental performance. *Science,* 178:708–713.
78. Stein, Z., Susser, M., Saenger, G., and Marolla, F. (1975): *Famine and Human Development. The Dutch Hunger Winter of 1944–1945.* Oxford University Press, New York.
79. Suchman, E. A. (1968): Sociocultural factors in nutritional studies. In: *Biology and Behavior: Environmental Influences,* edited by D. G. Glass. Rockefeller University Press and Russell Sage Foundation, New York.
80. Valman, H. B. (1974): Intelligence after malnutrition caused by neonatal resection of ileum. *Lancet,* 1:425–427.
81. Vuori-Christiansen, L., and Ortiz, N. (1974): Adaptacion de la prueba de desarrollo mental de Griffiths a la poblacion de Bogota: Reodenacion de los items. *Rev. Lat. Am. Psycol.,* 6:347–361.
82. Waterlow, J. C., and Alleyne, G. A. O. (1971): Protein malnutrition in children: Advances in knowledge in the last ten years. *Adv. Protein Chem.,* 25:117–241.
83. Waterlow, J. C., and Rutishauser, H. E. (1974): Malnutrition in man. In: *Early Malnutrition and Mental Development,* edited by J. Cravioto, L. Hambraeus, and B. Vahlquist. Almqvist & Wiksel, Uppsala.
84. Werner, E. E., Bierman, J. M., and French, F. E. (1971): *The Children of Kauai: A Longitudinal Study from the Prenatal Period to Age Ten.* University of Hawaii Press, Honolulu.
85. Winick, M., and Rosso, P. (1969): Head circumference and cellular growth of the brain in normal and marasmic children. *J. Pediatr.* 74:774–778.
86. Winick, M., Meyer, K., and Harris, R. (1975): Malnutrition and environmental enrichment by early adoption. *Science,* 190:1173–1175.
87. Wray, J. D., and Aguirre, A. (1969): Protein-calorie malnutrition in Candelaria, Colombia. I. Prevalence: social and demographic causal factors. *J. Trop. Pediatr.,* 15:76–98.
88. Yaktin, U. S., and McLaren, D. S. (1970): The behavioral development in infants recovering from severe malnutrition. *J. Ment. Defic. Res.,* 14:25–32.

## GLOSSARY[1]

**Bayley Infant Scales of Development:** Based on a revision and restandardization of the California First-Year Mental Scale, this test is composed of both a mental and a motor scale. The scale is applicable from birth to 15 months and includes items on sensory development, fine and large motor skills, and language development.

**Bettye Caldwell Home Inventory Scale:** Designed for infants 0 to 3 years of age, this scale assesses the quantity and quality of the social, emotional, and cognitive support given to the child in his home. The scale is completed by the examiner during a visit to the child's home.

**Binet:** See Stanford-Binet.

**Einstein Sensorimotor Development Scale:** This is a measure of cognitive functioning designed to assess levels of development based on the stages

---

[1]References 1, 24, and 32 were used to compile this glossary.

and substages of development as conceived by Jean Piaget. The test includes measures of object permanence and spatial relations.

**Gesell Developmental Schedules:** Items in this test are grouped into four categories: motor, adaptive, language, and personal-social. Those areas include items such as balance and locomotion, alertness, gestures and vocalizations, and feeding and play activity. Test items begin at approximately 1 month and extend to 72 months.

**Goodenough-Harris Drawing Test:** A 1963 revision of the original Goodenough Draw-a-Man Test, this test requires the child to draw a picture of a man, a woman, and him/herself. Pictures are rated on the child's accuracy of observation and on development of conceptual thinking. The test, appropriate for children in kindergarten through ninth grade, yields a standard score similar to the common deviation IQ.

**Griffiths Mental Development Scale:** Combining original items as well as some from the Gesell and other tests, this scale measures infant behavior in the areas of locomotor, personal-social, hearing-speech, eye-hand, and performance development. The test is appropriate for infants 0–2 years of age.

**Knox Cube Test:** This is one of a series of performance-type tests designed for administration without the use of language. The cube test assesses immediate memory by requiring the testee to reproduce a series of taps on four cubes as demonstrated by the examiner.

**Kohs Block Design:** This test was designed as a supplement to the Stanford-Binet and requires little use of language to administer. The test consists of a set of 1-inch cubes painted different colors with which the subject is required to reproduce a design appearing on a printed card.

**Lincoln-Oseretsky Motor Development Scale:** A 1955 revision of the Oseretsky Tests of Motor Proficiency originally published in Russia, this scale is appropriate for ages 6–14. It is constructed to measure all forms of body movement, from facial and finger musculature to postural reactions.

**Merrill-Palmer Scale of Mental Tests:** A preschool test in use since 1931, the emphasis of this scale is on performance items. The scale is applicable to children 18 months to 6 years of age.

**New South African Individual Scale:** Modeled after the Wechsler Intelligence Scale for Children, this test was devised for and standardized on South African children. It consists of five verbal (vocabulary, comprehension, verbal reasoning, problems, memory) and four nonverbal (pattern completion, block design, absurdities, form board) subscales.

**Ottawa School Behavior Checklist:** The evaluater (usually the teacher) rates a child's behavior on a multiple-item scale. Factor analysis of the checklist identifies four behavior areas: immaturity, overactivity, conduct, and personality.

**Peabody Picture Vocabulary Test:** This is an intelligence test appropriate for children 2–18 years old in which the child identifies, from among four illustrations, the stimulus word spoken by the examiner.

**Stanford-Binet:** A descendant of the first IQ test developed, the Binet-Simon, this test contains items appropriate for children from 2 years of age to superior adult level. Test items are grouped by age and yield a single deviation IQ score.

**The Progressive Matrices.** Developed by J. C. Raven in Great Britain, this test requires choosing the correct missing part from a matrix, from among six to eight possible answers. Used with individuals 8–14 and 20–65 years of age, this test is regarded as a measure of "g" (Spearman's general intelligence factor).

**Vineland Social Maturity Scale:** This test is designed to measure maturation and adjustment in the areas of self-help, self-direction, locomotion, occupation, communication, and socialization. It can be appropriately used on individuals from infancy to 30 years of age. The test items are grouped in age levels as in the Stanford-Binet, and the scale shows a high correlation (approximately .80) with intelligence scales.

**Wechsler Intelligence Scales for Children:** In addition to a full-scale IQ score, the WISC yields a separate score for verbal and performance scales. The items are grouped by content rather than by age levels, as in the Binet. The test is appropriate for children 5–15 years of age.

**Wechsler Preschool and Primary Scale:** Like the WISC, this scale yields a full-scale, a verbal, and a performance score. Items are grouped by content, but unlike the WISC, performance and verbal items are intertwined to increase test interest for the young child. The test, which consists of 10 subtests (11 possible) is designed for children 4–6.5 years of age.

**Wide Range Achievement Test:** This test measures children's competence in specific school subjects such as reading, spelling, and arithmetic.

**Yale Revised Developmental Exam:** A developmental scale based on the Gesell Schedules, this test provides a developmental quotient on various aspects of mental and motor development.

# Subject Index

## A

Absorption
  hormonal factors in, 16–18
  of nutrients, 14–18
Acetylcholine
  food intake and, 95
  in undernutrition, 171, 180–181
Acetylcholinesterase
  in malnutrition, 217
  in undernutrition, 171, 181
Age
  brain amino acids and, 219–222
  diet quality and, 38–39
  eating behavior and, 36–39
  homocarnosine and, 226
  protein synthesis and, 236
  protein turnover and, 239–240
Amino acids
  absorption of, 14–18
  age and, 219–222, 227
  of brain, 219–222, 225–227
  essential, 222
  excess levels of, 227–230, 242–243
  feeding behavior and, 38, 63–66
  hunger and, 51
  kwashiorkor and, 222–223, 245
  imbalance in, 63–64
  malnutrition and, 222–227
  of plasma, 38, 65, 219, 222–223, 227–230
  pools of
    age and, 219–222
    factors influencing, 219
    interpretation of, 219
    maturational changes, 219
    species differences, 219–222
  in protein deficiency, 222–227
  protein synthesis and, 242–245
Amphetamine
  catecholamines and, 94, 108
  hunger and, 79
  obesity and, 108–109
  ventromedial hypothalamus and, 79, 82

## B

Behavior
  in malnutrition, 265–300
  in neonatal disorders, 284, 286–287
  stature and, 299–300
  tests of, 269–283
  upgrading, 300
Body temperature
  environment and, 66–67

feeding behavior and, 66–70
  hypothalamus and, 68–69
  metabolism and, 67
Brain
  amino acid excess and, 227–230
  amino acids in, 219–222
  cell density in, 166–167, 207
  cholesterol, 201–203
  development and
    cholesterol content, 201–203
    DNA, 201–206, 207–213
    growth rate, 202–203
    protein synthesis and, 236
    region, 204–207
    species, 202–203
  DNA, 167, 201–206, 207–213
  energy sources of, 18–19
  histology, 166–168
  ketone body use in, 18
  in malnutrition, 193–246
  morphology, 166–177, 182–186
  myelination in, 165
  postnatal nutrition and, 165
  protein synthesis in
    components of, 234–235
    developmental changes, 236
    mechanism of, 230–234
    specificity of, 235–236
  protein turnover in, 236–240
  Purkinje cells in, 167
  size, 166
  in undernutrition, 164–186
  water content, 219–222
  weight, 201
Brain stem, development of, 204–206

## C

Caloric requirements, of man, 3
Carbohydrate, absorption of, 14–18
Carbohydrate metabolism, eating behavior
  and, 52–60
Catecholamines
  chemical lesions and, 100–104
  electrical lesions and, 100–104
  feeding behavior and, 94–104
  localization of, 93–94
  pharmacology of, 94, 96
  synthesis of, 92–93
  receptors of, 96–97
  in undernutrition, 171
Cerebellum
  development of, 204–206, 211
  in undernutrition, 164, 167, 168, 211

*307*